Cardiac Resynchronization Therapy

Cardiac Resynchronization Therapy

Edited by

MARTIN ST JOHN SUTTON MD FRCP

Professor, Cardiac Imaging Program
Hospital of the University of Pennsylvania
Philadelphia, PA
USA

JEROEN J BAX MD

Professor of Cardiology, Department of Cardiology
Leiden University Medical Center
Leiden
The Netherlands

MARIELL JESSUP MD

Medical Director, Heart Failure and Transplant Program
Hospital of the University of Pennsylvania
Cardiovascular Institute
Philadelphia, PA
USA

JOSEP BRUGADA MD

Professor and Director, Institut Clinic del Torax
University of Barcelona Hospital Clinic
Barcelona
Spain

MARTIN JAN SCHALIJ MD

Professor of Cardiology, Department of Cardiology
Leiden University Medical Center
Leiden
The Netherlands

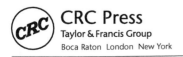

CRC Press
Taylor & Francis Group
Boca Raton London New York

CRC Press is an imprint of the
Taylor & Francis Group, an **informa** business

CRC Press
Taylor & Francis Group
6000 Broken Sound Parkway NW, Suite 300
Boca Raton, FL 33487-2742

First issued in paperback 2019

ISBN-13: 978-1-84184-637-8 (hbk)
ISBN-13: 978-0-367-38860-7 (pbk)

Visit the Taylor & Francis Web site at
http://www.taylorandfrancis.com

and the CRC Press Web site at
http://www.crcpress.com

Contents

Contributors

William T Abraham MD FACP FACC
Professor of Medicine
Chief, Division of Cardiovascular Medicine
Associate Director, Davis Heart and Lung
Research Institute
The Ohio State University
Columbus, OH
USA

Philip B Adamson MD FACC
The Heart Failure Institute at Oklahoma Heart
Hospital
Oklahoma Cardiovascular Associates
and
Department of Physiology
University of Oklahoma Health Sciences Center
Oklahoma City, OK
USA

Samuel J Asirvatham MD FACC
Consultant, Cardiovascular Diseases
Associate Professor of Medicine
Program Director Clinical Cardiac
Electrophysiology
Mayo Clinic and Mayo Clinic College of
Medicine
Division of Cardiology
Rochester, MN
USA

Jeroen J Bax MD
Department of Cardiology
Leiden
The Netherlands

Antonio Berruezo MD
Arrhythmia Section
Thorax Institute Hospital Clinic
University of Barcelona
Barcelona
Spain

Gabe B Bleeker MD
Leiden University Medical Center
Department of Cardiology
Leiden
The Netherlands

S Serge Barold MD
University of South Florida College of Medicine
and
Tampa General Hospital
Tampa, FL
USA

Ole-A Breithardt MD
Medizinische Klinik 2
Universitätsklinikum
Erlangen
Erlangen
Germany

Thomas Cappola MD SCM
Professor, University of Pennsylvania School
of Medicine
Philadelphia, PA
USA

Maria Rosa Costanzo MD
Medical Director, Center for Advanced Heart
Failure
Edward Hospital
Midwest Heart Foundation
Lombard, IL
USA

Anne B Curtis MD FHRS FACC FAHA
University of South Florida
Tampa, FL
USA

Alison Duncan MD
The Echocardiography Department
The Royal Brompton Hospital
London
UK

Arthur M Feldman MD PHD
Thomas Jefferson University Hospital
Jefferson Heart Institute PMA Building
Mezzanine
Philadelphia, PA
USA

Ignacio Fernández-Lozano MD
Unidad de Arritmias
Clínica Puerta de Hierro
Madrid
Spain

Jeffrey Wing-Hong FUNG MBCHB(CUHK) MRCP(UK)
FHKCP FHKAM(MEDICINE) FRCP(EDIN)
Director of Pacing and Electrophysiology
Services
Department of Medicine and Therapeutics
Prince of Wales Hospital
The Chinese University of Hong Kong
Hong Kong

Ignacio García-Bolao MD
Cardiac Electrophysiology Unit
Department of Cardiology and Cardiovascular
Surgery
University Clinic and School of Medicine
University of Navarra
Pamplona
Spain

Stéphane Garrigue MD
Clinique Saint-Augustin
Cardiologie
Bordeaux
France

Adriana C Gittenberger-de Groot MD
Department of Anatomy and Embryology
Leiden University Medical Center
Leiden
The Netherlands

John Gorcsan MD
University of Pittsburgh
Pittsburgh, PA
USA

Richard A Grimm DO FACC
Director, Echocardiography Laboratory
Section of Cardiovascular Imaging
Department of Cardiovascular Medicine
Cleveland Clinic
Cleveland, OH
USA

Edoardo Gronda MD
Heart Failure Unit
Istituto Clinico Humanitas
Rozzano, MI
USA

Garrie J Haas MD FACC
Associate Professor of Medicine
Director, Cardiovascular Clinical Research Unit
Heart Failure and Cardiac Transplant Program
Division of Cardiovascular Medicine
The Ohio State University Medical Center
The Richard M Ross Heart Hospital
Columbus, OH
USA

John Harding MD
Professor, Cardiovascular Division
Department of Medicine
University of Pennsylvania School of Medicine
Philadelphia, PA
USA

Michael Henein MD
The Echocardiography Department
The Royal Brompton Hospital
London
UK

Robert H Helm MD
Division of Cardiology
Department of Medicine
Johns Hopkins Medical Institutions
Baltimore, MD
USA

Bengt Herweg MD
University of South Florida College of Medicine
Tampa General Hospital
Tampa, FL
USA

J Thomas Heywood MD
Congestive Heart Failure Program
Scripps Clinic
La Jolla, CA
USA

Reginald T Ho MD
Thomas Jefferson University Hospital
Jefferson Heart Institute PMA Building
Mezzanine
Philadelphia, PA
USA

Mariell Jessup MD
Medical Director, Heart Failure/Transplant
Program
Hospital of the University of Pennsylvania
Cardiovascular Institute
Philadelphia, PA
USA

Arzu Ilercil MD
University of South Florida College of Medicine
and
Tampa General Hospital
Tampa, FL
USA

David A Kass MD
Department of Medicine
Johns Hopkins Medical Institutions
Baltimore, MD
USA

Fabio Leonelli MD
University of South Florida College of Medicine
and
Tampa General Hospital
Tampa, FL
USA

E Liodakis MD
Professor of Cardiology National Heart and
Lung Institute
Hammersmith Hospital
London
UK

Cecilia Linde MD
Department of Cardiology
Karolinska University Hospital
Solna
Sweden

Gustavo Lopera MD FACC
University of South Florida
MDC
Tampa, FL
USA

Mariell Jessup MD
Professor of Medicine
Cardiovascular Division,
Department of Medicine
University of Pennsylvania School of Medicine
Philadelphia, PA
USA

Monique RM Jongbloed MD PHD
Leiden University Medical Center
Department of Anatomy and Embryology
Department of Cardiology
Leiden
The Netherlands

Alfonso Macías MD
Cardiac Electrophysiology Unit
Department of Cardiology and Cardiovascular
Surgery
University Clinic and School of Medicine
University of Navarra
Pamplona
Spain

Lluis Mont MD
Department of Cardiology
Thorax Institute, Hospital Clínic
University of Barcelona
Catalonia
Spain

Petros Nihoyannopoulos MD
Professor of Cardiology National Heart and
Lung Institute
Hammersmith Hospital
London
UK

Behzad Pavri MD
Thomas Jefferson University Hospital
Jefferson Heart Institute
Mezzanine
Philadelphia, PA
USA

Daniela Pini MD
Heart Failure Unit
Istituto Clinico Humanitas
Rozzano, MI
USA

Jigar Patel DO
Congestive Heart Failure Program
Scripps Clinic
La Jolla, CA
USA

Ted Plappert CVT
University of Pennsylvania
Philadelphia, PA
USA

Hind Rahmouni MD
Department of Cardiology
University of Pennsylvania
Philadelphia, PA
USA

John Rogers MD
Congestive Heart Failure Program
Scripps Clinic
La Jolla, CA
USA

Martin J Schalij MD
Leiden University Medical Center
Department of Cardiology
Leiden
The Netherlands

Marta Sitges MD
Department of Cardiology
Thorax Institute
Hospital Clínic
University of Barcelona
Barcelona
Spain

David D Spragg MD
Division of Cardiology
Department of Medicine
Johns Hopkins Medical Institutions
Baltimore, MD
USA

Christoph Stellbrink MD
Department of Cardiology and Intensive Care
Medicine
Bielefeld Medical Center
Bielefeld
Germany

Martin St John Sutton MB FRCP
Professor, Cardiac Imaging Program
Hospital of the University of Pennsylvania
Philadelphia, PA
USA

Rajkumar K Sugumaran MD
Clinical Instructor
Division of Internal Medicine
The Ohio State University
Columbus, OH
USA

Bàrbara Vidal MD
Department of Cardiology
Thorax Institute
Hospital Clínic
University of Barcelona
Barcelona
Spain

Mary Norine Walsh MD
Director, Congestive Heart Failure
The Care Group
LLC
St Vincent Hospital
Indianapolis, IN
USA

Cheuk-Man Yu MBCHB(CUHK), MD(CUHK), FHKCP,
FHKAM(MEDICINE) FRACP, FRCP(EDIN/LONDON)
Professor
Head of Division of Cardiology
Department of Medicine and Therapeutics
Prince of Wales Hospital
The Chinese University of Hong Kong
Hong Kong

Qing Zhang BM PHD
Division of Cardiology
Department of Medicine and Therapeutics
Prince of Wales Hospital
The Chinese University of Hong Kong
Hong Kong
China

Preface

Cardiac resynchronization therapy (CRT) is one of the most exciting new advances in the treatment of chronic symptomatic heart failure despite optical medical treatment. In the large, randomized trials CRT has resulted in improvement in heart failure symptoms and left ventricular systolic performance in the majority of patients.

These symptomatic benefits are mediated by resynchronization of mainly the left ventricle by CRT, resulting in reverse left ventricular remodeling with a regression of LV mass, an improvement in left ventricular ejection fraction and a reduction in mitral regurgitation. These beneficial effects have recently been reported to translate in a better survival and reduced hospitalization for heart failure.

This book starts with an update on pathophysiology and treatment of heart failure, followed by an update on the results of CRT in the large, randomized trials. A specific part is dedicated to the "ABC" of CRT with chapters on implantation techniques, complications, pacemaker settings etc. Thereafter, the role of echocardiography in CRT is highlighted in various chapters. Particularly, the timely issue on the value of echocardiography in selecting patients who have a high likelihood to respond to CRT is addressed extensively. Various chapters discuss the value of new, sophisticated echocardiographic techniques to identify potential responders to CRT, including tissue Doppler imaging, strain imaging, and 3D echocardiography.

The role of echocardiography in optimization of pacemaker settings (including AV and VV optimization) is also addressed.

The final part of the book is focused on the future of CRT in expanding patient populations such as patients with atrial fibrillation, mild heart failure, or narrow QRS complex.

Cardiac Resynchronization Therapy is very clinically oriented. Particularly, the part on echocardiography is enriched with extensive cases to illustrate the theoretical basis of echocardiography and CRT.

The authors were selected on their knowledge and clinical experience in the field, and represent a broad panel of expertise both from a theoretical and clinical point-of-view. In particular, authors were selected on their leadership in heart failure, electrophysiology or echocardiography. Contributions have been provided by excellent scientists and clinicians from Europe, the United States and Asia.

The editors are grateful to all authors for their superb contributions. We feel that this book may be useful not only for specialists in heart failure, electrophysiology ot echocardiography, but also for the general clinical cardiologist. We sincerely hope that this book will provide a useful and practical handbook in the management of heart failure patients who are considered or selected for CRT.

Martin St John Sutton
Jeroen J Bax
Mariell Jessup
Josep Brugada
Martin Jan Schalij

1

Epidemiology of heart failure

Edoardo Gronda and Daniela Pini

Introduction • Intraventricular conduction delay in heart failure • Pathophysiological implications of Myocardial dyssynchrony • The issue of intraventricular dyssynchrony and QRS duration

INTRODUCTION

Heart failure is a clinical syndrome resulting from a structural or functional cardiac disorder that impairs the ability of the ventricle to fill with or eject blood commensurate with the needs of the body, or that precludes it from doing so in the absence of increased filling pressure. Heart failure is the end stage of all diseases of the heart and is a major cause of morbidity and mortality. Although heart failure may result from disorders of the pericardium, myocardium, endocardium or valve structures, or the great vessels of the heart, or from rhythm disturbances, it is usually discussed primarily in terms of myocardial dysfunction.

Based on left ventricular (LV) ejection fraction (LVEF), patients with heart failure can be divided into those with primarily systolic dysfunction and those with diastolic dysfunction. Patients with a low LVEF, usually <45%, are considered to have systolic dysfunction. Such patients typically have an enlarged left ventricle and a decreased cardiac output. In contrast, patients with signs and symptoms of heart failure but with a preserved LVEF are said to have diastolic dysfunction (or heart failure with preserved ejection fraction), which is a disease of impaired ventricular filling.

Heart failure affects approximately 4.9 million persons in the USA, and more than 500 000 new cases of heart failure are reported each year.[1,2] In the USA, approximately 300 000 persons die of heart failure each year.[3] Heart failure is predominantly a disease of the elderly, with prevalence rates ranging from 1% in persons younger than 50 years to 10% in those aged 80 years and older.[4] In the USA, approximately 80% of patients hospitalized with heart failure are older than 65 years.[3] Indeed, heart failure is the leading indication for hospitalization in older adults in industrialized countries.[5–7] Heart failure accounts for about 5% of annual hospital admissions, with more than 100 000 annual admissions in the UK and more than 2.5 million annual admissions in the USA.[8,9] Hospitalization for heart failure is not only common, but also prolonged. In the USA, the average length of stay has been estimated to be between 6 and 11 days.[10,11] In the UK, the mean length of stay is 11.4 days on acute medical wards and 28.5 days on acute geriatric wards.[12] In addition, hospital readmissions often occur soon after discharge. In elderly patients with heart failure, readmission rates range from 29% to 47% within 3–6 months of the initial hospital discharge.[9]

Heart failure is a considerable economic burden, and the costs of hospitalization represent 65–75% of the total cost of treating a patient.[6,13–17] In the USA, the annual expenditures for hospitalization for heart failure exceed $40 billion.[14] Reports from several countries suggest that approximately 1–2% of the total healthcare budget is spent on the management of heart failure.[13]

In western countries, coronary artery disease and hypertension – either alone or in combination – are the most common causes of heart failure.[18–21] Diabetes mellitus is also an important risk factor for heart failure.[22] Valvular heart disease remains an important cause of heart failure in many regions of the world.[23]

The prognosis of heart failure is poor, with mortality data that are comparable to data for the worst forms of malignant disease. Data derived from the Framingham cohort published in 1993 indicated that the overall 1-year survival rates in men and women were 57% and 64%, respectively. The overall 5-year survival rates were 25% in men and 38% in women. The mortality of heart failure appears to increase with age.[24] The underlying cause of heart failure also influences the prognosis. The presence of ischemic heart disease is associated with higher mortality, as compared with those patients with idiopathic dilated cardiomyopathy.[25,26] Patients with cardiomyopathy owing to amyloidosis, hemochromatosis, and doxorubicin therapy have an especially poor prognosis.[26] Renal impairment too, which is common in patients with heart failure, confers excess mortality.[27] A wide QRS complex (i.e., ≥120 ms), presumably reflecting left-sided intraventricular conduction delay, is also associated with increased all-cause mortality and possibly a higher incidence of sudden death.[28–33]

Advances in medical therapy seem to be improving survival in patients with heart failure. Among subjects in the Framingham study cohort, the 30-day, 1-year, and 5-year age-adjusted mortality rates among men declined from 12%, 30%, and 70%, respectively, in the period 1950–69 to 11%, 28%, and 59%, respectively, in the decade 1990–99. The corresponding rates among women were 18%, 28%, and 57% for the period 1950–69 and 10%, 24% and 45% for the decade 1990–99. Overall, there was an improvement in the survival rate after the onset of heart failure of 12% per decade.[2]

The limitations of medical therapy for heart failure have generated great interest in non-pharmacological treatments. The most efficacious non-pharmacological treatment so far has been cardiac resynchronization therapy (CRT), a device-based therapy that targets electromechanical ventricular dyssynchrony.

INTRAVENTRICULAR CONDUCTION DELAY IN HEART FAILURE

Disorders of the conduction system are often associated with myocardial dysfunction. Indeed, prolongation of QRS (≥120 ms) occurs in 14–47% of patients with heart failure and is generally accepted as occurring in approximately 30% of all patients with low-LVEF heart failure.[28–31,34–41] Left bundle branch block (LBBB) occurs more commonly than right bundle branch block (RBBB) (25–36% vs 4–6%, respectively).[28,42,43] Possible explanations for the varying reported incidence of QRS prolongation in the heart failure population include different definitions of QRS prolongation (some studies set the limit at 120 ms and others at 150 ms), and different methodologies to measure QRS duration.

Prolongation of QRS (≥120 ms) is a significant predictor of LV systolic dysfunction (low LVEF) in patients with heart failure.[29,31,36,37,44] In contrast, the significance of QRS prolongation has not yet been evaluated in heart failure with a normal LVEF and diastolic dysfunction. In patients with heart failure, an inverse correlation exists between QRS prolongation and LVEF.[28,31,36,37,45] In a study of nearly 3500 patients with heart failure, Shenkman et al[35] found a stepwise increase in the prevalence of systolic LV dysfunction as QRS complex duration increased progressively above 120 ms. A more recent study conducted in 343 patients with heart failure reported LVEF of 41%, 36%, 29%, and 25% in patients with QRS durations of <100 ms, 100–119 ms, 120–149 ms, and >150 ms, respectively.[37] These observations in patients with heart failure are consistent with the findings of Murkofsky et al,[46] who analyzed 226 patients (without typical bundle branch block, pacemaker or stated heart failure) referred for radionuclide exercise ventriculography. The study indicated a high likelihood of an abnormal LVEF <45% with a QRS >0.10 s. The specificity increased for each 0.01 s increase in QRS duration, so that it increased to over 99% with a QRS increment from >0.10 s to >0.12 s. Moderate or severe mitral regurgitation was seen in 8% and 20% of patients with heart failure with QRS <120 ms and ≥120 ms, respectively. Increasing QRS duration was also associated with more severe tricuspid regurgitation.[37]

As a rule, QRS duration increases as LV function worsens.[28,29,36,37,47] One heart failure study indicated that the incidence of QRS prolongation (>120 ms) increased from 10% to 32% and 53% when patients moved from New York Heart Association (NYHA) class I to classes II and III, respectively.[47] In a study of 5517 outpatients with heart failure, QRS prolongation was seen more frequently in patients with advanced NYHA functional class (32.8% of patients with complete LBBB vs 26.4% without complete LBBB were in NYHA class III–IV).[42] Gasparini et al[48] reported similar findings in a study of 158 patients with severe heart failure undergoing CRT implantation: 86% of patients with QRS >150 ms were in NYHA functional class III or IV versus 60% of patients with QRS <150 ms ($p = 0.002$). According to Xiao et al,[49] who analyzed a series of patients with dilated cardiomyopathy of various etiologies admitted to a tertiary care center, QRS prolongation progresses at an annual rate of 5 ms in a population presumed to have heart failure and who received appropriate therapy for it. Larger increases in QRS duration occur in patients with early mortality. In the same study,[49] the time from reaching a QRS of 160 ms to death was 9.8 ± 18 months in patients without an implanted pacemaker, versus 31 ± 16 months in patients with a pacemaker. A possible explanation for this observation is that in conventionally paced patients with normal or nearly normal systolic function, QRS prolongation is generated by the stimulation of the right apex, which is the major determinant of systolic dysfunction. Indeed, there is a strong association between the percentage of cumulative ventricular pacing and the progression of systolic dysfunction,[50,51] which may explain the delayed effect on prognosis observed in the study published by Xiao et al.[49]

One study of 56 patients with symptomatic heart failure (followup from 180–7660 days, mean 1755 days) and necropsy-proven idiopathic dilated cardiomyopathy documented an increase in QRS duration from an average of 0.10s to an average of 0.13s in 76% of patients before death.[43] These results are in keeping with those of other reports in cardiomyopathy (ischemic or non-ischemic) and patients with heart failure identifying QRS prolongation as a poor prognostic indicator.[29,49]

In patients with heart failure, mortality rates progressively increase as intraventricular conduction delay increases. In one study, QRS <0.12s, QRS 0.12–0.16s, and QRS >0.16s correlated with 20%, 36%, and 58% mortality at 36 months, respectively.[30] Kalra et al[36] investigated the optimal QRS duration separating patients with heart failure into those with a relatively benign versus a poor prognosis (i.e., increased mortality or heart transplantation). Patients with a QRS ≥0.12s had a threefold increased risk for the combined endpoint of death or transplantation. Also, 5-year survival was significantly lower in this patient population when compared with patients with heart failure with QRS <0.12s (47% vs 84%; $p <0.0001$).[36] In patients with B-type natriuretic peptide (BNP) levels >400 pg/ml, QRS prolongation was found to be a significant univariate and multivariate predictor of all-cause death, cardiac (i.e., sudden) death, and pump failure death.[52] In a study of 82 patients with heart failure and dilated cardiomyopathy, change in QRS duration over time (≥0.5 ms/month) was a multivariate predictor of cardiac death or need for heart transplant at 1 year.[53] In another study, QRS duration was the only electrocardiographic (ECG) parameter with independent prognostic value for adverse outcomes.[44] In 100 patients with heart failure referred for cardiac transplantation, 55% of patients with QRS duration ≥0.12s (vs 24% with QRS <0.12s) went on to transplantation or death.[31] In a substudy of the Multicenter Unsustained Tachycardia Trial (MUSTT),[54] Zimetbaum et al[55] analyzed ECGs from 1638 patients (approximately 70% had heart failure) who did not receive antiarrhythmic drugs or implantable cardioverter–defibrillators (ICDs). Multivariate analysis identified non-specific intraventricular conduction delay (defined as a QRS ≥0.11s but morphologically different from LBBB or RBBB) as a predictor of arrhythmic death or cardiac arrest (hazard ratio (HR) 1.44; 95% confidence interval (CI) 1.11–1.88) and total mortality (HR 1.47; 95% CI 1.22–1.78). LBBB was also a significant predictor of arrhythmic (HR 1.49; 95% CI 1.02–2.17) and total (HR 1.61; 95% CI 1.26–2.08) mortality. RBBB, however, was not associated with increased arrhythmic or total mortality.[55]

Prolongation of QRS and severe cardiomyopathy (defined as LVEF <30%) have an additive effect on mortality. The highest mortality rates are seen in patients with heart failure with QRS prolongation and LVEF <35% secondary to both ischemic and non-ischemic etiologies.[29,35]

PATHOPHYSIOLOGICAL IMPLICATIONS OF MYOCARDIAL DYSSYNCHRONY

The optimal contraction of the heart is the result of the coordinated, sequential activation of the atria and the ventricles. LV activation slightly anticipates right ventricular (RV) activation. Therefore, interventricular delay is usually defined as the time difference between the onset of aortic flow and the onset of pulmonary arterial flow with respect to the beginning of the QRS. An interventricular delay >40 ms is considered to represent interventricular dyssynchrony. Because the time to ejection of the RV and LV can be influenced by several factors, the predictive value of interventricular delay for responsiveness to CRT has been questioned, although improvement of interventricular dyssynchrony after CRT has been demonstrated by tissue Doppler imaging (TDI).[56] Possible explanations for the poor predictive value of interventricular delay are: (a) the magnitude of pre-pacing interventricular delay is relatively small compared with intraventricular delay; (b) physiologically, peak systolic contraction of the RV occurs later than that of the LV (the RV is a low-pressure chamber); (c) the correction of intraventricular delay should simultaneously improve interventricular delay through ventricular interdependence. The recently published CARE HF study[57] showed, indeed, an improved long-term survival with CRT in patients with interventricular dyssynchrony at enrolment.

Notwithstanding the above, intraventricular dyssynchrony is considered by the vast majority of authors to be the most important target of CRT. Intraventricular dyssynchrony may be defined as the mechanical dispersion of motion within the LV. In the intact myocardium, Purkinje cells build a diffuse network and propagate electrical impulses at high velocity in a uniform manner from the endocardium to the epicardium. In areas of diseased myocardium, rearrangement of extracellular matrix and of working myocytes results in intramural disarray, which may influence the entry, the direction, and ultimately the velocity of propagation of conducting impulses within the diseased area. It has been recognized for over 80 years that abnormalities of the ventricular activation sequence can adversely influence global contractility.[58] Of note, such an adverse effect is independent of whether the abnormality is due to natural causes (bundle branch block), local scarring in myocardial wall, or artificial causes such as ventricular pacing. Dyssynchronous contraction, indeed, causes a reduction in LV systolic function of up to 20% beyond that which exists as a consequence of intrinsic muscle dysfunction and chamber dilation.[59,60] This is because, in the presence of dyssynchrony, the mass of muscle that is activated early contracts against neighboring muscle in a weak (pre-existing) state. The early activated muscle shortens at the expense of stretching of the neighboring muscle, which reduces force generation, thus reducing pressure generation.[61,62] Ultimately, it has been proposed that a conduction defect reduces the effective mass of muscle contributing to pressure generation. However, the ineffective muscle mass still consumes oxygen at a rate equivalent to that consumed in a mechanically unloaded state. A dyscoordinated contraction leads to a metabolically inefficient state, as manifested by an increase in myocardial oxidative metabolism index in the lateral and posterior walls of the LV.[63] On the other hand, the electromechanical activation gradient between the septum and the lateral wall is associated with a local decrease in oxygen consumption in the early-activated septum, which generates systolic tension, without shortening,[64] mimicking a mechanical dysfunction quite similar to that resulting from the occlusion of the left anterior descending coronary artery.[65] Lastly, LV mechanical asynchrony in the failing heart generates a disparity in the regional expression of myocardial proteins involved with mechanical contraction and electrical activation. The transmural and transchamber expression gradients of calcium handling and gap junction proteins may worsen chamber function and arrhythmia susceptibility.[66]

Furthermore, recent electrophysiological mapping data[67] indicate that, when the activation sequence is abnormal, the physiological endocardium-to-epicardium depolarization gradient is lost and is replaced by a diffuse activation wavefront traveling throughout the myocardial wall. The disorganized depolarization creates local (endocardium, myocardium, and epicardium) abnormal loading conditions, thus favoring different degrees of transmural hypertrophy. Consequently, in the diseased ventricle, there may be large differences in hypertrophy and myocyte function. Finally, regional dyssynchrony may undermine the efficiency of the mitral valve apparatus,[68] leading to uncoordinated papillary muscle contraction, which impairs leaflet coaptation and promotes mitral regurgitation, a major component of LV dysfunction.[69]

THE ISSUE OF INTRAVENTRICULAR DYSSYNCHRONY AND QRS DURATION

Intraventricular dyssynchrony can be present even in patients without prolonged QRS.[70] Data on mechanical dyssynchrony in patients with narrow QRS duration are scarce. The incidence of intraventricular dyssynchrony in patients with QRS duration ≤120 ms ranges between 29% and 56% in different studies.[34,70,71] When mechanical dyssynchrony is present in patients with narrow QRS, systolic function is less impaired, although the effect of dyssynchrony is not negligible.[72] In a study by Auricchio et al,[73] the prevalence of CRT responders (as defined by demonstration of reverse remodeling) in the short term was lower in patients with a QRS duration of 120–150 ms, which was attributed to the less severe mechanical asynchrony, as reflected by a lower time to peak systolic contraction measured with TDI. In a subsequent study with a follow-up of 36 months, the same authors[74] found a higher number of responders to CRT (≥10% reduction of LV end-systolic volume) among patients with QRS ≤120 ms compared with patients with prolonged QRS. LV reverse remodeling was the best predictor of long-term survival. Similar results have recently been reported by Gasparini et al.[75] However, further data are needed before establishing whether dyssynchrony should be treated earlier than is currently accepted. Nevertheless, CRT results in improved survival only when reverse remodeling occurs.[74]

It follows that the restoration of coordinated ventricular contraction should provide the largest benefit by enhancing remodeling in the earlier phase of ventricular dysfunction. As has been suggested by an analysis of beta-blocker studies, reversibility of ventricular remodeling is strictly dependent on the extent of fibrosis, which may be viewed as an expression of ischemic injury.[76] Interestingly, data derived from the subset of patients with echocardiographic follow-up in the MIRACLE trial indicate that ischemic etiology of heart failure is the major independent factor limiting reverse remodeling after CRT.[77] On the other hand, Diaz-Iafante et al[78] showed in a careful multicenter observational study that extensive adverse remodeling, as well as severe mitral regurgitation and/or development of atrial fibrillation, are the main predictors of a poor response after CRT in both ischemic and non-ischemic patients.[78] In addition, Mangiavacchi et al[79] demonstrated that non-ischemic etiology and lower end-systolic volume are major predictors of reverse remodeling after CRT, with an increase in LVEF ≥10%.

Finally, dyssynchrony is frequently detectable in patients with isolated diastolic LV dysfunction, with increasing prevalence from diastolic dysfunction to diastolic heart failure to systolic heart failure.[45] This observation points to dyssynchrony as an independent mechanism involved in the decline of systolic function. On the other hand, it can also be hypothesized that dyscoordination of ventricular contraction is aggravated by progression of heart failure.

REFERENCES

1. Roger VL, Weston SA, Redfield MM, et al. Trends in heart failure: incidence and survival in a community based population. JAMA 2004;292:344–50.

2. Levy D, Kenchaiah S, Larson MG, et al. Long term trends in the incidence of and survival with heart failure. N Engl J Med 2002;347:1397–402.

3. Hunt SA, Baker D, Chin M, et al. ACC/AHA Guidelines for the Evaluation and Management of Chronic Heart Failure in the Adult: Executive Summary. A report of the

American College of Cardiology/American Heart Association Task Force on Practice Guidelines (Committee to Revise the 1995 Guidelines for the Evaluation and Management of Heart Failure). Developed in collaboration with the International Society for Heart and Lung Transplantation. Endorsed by the Heart Failure Society of America. J Am Coll Cardiol 2001;38:2101–13.

4. Kannel WB, Belanger AJ. Epidemiology of heart failure. Am Heart J 1991;121:951–7.

5. American Heart Association. 1998 Heart and Stroke Statistical Update. Dallas: American Heart Association, 1998.

6. Scott WG, Scott HM. Heart failure. A decision analytic analysis of New Zealand data using the published results of the SOLVD Treatment Trial. Studies of Left Ventricular Dysfunction. Pharmacoeconomics 1996; 9:156–7.

7. Ryden-Bergsten T, Andersson F. The health care costs of heart failure in Sweden. J Intern Med 1999;246: 275–84.

8. Haldeman GA, Croft JB, Giles WH, Rashidee A. Hospitalization of patients with heart failure: National Hospital Discharge Survey, 1985 to 1995. Am Heart J 1999;137:352–60.

9. Davis RC, Hobbs FDR, Lip GYH. ABC of heart failure: History and epidemiology (Clinical review). BMJ 2000;320:39–42.

10. Polanczyk CA, Rohde LE, Dec GW, DiSalvo T. Ten-year trends in hospital care for congestive heart failure: improved outcomes and increased use of resources. Arch Intern Med 2000;160:325–32.

11. Weingarten SR, Riedinger MS, Shinbane J, et al. Triage practice guideline for patients hospitalized with congestive heart failure: improving the effectiveness of the coronary care unit. Am J Med 1993;94:483–90.

12. McMurray J, McDonagh T, Morrison CE, Dargie HJ. Trends in hospitalization for heart failure in Scotland 1980–1990. Eur Heart J 1993;14:1158–62.

13. Cleland JGF. Health economic consequences of the pharmacological treatment of heart failure. Eur Heart J 1998;19(Suppl P):P32–9.

14. O'Connell JB, Bristow MR. Economic impact of heart failure in the United States: time for a different approach. J Heart Lung Transplant 1994;13:S107–12.

15. McMurray J, Hart W, Rhodes G. An evaluation of the cost of chronic heart failure to the National Health Service in the UK. Br J Med Econ 1993;6:99–110.

16. Launois R, Launois B, Reboul-Marty J, Battais J, Lefebvre P. The cost of chronic illness severity: the heart failure case. J Med Econ 1990;8:395–412.

17. van Hout BA, Wielink G, Bonsel GJ, Rutten FF. Effects of ACE inhibitors on heart failure in The Netherlands: a pharmacoeconomic model. Pharmacoeconomics 1993;3: 387–97.

18. Ho KK, Pinsky JL, Kannel WB, Levy D. The epidemiology of heart failure: the Framingham Study. J Am Coll Cardiol 1993;22(4 Suppl A):6A–13A.

19. McDonagh TA, Morrison CE, Lawrence A, et al. Symptomatic and asymptomatic left-ventricular systolic dysfunction in an urban population. Lancet 1997;350: 829–33.

20. Cowie MR, Wood DA, Coats AJ, et al. Incidence and aetiology of heart failure; a population-based study. Eur Heart J 1999;20:421–8.

21. McMurray JJ, Stewart S. Epidemiology, aetiology and prognosis of heart failure. Heart 2000;83:596–602.

22. Levy D, Larson MG, Vasan RS, Kannel WB, Ho KK. The progression from hypertension to congestive heart failure. JAMA 1996;275:1557–62.

23. Sharpe N, Doughty R. Epidemiology of heart failure and ventricular dysfunction. Lancet 1998;352(Suppl I): S3–7.

24. Ho KK, Anderson KM, Kannel WB, Grossman W, Levy D. Survival after the onset of congestive heart failure in Framingham Heart Study subjects. Circulation 1993;88: 107–15.

25. Adams KF, Jr., Dunlap SH, Sueta CA, et al. Relation between gender, etiology and survival in patients with symptomatic heart failure. J Am Coll Cardiol 1996; 28:1781–8.

26. Felker GM, Thompson RE, Hare JM, et al. Underlying causes and long-term survival in patients with initially unexplained cardiomyopathy. N Engl J Med 2000;342: 1077–84.

27. Smith GL, Lichtman JH, Bracken MB, et al. Renal impairment and outcomes in heart failure. Systematic review and meta-analysys. J Am Coll Cardiol 2006;47: 1987–96.

28. Baldasseroni S, Gentile A, Gorini M, et al. Intraventricular conduction defects in patients with congestive heart failure:left but not right bundle branch block is an independent predictor of prognosis. A report from the Italian Network on Congestive Heart Failure (IN-CHF database). Italian Heart Journal 2003; 4:607–13.

29. Iuliano S, Fisher SG, Karasik PE, Fletcher RD, Singh SN. QRS duration and mortality in patients with congestive heart failure. Am Heart J 2002;143:1085–91.

30. Shamim W, Francis DP, Yousufuddin M, et al. Intraventricular conduction delay: a prognostic marker in chronic heart failure. Int J Cardiol 1999;70:171–8.

31. Freudenberger R, Sikora JA, Fisher M, Wilson A, Gold M. Electrocardiogram and clinical characteristics of patients referred for cardiac transplantation: implications for pacing in heart failure. Clin Cardiol 2004;27: 151–3.

32. Huang X, Shen W, Gong L. Clinical significance of complete left bundle branch block in dilated cardiomyopathy. Chin Med Sci J 1995;10:158–60.

33. Silverman ME, Pressel MD, Brackett JC, Lauria SS, Gold MR, Gottlieb SS. Prognostic value of the signal-averaged electrocardiogram and a prolonged QRS in ischemic and nonischemic cardiomyopathy. Am J Cardiol 1995;75:460-4.

34. Bader H, Garrigue S, Lafitte S, et al. Intra-left ventricular electromechanical asynchrony. A new independent predictor of severe cardiac events in heart failure patients. J Am Coll Cardiol 2004;43:248-56.

35. Shenkman HJ, Pampati V, Khandelwal AK, et al. Congestive heart failure and QRS duration: establishing prognosis study. Chest 2002;122:528-34.

36. Kalra PR, Sharma R, Shamin W, et al. Clinical characteristics and survival of patients with chronic heart failure and prolonged QRS duration. Int J Cardiol 2002;86:225-31.

37. Sandhu R, Bahler RC. Prevalence of QRS prolongation in a community hospital cohort of patients with heart failure and its relation to left ventricular systolic dysfunction. Am J Cardiol 2004;93:244-6.

38. Shen AY, Wang X, Doris J, Moore N. Proportion of patients in a congestive heart failure care management program meeting criteria for cardiac resynchronization therapy. Am J Cardiol 2004;94:673-6.

39. Bode-Schnurbus L, Bocker D, Block M, et al. QRS duration: a simple marker for predicting cardiac mortality in ICD patients with heart failure. Heart 2003;89:1157-62.

40. Galizio NO, Pesce R, Valero E, et al. Which patients with congestive heart failure may benefit from biventricular pacing? Pacing Clin Electrophysiol 2003;26:158-61.

41. Grimm W, Sharkova J, Funck R, Maisch B. How many patients with dilated cardiomyopathy may potentially benefit from cardiac resynchronization therapy? Pacing Clin Electrophysiol 2003;26:155-7.

42. Baldasseroni S, Opasich C, Gorini M, et al. Left bundle-branch block is associated with increased 1-year sudden and total mortality rate in 5517 outpatients with congestive heart failure: a report from the Italian network on congestive heart failure. Am Heart J 2002;143:398-405.

43. Wilensky RL, Yudelman P, Cohen AI, et al. Serial electrocardiographic changes in idiopathic dilated cardiomyopathy confirmed at necropsy. Am J Cardiol 1988; 62:276-83.

44. Shamim W, Yousufuddin M, Cicoria M, et al. Incremental changes in QRS duration in serial ECGs over time identify high risk elderly patients with heart failure. Heart 2002;88:47-51.

45. Yu CM, Lin H, Zhang Q, Sanderson JE. High prevalence of left ventricular systolic and diastolic asynchrony in patients with congestive heart failure and normal QRS duration. Heart 2003;89:54-60.

46. Murkofsky RL, Dangas G, Diamond JA, et al. A prolonged QRS duration on surface electrocardiogram is a specific indicator of left ventricular dysfunction. J Am Coll Cardiol 1998;32:476-82.

47. Stellbrink C, Auricchio A, Diem B, et al. Potential benefit of biventricular pacing in patients with congestive heart failure and ventricular tachyarrhythmia. Am J Cardiol 1999;83:143D-50D.

48. Gasparini M, Mantica M, Galimbert P, et al. Beneficial effects of biventricular pacing in patients with a 'narrow' QRS. Pacing Clin Electrophysiol 2003;26:169-74.

49. Xiao HB, Roy C, Fujimoto S, Gibson DG. Natural history of abnormal conduction and its relation to prognosis in patients with dilated cardiomyopathy. Int J Cardiol 1996;53:163-70.

50. The DAVID Trial Investigators. Dual-chamber pacing or ventricular backup pacing in patients with an implantable defibrillator. The Dual Chamber and VVI Implantable Defibrillator (DAVID). JAMA 2002;288:3115-23.

51. Sweeney MO, Hellkamp AS, Ellenbogen KA, et al. Adverse effect of ventricular pacing on heart failure and atrial fibrillation among patients with normal baseline QRS duration in a clinical trial of pacemaker therapy for sinus node dysfunction. Circulation 2003;107:2932-7.

52. Vrtovec B, Delgado R, Zewail A, Thomas CD, Richartz BM, Radovancevic B. Prolonged QTc interval and high B-type natriuretic peptide levels together predict mortality in patients with advanced heart failure. Circulation 2003;107:1764-9.

53. Grigioni F, Carinci V, Boriani G, et al. Accelerated QRS widening as an independent predictor of cardiac death or of the need for heart transplantation in patients with congestive heart failure. J Heart Lung Transplant 2002;21:899-902.

54. Buxton AE, Lee KL, Fisher JD, et al. A randomized study of the prevention of sudden death in patients with coronary artery disease. Multicenter Unsustained Tachycardia Trial Investigators. N Engl J Med 1991;341:1882-990.

55. Zimetbaum PJ, Buxton AE, Batsford W, et al. Electrocardiographic predictos of arrhythmic death and total mortality in the multicenter unsustained tachycardia trial. Circulation 2004;110:766-9.

56. Yu CM, Chau E, Sanderson JE, et al. Tissue Doppler echocardiographic evidence of reverse remodeling and improved synchronicity by simultaneously delaying regional contraction after biventricular pacing therapy in heart failure. Circulation 2002;105:438-45.

57. Cleland JG, Daubert JC, Erdmann E, et al. The effect of cardiac resynchronization on morbidity and mortality in heart failure. N Engl J Med 2005;352:1539-49.

58. Wiggers CJ. The muscular reactions of the mammalian ventricles to artificial surface stimuli. Am J Physiol 1925;73:346-78.

59. Butter C, Auricchio A, Stellbrink C, et al. Clinical efficacy of one year cardiac resynchronization therapy in heart failure patients stratified by QRS duration: results of the PATH-CHF II trial. Eur Heart J 2003;24:363 (abst).

60. Nelson GS, Berger RD, Fetics BJ, et al. Left ventricular or biventricular pacing improves cardiac function at diminished energy cost in patients with dilated cardiomyopathy and left bundle-branch block. Circulation 2000;102:3053–9.

61. Burkhoff D, Oikawa RY, Sagawa K. Influence of pacing site on canine left ventricular contraction. Am J Physiol Heart Circ Physiol 1986;251:H428–35.

62. Curry CW, Nelson GS, Wyman BT, et al. Mechanical dyssynchrony in dilated cardiomyopathy with intraventricular conduction delay as depicted by 3D tagged magnetic resonance imaging. Circulation 2000;101:E2.

63. Ukkonen H, Beanlands RS, Burwash IG, et al. The effects of cardiac resynchronization on myocardial efficiency and regional oxidative metabolism. Circulation 2003;107:28–31.

64. Lindner O, Vogt J, Kammeier A, et al. Effect of cardiac resynchronization therapy on global and regional oxygen consumption and myocardial blood flow in patients with ischemic and non-ischemic cardiomyopathy. Eur Heart J 2005;26:70–6.

65. Verbeek XA, Vernooy K, Peschar M, Cornelussen RN, Prinzen FW. Intra-ventricular resynchronization for optimal left ventricular function during pacing in experimental left bundle branch block. J Am Coll Cardiol 2003;42:558–67.

66. Spragg DD, Leclercq C, Loghmani M, et al. Regional alterations in protein expression in the dyssynchronous failing heart. Circulation 2003;108:929–32.

67. Wyman BT, Hunter WC, Prinzen FW, Faris OP, McVeigh ER. Effects of single- and biventricular pacing on temporal and spatial dynamics of ventricular contraction. Am J Physiol Heart Circ Physiol 2002;282:H372–9.

68. Kanzaki H, Bazaz R, Schwartzman D, et al. A mechanism for immediate reduction in mitral regurgitation after cardiac resynchronization therapy: insights from mechanical activation strain mapping. J Am Coll Cardiol 2004;44:1619–25.

69. Koelling TM, Aaronson KD, Cody RJ, Bach DS, Armstrong WF. Prognostic significance of mitral regurgitation and tricuspid regurgitation in patients with left ventricular systolic dysfunction. Am Heart J 2002;144:524–9.

70. Bleeker GB, Schalij MJ, Molhoek SG, et al. Relationship between QRS duration and left ventricular dyssynchrony in patients with end-stage heart failure. J Cardiovasc Electrophysiol 2004;15:544–9.

71. Ghio S, Constantin C, Klersy C, et al. Interventricular and intraventricular dyssynchrony are common in heart failure patients, regardless of QRS duration. Eur Heart J 2004;25:571–8.

72. Auricchio A, Yu CM. Beyond the measurement of QRS complex toward mechanical dyssynchrony: cardiac resynchronisation therapy in heart failure patients with a normal QRS duration. Heart 2004;90:479–81.

73. Auricchio A, Stellbrink C, Butter C, et al. Clinical efficacy of cardiac resynchronization therapy using left ventricular pacing in heart failure patients stratified by severity of ventricular conduction delay. J Am Coll Cardiol 2003;42:2109–16.

74. Yu CM, Bleeker GB, Fung JW, et al. Left ventricular reverse remodeling but not clinical improvement predicts long-term survival after cardiac resynchronization therapy. Circulation 2005;112:1580–6.

75. Gasparini M, Galimberti P, Regoli F, et al. Long-term efficacy of cardiac resynchronization therapy (CRT) in patients with normal QRS duration. ESC Meeting Highlights 2005.

76. Bello D, Dipan J, Shahb D, Farah GM, et al. Gadolinium cardiovascular magnetic resonance predicts reversible myocardial dysfunction and remodeling in patients with heart failure undergoing beta-blocker therapy. Circulation 2003;108:1945–53.

77. St John Sutton MG, Plappert T, Hilpisch KE, et al. Sustained reverse left ventricular structural remodeling with cardiac resynchronization at one year is a function of etiology: quantitative Doppler echocardiographic evidence from the Multicenter InSync Randomized Clinical Evaluation (MIRACLE). Circulation 2006;113:266–72.

78. Diaz-Infante E, Mont L, Leal J, et al. Predictors of lack of response to resynchronization therapy. Am J Cardiol 2005;95:1436–40.

79. Mangiavacchi M, Gasparini M, Faletra F, et al. Clinical predictors of marked improvement in left ventricular performance after cardiac resynchronization therapy in patients with chronic heart failure. Am Heart J 2006;15:477. e1–e6.

2

Pathobiology of left ventricular dyssynchrony

David D Spragg, Robert H Helm, and David A Kass

Introduction • Dyssynchrony and heart failure: epidemiology • Chamber dysfunction from dyssynchrony • Electrophysiology of dyssynchrony • Dyssynchrony and molecular polarization • Chamber effects of cardiac resynchronization • Factors that can influence CRT efficacy • Non-responders and electrical versus mechanical dyssynchrony • Conclusions

INTRODUCTION

Heart failure combines multiple abnormalities, including molecular and structural cardiac remodeling, neurohormonal stimulation, excessive loading, and vascular insufficiency – all conspiring to limit cardiac pump performance. Typically, heart failure therapy has relied on moderating fluid balance, and blocking both the rennin–angiotensin–aldosterone and β-adrenergic systems (see recent reviews[1,2]). However, mechanical factors also play a role in the pathophysiology of heart failure, particularly those affecting the intrachamber synchrony of contraction and atrial and ventricular timing intervals. Atrial activation that occurs too close or well prior to ventricular activation results in suboptimal cardiac filling and a net fall in ejection.[3-5] Initial clinical trials with pacing therapy in heart failure focused on this effect, and tried to optimize atrioventricular (AV) delay time using right ventricular (RV) single-site pacing.[6] However, this was soon found to be ineffective in a majority of patients.[7-9] Attention shifted to problems with dyscoordinate ventricular contraction, typically the result of disparities in timing of electrical activation between one region of the heart and another. Such dyssynchrony can be reflected by prolongation of the surface QRS complex, which has been shown to be an independent and major contributor to heart failure morbidity and mortality.[10-13] In 1994, Cazeau et al[14] reported on the use of multisite cardiac pacing to re-establish coordinate contraction in a patient with dilated heart failure. In the years leading up to this, there were barely a handful of studies reporting on cardiac dyssynchrony or resynchronization. There are now more than a thousand. Cardiac resynchronization therapy (CRT) is now an important, approved therapy for a subset of heart failure patients, having been shown to improve overall survival, clinical symptoms, and hospitalization rates.[15-20]

Left ventricular (LV) mechanical dyssynchrony is fairly common, due either to intrinsic conduction delays or to artificial ventricular stimulation from pacemakers. Estimates of the incidence of left bundle branch block (LBBB) in congestive heart failure (CHF) patients range around 25–35%,[10,21-23] or over 150 000 patients in the USA alone. While the relationship between LBBB-type conduction delay and mechanical dyssynchrony of the LV is not straightforward (as discussed in more detail below), QRS widening has served as a surrogate marker for dyssynchrony in most large patient studies. There were nearly

200 000 permanent pacemakers and 63 000 internal defibrillators (with pacemakers) implanted in the USA in 2002, and clinical and experimental data have now shown that sustained single-site pacing can itself trigger the development of heart failure and worsened ventricular dysfunction.[24-27]

In this chapter, we discuss the pathobiology of LV dyssynchrony, as well as the acute and chronic physiological effects of cardiac resynchronization. The mechanics of dyssynchrony and its assessment are also discussed, particularly as they relate to CRT implementation and identification of suitable patients. Lastly, we note unresolved issues and controversies related to CRT mechanisms and pathophysiology.

DYSSYNCHRONY AND HEART FAILURE: EPIDEMIOLOGY

Cardiac dyssynchrony has now taken its place as an important independent predictor of poor outcome in patients with CHF. In addition to well-established predictors of mortality – age, degree of systolic impairment, ejection fraction, New York Heart Association (NYHA) function class – data now show QRS prolongation and/or evidence of mechanical contractile dyssynchrony to be independent predictors as well. The mortality risk increased by 45% in the CHF-STAT cohort of 669 dilated cardiomyopathy patients if their QRS duration exceeded 120 ms.[12] The larger Italian Network on CHF Registry (5500 subjects) found that the presence of a LBBB (which occurred in 25% of the cohort) was an independent predictor of both annual overall mortality and mortality from sudden cardiac death. Furthermore, having an LBBB chronically increases risk. In a case–control study of more than 17 000 subjects (from 1958 to 2002), Imanishi et al[21] found LBBB occurring in less than 1%, typically older subjects, but that it raised their risk of dying from heart failure. Patients receiving pacemakers and developing de novo LV mechanical dyssynchrony are at risk as well. In a study of 11 656 patients without known heart failure, Freudenberger et al[28] showed 20% of paced patients suffered a new hospitalization for heart failure, compared with 12.5% of controls, and deaths from heart failure were 53%

higher in the paced group. In addition to surface electrocardiography, mechanical dyssynchrony has also been assessed using newer tissue Doppler imaging methods. This has been shown to be a predictor of worsened outcome in heart failure patients, independent of QRS duration and other conventional factors.[29]

CHAMBER DYSFUNCTION FROM DYSSYNCHRONY

For the most common pattern of LV dyssynchrony, the septal region is stimulated first, followed by delayed activation of the lateral LV free wall. Early septal contraction does not generate pressure rapidly, since the force is largely converted into prestretch of the still-quiescent lateral wall. The result is a delay in rate of intracavitary pressure rise (dP/dt_{max}) and suboptimal mitral valve closure, causing mitral regurgitation.[30] Late-systolic activation of the LV lateral free wall, in turn, stretches the anteroseptal region, competing with aortic ejection and reducing net cardiac output. One can consider this mechanical process as the result of a phase delay in muscle stiffening (activation). In Figure 2.1(a), we depict two time-varying elastance curves representing activation of muscle. The lateral wall (dotted line) is shifted rightward (i.e., delayed activation) relative to the tracing of septal activation (solid line). When there is a vertical difference between the curves, one part of the wall is stiffer than the other, resulting in a shift of volume into the latter. This is substantial very early in systole (isovolumic contraction – hence the sensitivity of dP/dt_{max} to dyssynchrony), and in very late systole/early relaxation (underlying the common observation of motion abnormalities after aortic valve closure). The net result is mechanical inefficiency, with transmission of the ventricular blood pool between two intracavitary sinks (the stretched lateral wall in early systole and the anteroseptal region in late systole) rather than into the arterial system.[31,32]

The acute effects of LV dyssynchrony on global systolic function have been revealed by pacing studies in both ex vivo and in vivo models. Compared with atrial pacing and activation of the LV through the His–Purkinje

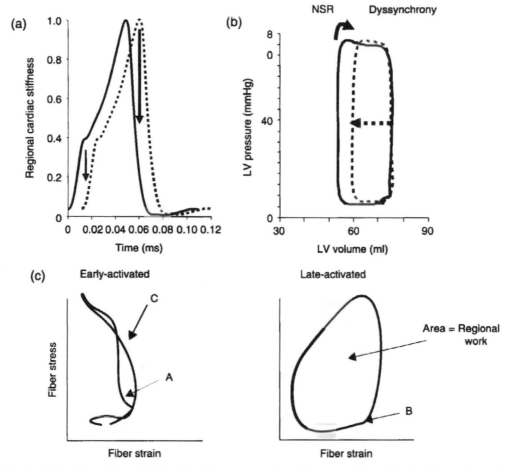

Figure 2.1 (a) Septal (solid) and lateral (dotted) LV stiffness versus time. Pronounced disparities in stiffness (vertical difference at a given time point) are present early and late in systole (arrows). (b) Pressure–volume loops showing the effect of LV dyssynchrony induced by RV pacing. Stroke volume is reduced, the LV end-systolic pressure–volume relationship (ESPVR) is shifted to the right, and end-systolic volume and stress are increased. NSR, normal sinus rhythm. (c) Stress–strain loops from early- and late-activated myocardial regions in dyssynchronous hearts. In early-activated regions, contraction initially occurs at low stress levels (A) as quiescent, late-activated regions undergo passive stretch. Later in systole, early-activated regions undergo reciprocal deformation as the late-activated territories contract (C). The small net area of the stress–strain loop in early-activated regions reflects reduced regional work performed. In late-activated territories, passive stretch in early systole generates increased stress prior to contraction (B). The increased stress–strain loop area reflects increased work performed by late-activated territories.

network, univentricular pacing from various RV and LV sites reduces developed LV pressure,[33] dP/dt_{max},[34] and stroke volume,[35] and induces a rightward shift of the end-systolic pressure–volume relationship (ESPRV).[35] Figure 2.1(b) depicts the effects of dyssynchrony on global chamber function as a pressure–volume loop. Relative to normal sinus rhythm (NSR: solid loop), pacing-induced dyssynchrony (dotted loop) results in a reduction in stroke volume (loop width), and a rightward shift of the end-systolic pressure–volume point and thus a rise in the end-systolic wall stress. From tagged magnetic resonance imaging (MRI), one can estimate regional workload in the early- and late-activated territories, as was done by Prinzen et al.[36]

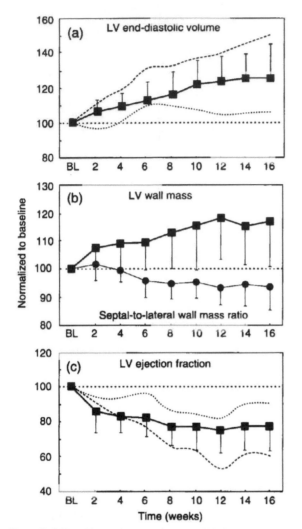

Figure 2.2 The effects of dyssynchrony on LV chamber properties over time. After 16 weeks of dyssynchrony, significant increases were seen in LV end-diastolic volumes (a) and CV wall mass (6; squares). Septal-to-lateral mass ratios decreased (B; circles), as did global LV systolic function (assessed by EF;C).

Work is indexed by the area of a stress–strain loop in each territory. It is substantially reduced in the early-activated region as compared with the late one (Figure 2.1c). This is thought to underlie the matching disparities in regional blood flow and metabolic demand demonstrated by several investigators[26,37,38] and to reduce mechanical efficiency.[31,39,40]

Mechanical dyssynchrony alone induces deleterious effects even in the absence of underlying heart failure. In dogs subjected to left bundle ablation and followed for 16 weeks,

ejection fraction gradually declined by 23%, while chamber dimensions and LV mass rose (Figure 2.2). This suggests that discoordinated contraction itself leads to regional stress maladaptations and in the long term contributes to cardiac dysfunction. Using more complex tissue analysis based on MRI, Helm et al[41] found similar regional changes in wall thickness and chamber dilation, as well as regional effects on fiber architecture and orientation. In particular, the transmural fiber gradient and laminar sheet orientation increased in the early-activated septum – changes thought to be a result of heterogeneous mechanical and electrical properties of the dyssynchronous heart.

ELECTROPHYSIOLOGY OF DYSSYNCHRONY

Cardiac dyssynchrony is also accompanied by regional heterogeneity of ventricular electrophysiology, including conduction velocity and refractoriness.[42] Using a canine model of LBBB-induced dyssynchrony (without superimposed heart failure), we found that zones in the highest-stress lateral LV endocardium displayed changes in connexin43 protein distribution, with lateralization of protein away from its usual location at the terminal intercalated disks (Figure 2.3a). In addition, while the normal ventricle displays more rapid conduction velocity (CV) in the endocardium versus overlying epicardium, we found that CV in the late-contracting region was significantly reduced (Figure 2.3b). The septal zone retained normal transmural patterns of CV. Neither of these changes were observed in controls. We also observed changes in refractoriness – indexed by action potential duration (APD) and tissue refractoriness. APD is normally somewhat longer in endocardium versus epicardium – a finding seen throughout the ventricle. However, in chronic LBBB hearts, while the epi/endo pattern was more or less preserved, there was striking regional shortening of APD in the late-contracting region (Figure 2.3c). The combination of both prolonged conduction velocity and shorter APD provides an intriguing and worrisome substrate for arrhythmia, and could contribute to the risk of sudden cardiac death in patients with dyssynchrony.

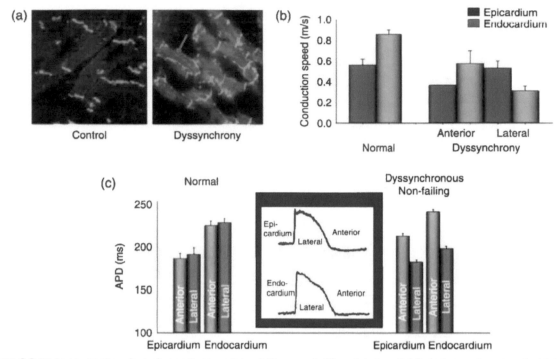

Figure 2.3 (a) In myocardium from dyssynchronous lateral LV, connexin43 protein is redistributed away from terminal interca-lated discs to the lateral myocyte border. (b) Regional patterns of conduction velocity (endocardium > epicardium in normal controls) are preserved in anterior segments of the dyssynchronous LV, but reversed in the lateral wall. (c) Marked reductions in endocardial and epicardial action potential duration (APD) were seen in lateral segments of dyssynchronous LV compared with anterior segments; no regional difference was seen in controls.

DYSSYNCHRONY AND MOLECULAR POLARIZATION

Given the substantial regional changes in mechanical stress and electrical remodeling seen in the dyssynchronous LV, it is perhaps not surprising that there are substantial local molecular signaling changes that occur as well. We have termed this 'molecular polarization', where localized alterations target to early-versus late-stimulated territories. In dyssynchro-nous failing hearts, we reported[43] a marked local decline in lateral LV expression of the gap junction protein connexin43 (Figure 2.4a) and the calcium cycling protein phospholamban (Figure 2.4b); a more modest reduction in sar-coplasmic reticular ATPase2a in the lateral LV was seen as well. Finally, regional changes in stress response kinases have been also been observed, including the mitogen-activated

protein (MAP) kinase ERK1/2[43] (Figure 2.4c), as well as calcium calmodulin kinase II, the MAP kinases p38 and JNK, and tumor necrosis factor α (TNF-α).[44] From new data, we have evi-dence that local amplifications of these stress responses in the late-contracting lateral wall are offset by CRT treatment,[44] and the mechanisms underlying these changes are being studied.

Another recent study examined regional gene expression changes induced by cardiac dys-synchrony. This investigation required the development of a miniature pacemaker for mice, and implantation of the chronic pacer to gener-ate dyssynchrony for 1–2 weeks (Figure 2.5a). As shown, pacing the RV free wall resulted in widening of the QRS and dyssynchronous wall motion revealed by M-mode echocardiography. Microarray analyis revealed that out of nearly 17 000 genes, relatively few were differentially affected at this early time point. The changes

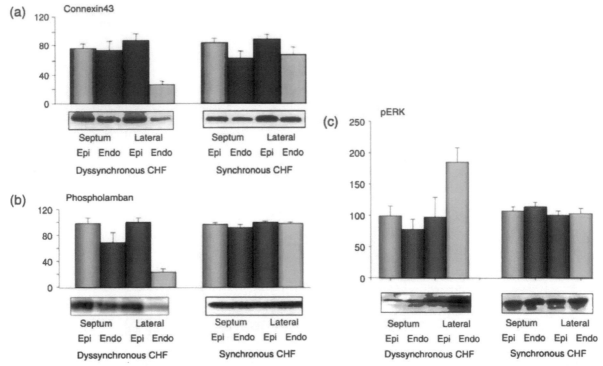

Figure 2.4 Molecular polarization of the dyssynchronous, failing LV includes significant LV endocardial reduction in connexin43 (a) and phospholamban (b) expression, and an increase in phosphorylated ERK (pERK) expression (c). Epi, epicardium; Endo, endocardium.

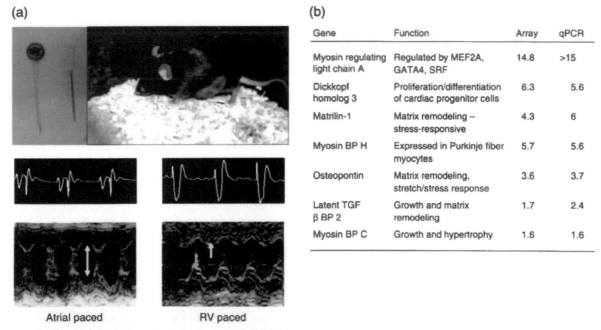

Gene	Function	Array	qPCR
Myosin regulating light chain A	Regulated by MEF2A, GATA4, SRF	14.8	>15
Dickkopf homolog 3	Proliferation/differentiation of cardiac progenitor cells	6.3	5.6
Matrilin-1	Matrix remodeling – stress-responsive	4.3	6
Myosin BP H	Expressed in Purkinje fiber myocytes	5.7	5.6
Osteopontin	Matrix remodeling, stretch/stress response	3.6	3.7
Latent TGF β BP 2	Growth and matrix remodeling	1.7	2.4
Myosin BP C	Growth and hypertrophy	1.6	1.6

Figure 2.5 (a) Sustained dyssynchrony in a mouse model has been achieved through the development of minature permanent pacemakers. Atrial pacing preserves LV synchrony, while RV pacing results in dyssynchrony (M-mode panels). (b) A variety of genes are differentially expressed in the dyssynchronous mouse model relative to controls. (Reproduced from Bilchick KC, Saha SK, Mikolajczyk E, et al. Differential regional gene expression from cardiac dyssynchrony induced by chronic right ventricular free wall pacing in the mouse. Physiol Genomics. 2006 Jul 12; 26(2):109–15[63].)

observed (Figure 2.5b) were intriguing, however, as they reflected genes that regulate muscle and electrical tissue development and differentiation, stem cell differentiation, and growth responses. Ongoing efforts to expand this to more chronic dyssynchrony in a large-animal model are presently underway.

CHAMBER EFFECTS OF CARDIAC RESYNCHRONIZATION

Mechanical and energetic consequences of intraventricular dyssynchrony can be mitigated by either biventricular or LV-only pacing. Early stimulation of the lateral LV free wall leads to mechanical re-coordination of contraction,[45,46]

as shown by MRI tagged imaging (Figure 2.6a). This effect results in a nearly instantaneous improvement in systolic function, demonstrated by the rapid rise in dP/dt_{max}, aortic systolic pressure, and stroke volume in a patient with CHF and LBBB, observed within one beat of LV pacing onset (Figure 2.6b,c). Improved systolic function has traditionally come with an energetic cost. This is shown from a study in 10 CHF patients subjected to dobutamine stress (Figure 2.6d). In contrast, CRT-induced systolic improvement occurs with a decline in energy demand (myocardial oxygen consumption) due to improved efficiency[32] (Figure 2.6d). Both acute mechanical and energetic benefits of CRT appear similar whether the stimulation is

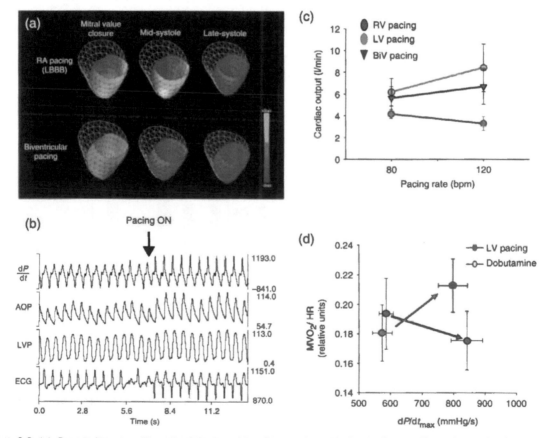

Figure 2.6 (a) Dyssynchronous LV activation (transition from red to blue) can be rectified with biventricular pacing. (b) Resynchronization results in immediate hemodynamic effects, including increase in dP/dt_{max}, aortic pressure (AOP), and LV pressure (LVP). (c) Cardiac ouput is increased with either biventricular (BiV) or LV-only pacing, but reduced with RV apical pacing. (d) The increase in LV systolic performance during CRT reduces myocardial energy consumption, in contrast to inotropic therapy, MVO_2/HR, myocardial oxygen consumption/heart rate.

biventricular or based solely on a single LV lead.[32,47,48] However, some changes, such as shortening of ventricular relaxation time and improvement in LV diastolic filling, appear better with biventricular rather than LV-only pacing.[49–51] In addition, biventricular pacing improves mechanical synchrony both in systole and in diastole, unlike LV-only pacing, which was less efficacious in diastole.[52] This disparity may reflect differences in the duration of myocardial activation between the two pacing patterns, with biventricular activation leading to more rapid contraction and earlier relaxation. When the LV alone is paced, contraction is slower in duration and can limit the diastolic period and relaxation rates. Whether chronic treatment with both approaches yields similar responses remains unclear, but studies are underway.

Chronic CRT leads to secondary reverse remodeling. In a study of 25 patients with class III–IV CHF and QRS widths >140 ms, Yu et al[53] found reductions in both end-systolic and end-diastolic volumes after 3 months of biventricular pacing. Importantly, when pacing was stopped acutely, these volumes remained low while systolic function (indexed by dP/dt_{max}) immediately declined (Figure 2.7a), suggesting true tissue remodeling, rather than a reflection of LV filling pressure or function. Leaving pacing off for 1 month resulted in gradual re-dilation, again further supporting true reverse remodeling. Reverse remodeling has also been observed in larger placebo-controlled trials, including MIRACLE[19] and Vigor-CHF,[54] with roughly 10% reductions in both end-systolic and end-diastolic volumes after 6 months of CRT treatment. Recent data from MIRACLE have extended these observations to 1 year (Figure 2.7b). While the data remain positive (sustained reverse remodeling) in patients with non-ischemic dilated cardiomyopathy, the results appear less sustained in ischemic heart disease patients.

It remains largely unknown whether CRT can reverse electrophysiological or molecular changes reported with chronic dyssynchrony.

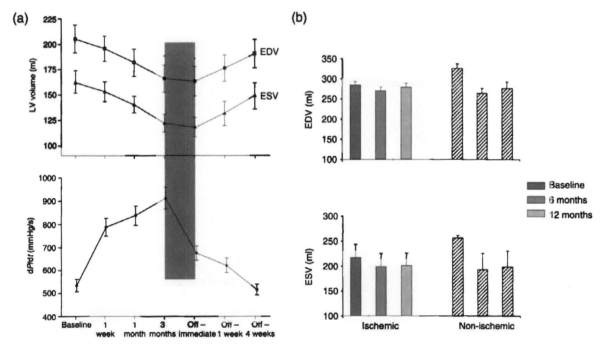

Figure 2.7 (a) Chronic CRT results in reverse remodeling (top: with reduced LV end-systolic volume (ESV) and end-diastolic volume (EDV)) during therapy; increased LV systolic function decreases immediately with cessation of CRT (bottom), while remodeling changes occur more slowly (orange highlight). (b) Remodeling is seen more in non-ischemic than in ischemic patients undergoing CRT.

Some investigators have expressed concerns that use of epicardial pacing is itself arrhythmogenic due to differences in transmural conduction and repolarization.[55] However, the recent CARE-HF trial supports improved mortality both from pump function and from sudden death with CRT only, and would argue against CRT augmenting arrhythmia susceptibility.[17] Ongoing studies are examining electrophysiological and molecular changes.[44]

FACTORS THAT CAN INFLUENCE CRT EFFICACY

There are four major components of implementing CRT that can impact how therapy influences heart function: AV delay time, interventricular delay time (i.e., delay between RV and LV), the location of the RV lead (i.e., septum versus apex), and the position of the LV lead.

Current biventricular pacing devices allow for modification of the AV delay during sequential AV pacing. Aurrichio et al[48] demonstrated that comparable mechanical benefits are achieved across a moderate range of AV delays, with optimal ventricular function at roughly half of the patient's native PR interval less 30 ms (Figure 2.8a). Some patients with particularly long intrinsic delays require customization, but most will gain a similar CRT effect by using a nominal AV delay of roughly 120 ms. Importantly, all of the major clinical trials of CRT utilized a mode of pacing in which the atria were not paced. Rather, atrial sensing was used to trigger pre-excited RV and LV pacing. Atrial pacing is suggested only in those individuals in whom symptomatic bradycardia due to sinus node dysfunction is present.

A more recent advance available in CRT devices is variable interventricular stimulation delay (i.e., RV–LV delay). Early reports have suggested that patients generally benefit from slightly premature LV activation, although

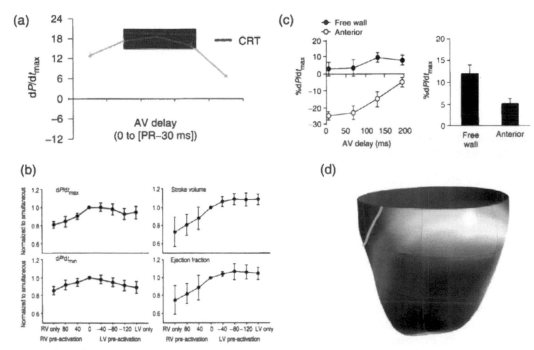

Figure 2.8 (a) LV systolic function as it relates to varying AV delay, with optimal function seen across a moderate range of AV delays. (b) LV systolic function varies with RV versus LV activation timing, with optimal LV dP/dt$_{max}$ and stroke volumes seen with LV-early or simultaneous RV/LV activation. (c) The effects of LV lead position (anterior or free wall) across a range of AV delays; optimal LV systolic function depends on lateral LV lead position. (d) MRI-guided map of optimal LV pacing site, with increased LV stroke work in red (lateral wall and apex).

this advance timing is rather small (namely, 10–15 ms).[56] Some patients were also found to have optimal LV systolic function with simultaneous or even premature RV activation (Figure 2.8b).[56] In subjects with atrial fibrillation and high-degree AV so that no supraventricular stimuli are present, there was no benefit of RV pre-activation, and minimal gain from LV pre-excitation.[50] Importantly, the simultaneous RV–LV stimulation used in all the major clinical trials appears very similar (within 10%) to the best results from optimized interventricular delay stimulation.

One of the most important aspects of effective CRT appears to be LV lead placement.[57] Butter et al[57] explored the acute effects of LV pacing site (anterior versus free wall) on net change in global systolic function (Figure 2.8c). In a series of 30 CHF patients (NYHA II–III) with a mean QRS width of 152 ms, biventricular pacing using lateral LV pacing sites consistently induced greater increases in dP/dt_{max} and aortic pulse pressure than anterior sites. In one-third of patients, anterior LV pacing reduced global systolic function, whereas this was not observed with later LV pacing. Experimental data suggests pacing at the mid to apical lateral wall may be superior than at the lateral base[58] (Figure 2.8d), but this has yet to be demonstrated clinically.

NON-RESPONDERS AND ELECTRICAL VERSUS MECHANICAL DYSSYNCHRONY

While generally effective, CRT does not have an appreciable clinical benefit in approximately 30% of patients, and substantial efforts have been made to better identify responders before implantation. This area is reviewed in other chapters in this volume, but here we focus on some of the reasons likely underlying poor response. One is the somewhat indirect relationship between QRS duration on surface electrocardiogram and mechanical LV dyssynchrony (Figure 2.9). Prolonged electrical activation, typically defined as a QRS width >120 ms remains the standard by which patients are selected, having been used in all major clinical trials. However, QRS width is a poor predictor of CRT efficacy, and studies have further shown

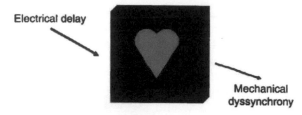

- Muscle fibrosis
- Heterogeneous scar/ischemia
- Heterogeneous contractile function
- Pulmonary hypertension
- Intramyocardial conduction delay
- Wall geometry/size

Figure 2.9 The 'black box' model of the complexity linking electrical activation delay and ultimate mechanical dyssynchrony. There are numerous factors that can alter the impact of the electrical timing delay as noted. Thus, examination of solely the ECG duration can be deceptive for predicting whether CRT efficacy will be achieved.

that it is poorly correlated with measures of LV mechanical dyssynchrony[59-61] based on tissue Doppler echocardiography.[60,61] Importantly, ventricular response to CRT correlates better with mechanical dyssynchrony than ECG duration (Figure 2.10a, b). This suggests that screening heart failure patients for CRT by QRS width alone may include a significant number who do not have sufficient mechanical dyssynchrony, while also missing many who might benefit from CRT.

The primary methodology being used to assess mechanical dyssynchrony is presently tissue Doppler, mostly based on longitudinal motion analysis. However, it should be remembered that this is not the orientation of the vast majority of myocardial fibers. As shown by the diffusion tensor MRI fiber analysis (Figure 2.10c), nearly 80% of myocardial fibers run in the circumferential orientation. Importantly, analysis of dyssynchrony based on motion in the two different orientations does not yield equivalent results. This was shown in an experimental animal model where MRI tags were used to simultaneously derive dyssynchrony indexes based on longitudinal versus circumferential strains. The latter provided clear delineation of the development of dyssynchrony during systole and marked separation between synchronization by CRT and baseline (Figure 2.10d).

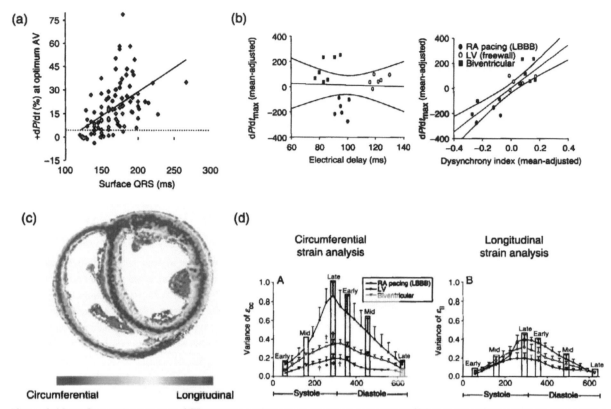

Figure 2.10 (a) Correlation between QRS duration and acute mechanical response to CRT in heart failure patients. While there is an over-significant relation, there is substantial scatter and the predictive value of the basal QRS duration is poor. (b) Experimental data from a canine model of heart failure and dyssynchrony demonstrating poor correlation between mechanical response and electrical delay, but a good relation between response and mechanical dyssynchrony in the same animals.[45] (c) Diffusion tensor MRI showing that the dominant orientation of myocardial fibers is circumferential (blue), with only small zones of epi- and endocardium oriented in more longitudinal directions. (d) Differential analysis of dyssynchrony depending on the orientation of the strain (circumferential versus longitudinal). The dyssynchrony index shows a gradual rise and decline in the basal state (LBBB + CHF), and this is markedly improved by CRT, particularly when viewed in the circumferential orientation. However, longitudinal strain analysis provides a far lower amplitude of change and greater variance, with little apparent effect from CRT, particularly during systole. (Part (b) reproduced from Leclercq C et al. Circulation 2002; 106: 1760–3.[45])

This contrasts to longitudinal analysis, which generated little differences during systole and an overall less disparity between conditions. (Figure 2.10d)[52]

With the growing emphasis on mechanical dyssynchrony analysis, it is important not to overestimate potential CRT response in candidates who may indeed have discoordinate wall motion, but an underlying mechanism not amenable to electrical stimulation therapy. This is depicted in Figure 2.11. Recall that with the activation delay (Figure 2.11a), regions develop stiffening at different times and effectively push and stretch upon each other. The vertical distance between the two stiffness curves describes this shift and is shown by the green curve – this would be perceived as dyssynchrony by tissue Doppler. However, suppose that the heart is heterogeneous and while it is stimulated simultaneously, one region is stronger and thus can stiffen more than the other (Figure 2.11b). This will also generate an apparent dyssynchrony pattern on tissue Doppler, but this is not treatable by CRT, since activation is simultaneous. As we move forward, combining both electrical

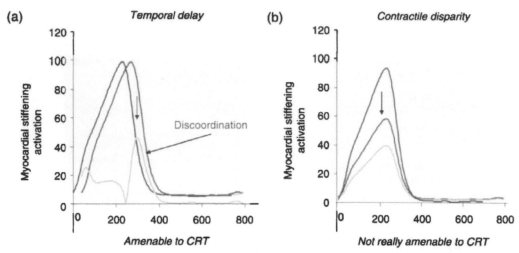

Figure 2.11 Dyssynchrony that can – or cannot – be ameliorated by CRT. (a) Basic model where electrical delay results in stiffening of one part of the heart later than the other. The difference between the two stiffness curves provides a time course of apparent dyssynchrony where one wall will stretch the other as it contracts. (b) This relation shows what would happen if one region of the heart were weaker than the other, but activated synchronously. There are again differences in stiffening that will result in stretch and contraction and apparent dyssynchrony. However, this is not amenable to electrical stimulation treatment. Reliance of purely mechanical analysis may also result in CRT implemented in patients who will not respond since the problem was not treatable by electrical stimulation.

and mechanical activation data will likely provide the best methods to identify responder patients.

CONCLUSIONS

LV mechanical dyssynchrony has multiple deleterious effects on the failing heart, altering molecular and electrophysiological behavior, altering regional stress, and inducing heterogeneous remodeling. Global contraction is depressed and there is impairment of energetic efficiency. CRT effectively re-coordinates contraction and likely reverses many of these abnormalities. Ongoing basic studies will further define just how this apparently simple yet ultimately complex interaction of mechanical contraction timing and myocardial failure works to alter heart failure pathophysiology.

REFERENCES

1. Gheorghiade M, De Luca L, and Bonow R O. Neurohormonal inhibition in heart failure: insights from recent clinical trials. Am J Cardiol 2005;96:3L–9L.
2. Jessup M, and Brozena S. Heart failure. N Engl J Med 2003;348:2007–18.
3. Capucci A, Romano S, Pugliesi A, et al. Dual chamber pacing with optimal AV delay in congestive heart failure: a randomized study. Europace 1999;1:174–8.
4. Scharf C, Li P, Muntwyler J, et al. Rate-dependent AV delay optimization in cardiac resynchronization therapy. Pacing Clin Electrophysiol 2005;28:279–84.
5. Meisner JS, McQueen DM, Ishida Y, et al. Effects of timing of atrial systole on LV filling and mitral valve closure: computer and dog studies. Am J Physiol. 1985;249:H604–19.
6. Brecker SJ, Xiao HB, Sparrow J, Gibson DG. Effects of dual-chamber pacing with short atrioventricular delay in dilated cardiomyopathy. Lancet 1992;340:1308–12.
7. Gold MR, Feliciano Z, Gottlieb SS, Fisher ML. Dual-chamber pacing with a short atrioventricular delay in congestive heart failure: a randomized study. J Am Coll Cardiol 1995;26:967–73.
8. Nishimura RA, Symansti JD, Hurrell DG, et al. Dual-chamber pacing for cardiomyopathies: a 1996 clinical perspective. Mayo Clin Proc 1996;71:1077–87.
9. Nishimura RA, Trusty JM, Hayes DL, et al. Dual-chamber pacing for hypertrophic cardiomyopathy: a randomized, double-blind, crossover trial. J Am Coll Cardiol 1997;29:435–41.
10. Baldasseroni S, Opasich C, Gorini M, et al. Left bundle-branch block is associated with increased 1-year sudden and total mortality rate in 5517 outpatients with

congestive heart failure: a report from the Italian network on congestive heart failure. Am Heart J 2002;143:398–405.

11. Murkofsky RL, Dangas G, Diamond JA, et al. A prolonged QRS duration on surface electrocardiogram is a specific indicator of left ventricular dysfunction. J Am Coll Cardiol 1998;32:476–82.

12. Iuliano S, Fisher SG, Karasik PE, Fletcher RD, Singh, SN. QRS duration and mortality in patients with congestive heart failure. Am Heart J 2002;143:1085–91.

13. Kashani A, Barold SS. Significance of QRS complex duration in patients with heart failure. J Am Coll Cardiol 2005;46:2183–92.

14. Cazeau S, Ritter P, Bakdaeh S, et al. Four chamber pacing in dilated cardiomyopathy. Pacing Clin Electrophysiol 1994;17:1974–9.

15. Bristow MR, Saxon LA, Boehmer J, et al. Cardiac-resynchronization therapy with or without an implantable defibrillator in advanced chronic heart failure. N Engl J Med 2004;350:2140–50.

16. Rivera DA, Bristow MR. Cardiac resynchronization – a heart failure perspective. Ann Noninvasive Electrocardiol 2005;10:16–23.

17. Cleland JG, Daubert JC, Erdmann E, et al. The effect of cardiac resynchronization on morbidity and mortality in heart failure. N Engl J Med 2005;352:1539–49.

18. Abraham WT. Cardiac resynchronization therapy. Prog Cardiovasc Dis 2006;48:232–8.

19. Abraham WT, Fisher WG, Smith AL, et al. Cardiac resynchronization in chronic heart failure. N Engl J Med 2002;346:1845–53.

20. Cazeau S, Leclercq C, Lavergne T, et al. Effects of multisite biventricular pacing in patients with heart failure and intraventricular conduction delay. N Engl J Med 2001;344:873–80.

21. Imanishi R, Seto S, Ichimaru S, et al. Prognostic significance of incident complete left bundle branch block observed over a 40-year period. Am J Cardiol 2006;98:644–8.

22. Baldasseroni S, Gentle A, Gorini M, et al. Intraventricular conduction defects in patients with congestive heart failure: left but not right bundle branch block is an independent predictor of prognosis. A report from the Italian Network on Congestive Heart Failure (IN-CHF database). Ital Heart J 2003;4:607–13.

23. Shamim W, Francis DP, Yousufuddin M, et al. Intraventricular conduction delay: a prognostic marker in chronic heart failure. Int J Cardiol 1999;70:171–8.

24. Wilkoff BL, Cook JR, Epstein AE, et al. Dual-chamber pacing or ventricular backup pacing in patients with an implantable defibrillator: the Dual Chamber and VVI Implantable Defibrillator (DAVID) Trial. JAMA 2002; 288:3115–23.

25. Sweeney MO, Hellkamp AS, Ellenbogen KA, et al. Adverse effect of ventricular pacing on heart failure and atrial fibrillation among patients with normal baseline QRS duration in a clinical trial of pacemaker therapy for sinus node dysfunction. Circulation 2003; 107:2932–7.

26. Vernooy K, Varbeek XA, Peschar M, et al. Left bundle branch block induces ventricular remodelling and functional septal hypoperfusion. Eur Heart J 2005;26: 91–8.

27. Vernooy K, Dijkman B, Cheriex EC, Prinzen FW, Crijns HJ. Ventricular remodeling during long-term right ventricular pacing following His bundle ablation. Am J Cardiol 2006;97:1223–7.

28. Freudenberger RS, Wilson AC, Lawrence-Nelson J, Hare JM, Kostis JB. Permanent pacing is a risk factor for the development of heart failure. Am J Cardiol 2005;95: 671–4.

29. Bader H, Garrique S, Lafitte S, et al. Intra-left ventricular electromechanical asynchrony. A new independent predictor of severe cardiac events in heart failure patients. J Am Coll Cardiol 2004;43:248–56.

30. Breithardt OA, Sinha AM, Schwammenthal E, et al. Acute effects of cardiac resynchronization therapy on functional mitral regurgitation in advanced systolic heart failure. J Am Coll Cardiol 2003;41:765–70 [Erratum 1852].

31. Baller D, Wolpers HG, Zipfel J, Bretschneider HJ, Hellige G. Comparison of the effects of right atrial, right ventricular apex and atrioventricular sequential pacing on myocardial oxygen consumption and cardiac efficiency: a laboratory investigation. Pacing Clin Electrophysiol 1988;11:394–403.

32. Nelson GS, Berger RD, Fetics BJ, et al. Left ventricular or biventricular pacing improves cardiac function at diminished energy cost in patients with dilated cardiomyopathy and left bundle-branch block. Circulation 2000;102:3053–9 [Erratum 2001;103:476].

33. Burkhoff D, Oikawa RY, Sagawa K. Influence of pacing site on canine left ventricular contraction. Am J Physiol 1986;251:H428–35.

34. Liu L, Tackman B, Girouard S, et al. Left ventricular resynchronization therapy in a canine model of left bundle branch block. Am J Physiol Heart Circ Physiol 2002;282:H2238–44.

35. Park RC, Little WC, O'Rourke RA. Effect of alteration of the left ventricular activation sequence on the left ventricular end-systolic pressure–volume relation in closed-chest dogs. Circ Res 1985;57:706–17.

36. Prinzen FW, Hunter WC, Wyman BT, McVeigh ER. Mapping of regional myocardial strain and work during ventricular pacing: experimental study using magnetic resonance imaging tagging. J Am Coll Cardiol 1999;33:1735–42.

37. van Oosterhout MF, Arts T, Bassingthwaighte JB, Reneman RS, Prinzen FW. Relation between local myocardial growth and blood flow during chronic ventricular pacing. Cardiovasc Res 2002;53:831–40.

38. Nowak B, Sinha AM, Schaefer WM, et al. Cardiac resynchronization therapy homogenizes myocardial glucose metabolism and perfusion in dilated cardiomyopathy and left bundle branch block. J Am Coll Cardiol 2003; 41:1523–8.

39. Baller D, Wolpers HG, Zipfel J, Hoeft A, Hellige G. Unfavorable effects of ventricular pacing on myocardial energetics. Basic Res Cardiol 1981;76:115–23.

40. Owen CH, Esposito DJ, Davis JW, Glower DD. The effects of ventricular pacing on left ventricular geometry, function, myocardial oxygen consumption, and efficiency of contraction in conscious dogs. Pacing Clin Electrophysiol 1998;21:1417–29.

41. Helm PA, Younes L, Beg MF, et al. Evidence of structural remodeling in the dyssynchronous failing heart. Circ Res 2006;98:125–32.

42. Spragg DD, Akar FG, Helm RH, et al. Abnormal conduction and repolarization in late-activated myocardium of dyssynchronously contracting hearts. Cardiovasc Res 2005;67:77–86.

43. Spragg DD, Leclercq C, Loghmani M, et al. Regional alterations in protein expression in the dyssynchronous failing heart. Circulation 2003;108:929–32.

44. Chakir K, et al. Regional and global reverse molecular remodeling from cardiac resynchronization therapy despite persistent heart failure in the dog. Circulation (in press).

45. Leclercq C, Faris O, Tunin R, et al. Systolic improvement and mechanical resynchronization does not require electrical synchrony in the dilated failing heart with left bundle-branch block. Circulation 2002;106: 1760–3.

46. Kawaguchi M, Murabayashi T, Fetics BJ, et al. Quantitation of basal dyssynchrony and acute resynchronization from left or biventricular pacing by novel echo-contrast variability imaging. J Am Coll Cardiol 2002;39:2052–8.

47. Kass DA, Chen CH, Carry C, et al. Improved left ventricular mechanics from acute VDD pacing in patients with dilated cardiomyopathy and ventricular conduction delay. Circulation 1999;99:1567–73.

48. Auricchio A, Stellbrink C, Block M, et al. Effect of pacing chamber and atrioventricular delay on acute systolic function of paced patients with congestive heart failure. The Pacing Therapies for Congestive Heart Failure Study Group. The Guidant Congestive Heart Failure Research Group. Circulation 1999;99:2993–3001.

49. Kass D. Left ventricular versus biventricular pacing in cardiac resynchronization therapy: the plot in this tale of two modes. J Cardiovasc Electrophysiol 2004;15:1348–9.

50. Hay I, Melenovsky V, Fetics BJ, et al. Short-term effects of right-left heart sequential cardiac resynchronization in patients with heart failure, chronic atrial fibrillation, and atrioventricular nodal block. Circulation 2004;110: 3404–10.

51. Bordachar P, Lafitte S, Reuter S, et al. Biventricular pacing and left ventricular pacing in heart failure: similar hemodynamic improvement despite marked electromechanical differences. J Cardiovasc Electrophysiol 2004;15:1342–7.

52. Helm RH, Leclercq C, Faris UP, et al. Cardiac dyssynchrony analysis using circumferential versus longitudinal strain: implications for assessing cardiac resynchronization. Circulation 2005;111:2760–7.

53. Yu CM, Chau E, Sanderson JE, et al. Tissue Doppler echocardiographic evidence of reverse remodeling and improved synchronicity by simultaneously delaying regional contraction after biventricular pacing therapy in heart failure. Circulation 2002;105:438–45.

54. Saxon LA, De Marco T, Schafer J, et al. Effects of long-term biventricular stimulation for resynchronization on echocardiographic measures of remodeling. Circulation 2002;105:1304–10.

55. Fish JM, Brugada J, Antzelevitch C. Potential proarrhythmic effects of biventricular pacing. J Am Coll Cardiol 2005;46:2340–7.

56. Sogaard P, Egeblad H, Pedersen AK, et al. Sequential versus simultaneous biventricular resynchronization for severe heart failure: evaluation by tissue Doppler imaging. Circulation 2002;106:2078–84.

57. Butter C, Auricchio A, Stellbrink C, et al. Effect of resynchronization therapy stimulation site on the systolic function of heart failure patients. Circulation 2001;104: 3026–9.

58. Helm RH, et al. Three dimensional mapping of optimal left ventricular pacing site for cardiac resynchronization. Circulation. 2007 Feb 27;115(8):953–61.

59. Schuster P, Faerestrand S, Ohm OJ. Color Doppler tissue velocity imaging can disclose systolic left ventricular asynchrony independent of the QRS morphology in patients with severe heart failure. Pacing Clin Electrophysiol 2004;27:460–7.

60. Bleeker GB, Schalij MJ, Molhoek SG, et al. Relationship between QRS duration and left ventricular dyssynchrony in patients with end-stage heart failure. J Cardiovasc Electrophysiol 2004;15:544–9.

62. Bleeker GB, Schalij MJ, Molhoek SG, et al. Frequency of left ventricular dyssynchrony in patients with heart failure and a narrow QRS complex. Am J Cardiol 2005; 95:140–2.

63. Bilchick KC, et al. Differential regional gene expression from cardiac dyssynchrony induced by chronic right ventricular free wall pacing in the mouse. Physiol Genomics. 2006 Jul 12;26(2):109–15.

3

Optimal medical therapy for heart failure with low ejection fraction: When to consider cardiac resynchronization therapy?

Mariell Jessup

Introduction • Neurohormonal antagonism: the foundation of medical therapy for dilated cardiomyopathy • Observations on optimal medical therapy • What else to consider before CRT? • Conclusions

INTRODUCTION

Heart failure is a complex clinical syndrome that can result from any structural or functional cardiac disorder that impairs the ability of the ventricle to fill with or eject blood.[1] The classic symptoms of heart failure are fatigue and dyspnea, which serve to limit exercise tolerance. In addition, the cardinal sign of heart failure is fluid retention, leading to congestion of the lungs and edema of the abdomen or extremities. There are many causes of heart failure, including disorders of the myocardium (the focus of this textbook), as well as abnormalities of the pericardium, endocardium, valves, or great vessels. The lifetime risk of developing heart failure is 20% in both men and women; this risk changes with age and time.[2]

There have been a number of recent comprehensive practice guidelines that outline an approach to the patient with suspected heart failure.[1,3–5] Most also emphasize an opportunity to identify patients at risk for heart failure, and institute a prevention strategy with the goal of minimizing ventricular remodeling. The American College of Cardiology/American Heart Association (ACC/AHA) Guidelines for the Evaluation and Management of Chronic Heart Failure in the Adult have been instrumental in more clearly articulating the early stages of heart failure, or the preclinical phase of the disease, and the patterns of disease associated with subsequent progression to clinical symptoms. (Figure 3.1). Nevertheless, there are no endorsed screening efforts to detect the disease at its earlier stages, and most countries are just now beginning to understand the economic impact of heart failure on national healthcare budgets.[6–9]

Myocardial dysfunction in heart failure is exhibited as a wide spectrum of phenotypes: from the patient with normal left ventricular (LV) volume and preserved ejection fraction (LVEF) to those with marked ventricular dilation and an associated low LVEF. The overwhelming numbers of clinical trials performed in a heart failure population have been in those patients with a dilated LV that is poorly contracting – a syndrome often referred to as systolic dysfunction. Although there is a growing recognition that as many as 30–50% of all hospitalized patients with heart failure have normal cardiac contractility, or a preserved LVEF, there remains a paucity of

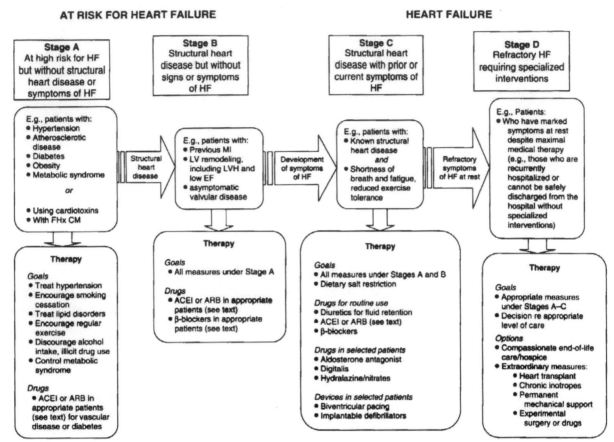

Figure 3.1 Stages in the development of heart failure (HF)/recommended therapy by stage. ACEI, angiotensin-converting enzyme inhibitor; ARB, angiotensin receptor blocker; EF, ejection fraction; FHx CM, family history of cardiomyopathy; LV, left ventricular; LVH, LV hypertrophy; MI, myocardial infarction. (Reproduced from Hunt SA et al. Circulation 2005;112:e154–235.[1])

evidence-based recommendations for this group.[10,11] (This syndrome has been given a variety of names, including diastolic heart failure and non-dilated heart failure.) Thus, in Figure 3.2, the greater part of the algorithm for the approach to the patient with the clinical syndrome of heart failure concerns systolic dysfunction.

Cardiac resynchronization therapy (CRT) is a well-accepted, device-based intervention for patients with dilated cardiomyopathy and heart failure symptoms.[12–15] The efficacy of CRT in improving morbidity and mortality in such patients has been explored through scores of large and small trials. Accordingly, the most recent recommendations from some of the

major cardiac societies have been to strongly endorse CRT in a selected population, as reproduced in Table 3.1. A high level of evidence supports CRT in patients with systolic dysfunction, for example, an LVEF ≤35%, a QRS complex duration >120 ms, in sinus rhythm, and who remain symptomatic (as in New York Heart Association (NYHA) functional class III or IV) despite *optimal* or *maximal medical therapy*. Unfortunately, there are no additional clues in any of the guidelines as to what constitutes optimal medical therapy before CRT should be considered. Clinicians must make reasonable judgments not only about the kind of medications on which their individual patients should be maintained, but also for how long the patients

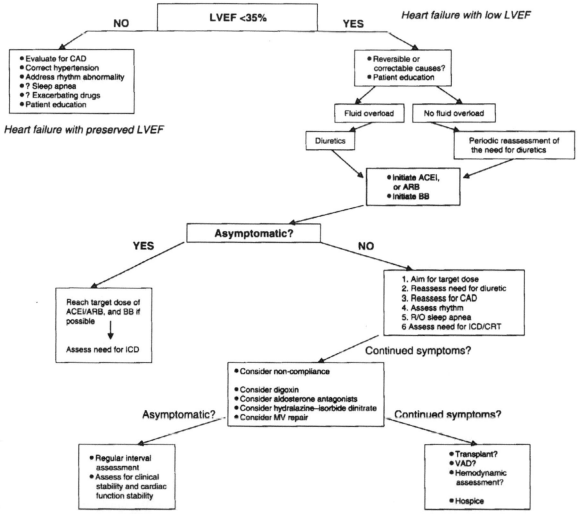

Figure 3.2 Management of the patient with the heart failure syndrome. This flow diagram represents an approach to the patient with symptomatic heart failure. ACEI angiotensin-converting enzyme inhibitor; ARB, angiotensin receptor blocker; BB, beta-blocker; CAD, coronary artery disease; CRT, cardiac resynchronization therapy; ICD, implantable cardioverter–defibrillator; LVEF, left ventricular ejection fraction; MV, mitral valve; VAD, ventricular assist device.

should be observed on medical therapy alone. Furthermore, it is not clear what criteria should be used to determine failed medical therapy.

This chapter outlines a reasonable (but not necessarily evidence-based) approach to patients with dilated cardiomyopathy who may become candidates for CRT. Clinicians must develop and use a clinical skill set in a systematic manner for all patients with heart failure, with regular reassessment tools to determine when therapy must be expanded. Figure 3.2 depicts this approach in a flow diagram.

If the patient has heart failure in the setting of a dilated LV and a low LVEF as determined by an echocardiogram, nuclear ventriculography, or angiography, the next step is to pursue, by means of a complete history and physical examination and a few simple diagnostic tests, a search for reversible or correctable causes of the cardiomyopathy. In the USA, the most common cause of dilated cardiomyopathy is chronic ischemia related to coronary artery obstruction.[16] A complete list of potentially correctable etiologies is beyond the scope of

Table 3.1 Indications for CRT according to recent guidelines.

ACC/AHA 2005: Guidelines for the Diagnosis and Management of Chronic Heart Failure in the Adult[1]
Patients with LVEF ≤35%, sinus rhythm, and NYHA functional class III or ambulatory class IV symptoms despite recommended, optimal medical therapy and who have cardiac dyssynchrony, which is currently defined as a QRS duration >0.12 ms, should receive cardiac resynchronization therapy unless contraindicated (level of evidence A)

HFSA 2006: Comprehensive Heart Failure Practice Guideline[3]
Biventricular pacing therapy should be considered for patients with sinus rhythm, a widened QRS interval (≥120 ms) and severe LV systolic dysfunction (LVEF ≤35% with LV dilation >5.5 cm) who have persistent, moderate to severe heart failure (NYHA class III) despite optimal medical therapy. (strength of evidence A)

ESC 2005: Guidelines for the Diagnosis and Treatment of Chronic Heart Failure[5]
Resynchronization therapy using biventricular pacing can be considered in patients with reduced ejection fraction and ventricular dyssynchrony (QRS width >120 ms), who remain symptomatic (NYHA class III–IV) despite optimal medical therapy to improve symptoms (class of recommendation I, level of evidence A), hospitalizations (class of recommendation I, level of evidence A), and mortality (class of recommendation I, level of evidence B)

this review, but may include illicit drug use or alcohol abuse, thyroid disorders, or uncontrolled hypertension. There is an increased understanding of the role of familial cardiomyopathy in the epidemiology of this disorder.[17–20]

Fundamental to the care algorithm, and to the successful management of the heart failure patient, is the initiation of patient (and family) education.[21] There are some key principles to cover with the patient, including the potential seriousness of the diagnosis; recommendations about diet (i.e., whether the patient needs to restrict fluid or sodium); recommendations about exercise; the development of a routine for the patient to self-monitor his or her volume status at home (usually done by daily weights); counseling about alcohol and/or nicotine use; an action plan for the patient who may develop increasing symptoms; and, finally, the discussion of end-of-life wishes. Although these instructions do take time initially, they will serve both the office staff and the patient well in the future. Moreover, there are an increasing number of interactive educational sites available on the Internet that will reinforce the instructions and teaching done in the office.

A great many of the symptoms experienced by patients with heart failure are a result of fluid retention and volume expansion. Breathlessness, abdominal bloating, peripheral edema, orthopnea, and dyspnea on exertion are often relieved with judicious use of diuretic agents. Indeed, diuretics produce symptomatic benefits more rapidly than any other drug used for heart failure; they can relieve peripheral or pulmonary edema within hours or days.[22–24] Currently, diuretics are the only drugs used in the outpatient management of heart failure that can adequately control fluid retention. Clinicians need to look for evidence of jugular venous distension, hepatic congestion, or edema during each patient encounter.[25] These simple items from a more extensive physical examination can be extremely helpful in the determination of fluid overload in an individual patient, and can be the first indication that drug therapy may need to be altered or added. Although some patients with dilated cardiomyopathy who have been stabilized on a standard regimen of neurohormonal antagonists may be effectively managed without diuretics, the large majority of patients will need a regular dose of diuretic (usually daily). Diuretic dosage may need to be adjusted as time and other circumstances change. Periodic physical examinations coupled with home weight monitoring and laboratory testing should be done to avoid azotemia or electrolyte imbalances. A key reason for follow-up office visits of the heart failure patient is to assess the need for diuretic dose adjustment.

Although illustrated as a separate step in Figure 3.2, the assessment for excessive volume, and the treatment of the same, is done simultaneously with the institution of the basic pharmacological weapons available for patients with systolic dysfunction.

NEUROHORMONAL ANTAGONISM: THE FOUNDATION OF MEDICAL THERAPY FOR DILATED CARDIOMYOPATHY

Every guideline published for the management of heart failure with low LVEF has reached concordance on recommendations mandating the use of angiotensin-converting enzyme inhibitors (ACEIs) and beta-blockers.[1,5,26] These two classes of agents have been unequivocally established to significantly improve both morbidity and mortality in this population. Likewise, review of mortality trials has suggested that there is no specific, preferred ACEI, in contrast to specific counsel about evidence-based beta-blockers.

All patients with a low LVEF (in the absence of aortic outflow obstruction) should be initiated and maintained on both an ACEI and a beta-blocker. For historical reasons, clinicians commonly start an ACEI first and add a beta-blocker as a second agent, but recent data suggest that starting a beta-blocker as initial therapy may have some advantages.[27] Clinicians need to keep in focus that their ultimate task is to maintain patients on both drugs at the highest tolerated dosages. Thus, it is reasonable to start both drugs at very low doses and then up-titrate each drug alternately until target doses are reached or patients become intolerant. If hypotension or azotemia develops, reducing diuretics or staggering the dosing time of the drugs may alleviate symptoms.

Clinicians, in their eagerness, may simultaneously start a patient with newly diagnosed dilated cardiomyopathy and heart failure on diuretics, ACEIs, and beta-blockers, all within a 12-hour period. The result is often hypotension, azotemia, or both, and the clinician may wrongly conclude that the patient is intolerant of these lifesaving drugs. Once a patient is euvolemic, there is no specific time course that necessitates rushing to get a patient on both drugs. A slow steady approach over several weeks is usually more successful. Many times, this can be done without an office visit, but rather through a nurse-administered titration protocol supervised by phone calls.

Patients with an intractable cough secondary to an ACEI should be placed on an angiotensin-receptor antagonist (ARB). On the other hand, patients with a rapid increase in creatinine, blood urea nitrogen (BUN), or potassium after an ACEI has been initiated will likely not tolerate an ARB either.[28,29] ARBs are appropriate substitutes for the patient intolerant of ACEI, but the available data suggest that there are no good substitutes for the benefits accrued by beta-blockade in these patients.[30-32] Every effort should be made to maintain patients with dilated cardiomyopathy on beta-blockers, even in the majority of patients with some degree of lung disease, and most certainly in diabetic patients.[33]

OBSERVATIONS ON OPTIMAL MEDICAL THERAPY

It takes time for the beneficial effects of the ACEI and beta-blocker combination to be quantifiable, especially when observing for evidence of reverse LV remodeling.[34] After target dosages of the two neurohormonal antagonists have been maintained for approximately 3–4 months, it is appropriate to reassess the functional status of the patient. If the patient is able to perform an acceptable level of daily living activities and is free from fluid retention (equivalent to an NYHA functional class I or II), the only remaining task is to assess whether the patient should be considered for an implantable cardioverter–defibrillator (ICD).[35-37] These patients should then be followed at intervals often enough to detect any worsening of symptoms or the addition of comorbid conditions.

It is important to assess a patient in a routine manner at each visit to accurately determine their symptomatic status. Patients with heart failure often begin to decrease their attempts at physical activity (usually subconsciously), so that over time their subjective complaints may diminish despite progressive cardiac deterioration. It is useful to inquire about one or two items that a patient must do on a regular basis, such as making a bed or showering and dressing without stopping, as a routine at each visit. Questions to patients about social outings or visits with family members can also be revealing, as patients with severe heart failure or profound fatigue will stop undertaking even pleasurable encounters but may not volunteer this information. Many clinicians incorporate some simple assessment of submaximal exercise into an office visit periodically. This may involve watching the patient walk in place, a measured walk in a hall, or a more formal treadmill test.[38] The amount of information gained, including the possibility of noting marked increases in blood pressure, failure of heart rate to augment, or the aggravation of arrhythmias, can often justify the time and expense of the test. There are also some standardized questionnaires that assess quality of life in patients with heart failure that can be self-administered in the office and maintained in the office file.[39,40]

If the patient continues to complain of fatigue, breathlessness, and fluid retention, there are some steps to consider before additional drug classes are initiated, or CRT is proposed. These considerations, as shown in Figure 3.2, include the following. Is it possible to try again to reach target doses of the ACEI and beta-blocker. Perhaps the patient will benefit from an increased dose or frequency of diuretics, or a combination of loop and distal tubule diuretics. Is there evidence of new or exacerbated ischemia that accounts for the patient's symptoms, and should a re-evaluation for coronary artery disease be undertaken?[41] Is the rhythm appropriate for the patient, and have both undue bradycardia or tachycardia been excluded? Is the patient's fatigue and nocturnal restlessness a manifestation of sleep apnea rather than worsening heart failure with orthopnea?[42,43] Is the patient's depression mimicking heart failure symptoms?[44,45] Finally, an effort should be made to ensure that the patient is indeed taking their prescribed medications. Non-compliance with a medical regimen is a frequent cause for heart failure decompensation.[46,47]

The above questions and considerations are challenging, and require time and diligence on the part of the clinician *and* the patient. Nevertheless, the differential diagnoses for a patient who is functioning poorly must include these alternative explanations. Despite the remarkable success of CRT, it continues to be evident that about one-third of all patients will derive very little clinical benefit after implantation.[15] Part of this failure to respond to CRT may be related to comorbid conditions such as arrhythmias, ischemia, sleep apnea, or depression that were not adequately addressed before implantation.

WHAT ELSE TO CONSIDER BEFORE CRT?

If a patient with dilated cardiomyopathy continues to have symptomatic heart failure despite all of the measures outlined above, they fall into unchartered territory as to the proper sequence of device or pharmacotherapy. There are a number of drugs that can be added to baseline ACEI and beta-blocker, but the relative value of one additional drug class over another cannot be compared.[33] Currently, there are three possible therapeutic alternatives that have been explored in randomized clinical trials: (i) the addition of an ARB;[48,49] (ii) the addition of an aldosterone antagonist;[50-52] or (iii) the addition of the drug combination hydralazine–isosorbide dinitrate.[53,54] All three approaches, when added to patients already on diuretics, ACEIs and beta-blockers, have been shown to have a meaningful and beneficial impact on outcome. Less well studied in a population already on ACEI and beta-blocker therapy is the addition of digoxin, but this drug has historically been a mainstay of heart failure treatment.[55-57] Nevertheless, clinicians should make every effort to add one of the above therapies to a patient with ongoing symptoms, with a preference for the use of one of the first three regimens, as they have been shown to significantly reduce morbidity and mortality.

It is at this point, however, that strong consideration for CRT in eligible patients should be undertaken. Indeed, there are virtually no data comparing the utility of implanting CRT to the patient already on the foundation of neurohormonal antagonists as compared with the addition of any of the drugs indicated above. The vast majority of patients enrolled in the large CRT trials were maintained on diuretics, ACEIs or ARBs, and beta-blockers. More recently, about half of the patients enrolled in CRT trials were also on aldosterone antagonists. Some patients had digoxin as part of their treatment regimen as well. As an example, in the CARE-HF trial, 95% of patients were either on an ACEI or an ARB, beta-blockers were maintained in roughly 75%, and approximately 55% of patients had the concomitant use of aldosterone antagonists; only 40% were using digoxin.[58] Likewise, in the COMPANION trial, 90% of patients were on either an ACEI or ARB, approximately 68% were using beta-blockers, and only 55% were on aldosterone antagonists.[59] Ultimately, clinicians have to decide, in the absence of trial data, whether the cost and potential efficacy of CRT is a superior choice over the employment of additional medications.

Further complicating this decision process are those factors that would mandate implantation of an ICD. As can be seen in Figure 3.2, the assessment for the need of an ICD is, for the most part, *independent of symptoms*. Thus, the current reality for most patients is that, after they have been stabilized on ACEIs and beta-blockers, and followed for 3–9 months, a repeat measure of LV function is typically performed. If, at that time, LVEF continues to be depressed, then strong consideration for ICD implantation is recommended for many patients.[34] Many clinicians are tempted, in selected patients with left bundle branch block, to implant CRT concomitant with the ICD surgery, even if optimal therapy has not been attained or the patient is symptom-free. The wisdom of this strategy is currently being investigated in a randomized trial.

CONCLUSIONS

Every consensus and guideline panel agrees that appropriate selection of the CRT candidate include an optimization of medical therapy prior to implantation. There is also unequivocal data to support the use of ACEIs or ARBs, in combination with beta-blockers, for all patients with dilated cardiomyopathy. Most clinicians recognize the signs and symptoms of a volume-overloaded patient, and the necessity to initiate diuretic therapy. The issue that remains problematic, and continues to be explored in clinical trials, is the extent to which medical therapy must fail before CRT is applied. If CRT proves to be useful in the stage B patient[60] – the patient who has never had symptoms of heart failure despite significant adverse remodeling of the

myocardium – then the future will bring a very different algorithm of care.

REFERENCES

1. Hunt SA, Abraham WT, Chin MH, et al. ACC/AHA 2005 Guideline Update for the Diagnosis and Management of Chronic Heart Failure in the Adult: a report of the American College of Cardiology/American Heart Association Task Force on Practice Guidelines (Writing Committee to Update the 2001 Guidelines for the Evaluation and Management of Heart Failure): developed in collaboration with the American College of Chest Physicians and the International Society for Heart and Lung Transplantation: endorsed by the Heart Rhythm Society. Circulation 2005;112:e154–235.

2. Lloyd-Jones DM, Larson MG, Leip EP, et al. Lifetime risk for developing congestive heartfailure: the Framingham Heart Study. Circulation 2002;106:3068–72.

3. Adams K, Lindenfeld J, Arnold J, et al. Executive Summary: HFSA 2006 Comprehensive Heart Failure Practice Guidelines. J Card Fail 2006;12:10–38.

4. Bocchi EA, Vilas-Boas F, Perrone S, et al. I Latin American Guidelines for the Assessment and Management of Decompensated Heart Failure. Arq Bras Cardiol 2005;85 (Suppl 3):49–94; 1–48.

5. Krum H. The Task Force for the Diagnosis and Treatment of Chronic Heart Failure of the European Society of Cardiology. Guidelines for the Diagnosis and Treatment of Chronic Heart Failure: full text (update 2005). Eur Heart J 2005;26:2472; author reply 3–4.

6. Boyd CM, Darer J, Boult C, et al. Clinical practice guidelines and quality of care for older patients with multiple comorbid diseases: implications for pay for performance. JAMA 2005;294:716–24.

7. Cleland JGF. Health economic consequences of the pharmacological treatment of heart failure. Euro Heart J 1998;19(Suppl P):P32–9.

8. Masoudi FA, Baillie CA, Wang Y, et al. The complexity and cost of drug regimens of older patients hospitalized with heart failure in the United States, 1998–2001. Arch Intern Med 2005;165:2069–76.

9. Masoudi FA, Havranek EP, Krumholz HM. The burden of chronic congestive heart failure in older persons: magnitude and implications for policy and research. Heart Fail Rev 2002;7:9–16.

10. Bhatia R, Tu J, Lee D, et al. Outcome of heart failure with preserved ejection fraction in a population-based study. N Engl J Med 2006;355:260–9.

11. Owan T, Hodge D, Herges R, et al. Trends in prevalence and outcome of heart failure with preserved ejection fraction. N Engl J Med 2006;355:251–9.

12. Bax JJ, Abraham T, Barold SS, et al. Cardiac resynchronization therapy: Part 2 – Issues during and after device implantation and unresolved questions. J Am Coll Cardiol 2005;46:2168–82.

13. Bax JJ, Abraham T, Barold SS, et al. Cardiac resynchronization therapy: Part 1 – Issues before device implantation. J Am Coll Cardiol 2005;46:2153–67.

14. Strickberger SA, Conti J, Daoud EG, et al. Patient selection for cardiac resynchronization therapy: from the Council on Clinical Cardiology Subcommittee on Electrocardiography and Arrhythmias and the Quality of Care and Outcomes Research Interdisciplinary Working Group, in collaboration with the Heart Rhythm Society. Circulation 2005;111:2146–50.

15. Jarcho J. Biventricular pacing. N Engl J Med 2006;355: 288–94.

16. Maron BJ, Towbin JA, Thiene G, et al. Contemporary definitions and classification of the cardiomyopathies: an American Heart Association Scientific Statement from the Council on Clinical Cardiology, Heart Failure and Transplantation Committee; Quality of Care and Outcomes Research and Functional Genomics and Translational Biology Interdisciplinary Working Groups; and Council on Epidemiology and Prevention. Circulation 2006;113:1807–16.

17. Caforio AL, Mahon NJ, Tona F, McKenna WJ. Circulating cardiac autoantibodies in dilated cardiomyopathy and myocarditis: pathogenetic and clinical significance. Eur J Heart Fail 2002;4:411–17.

18. Kies P, Bootsma M, Bax J, Schalij MJ, van der Wall EE. Arrhythmogenic right ventricular dysplasia/cardiomyopathy: screening, diagnosis, and treatment. Heart Rhythm 2006;3:225–34.

19. Matsumura Y, Elliott PM, Mahon NG, et al. Familial dilated cardiomyopathy: assessment of left ventricular systolic and diastolic function using Doppler tissue imaging in asymptomatic relatives with left ventricular enlargement. Heart 2006;92:405–6.

20. Portig I, Wilke A, Freyland M, et al. Familial inflammatory dilated cardiomyopathy. Eur J Heart Fail 2006;8: 816–25.

21. Colonna P, Sorino M, D'Agostino C, et al. Nonpharmacologic care of heart failure: counseling, dietary restriction, rehabilitation, treatment of sleep apnea, and ultrafiltration. Am J Cardiol 2003;91(9A): 41F–50F.

22. Brater DC. Drug therapy: diuretic therapy. N Engl J Med 1998;339:387–95.

23. Haller H. Diuretics in congestive heart failure: new evidence for old problems. Nephrol Dial Transplant 1999;14:1358–60.

24. Kramer BK, Schweda F, Riegger GAJ. Diuretic treatment and diuretic resistance in heart failure. Am J Med 1999;106:90–6.

25. Drazner M, Rame E, Stevenson L, Dries DL. Prognostic importance of elevated jugular venous pressure and a third heart sound in patients with heart failure. N Engl J Med 2001;345:574–81.

26. Adams J, Lindenfeld J, Arnold JM, et al. HFSA 2006 Comprehensive Heart Failure Practice Guideline. J Card Fail 2006;12:e1–e119.

27. Sliwa K, Norton GR, Kone N, et al. Impact of initiating carvedilol before angiotensin-converting enzyme inhibitor therapy on cardiac function in newly diagnosed heart failure. J Am Coll Cardiol 2004;44: 1825–30.

28. Gring CN, Francis GS. A hard look at angiotensin receptor blockers in heart failure. J Am Coll Cardiol 2004;44:1841–6.

29. Jong P, Demers C, McKelvie RS, Liu PP. Angiotensin receptor blockers in heart failure: meta-analysis of randomized controlled trials. J Am Coll Cardiol 2002;39:463–70.

30. Abraham WT, Iyengar S. Practical considerations for switching beta-blockers in heart failure patients. Rev Cardiovasc Med 2004;5(Suppl 1):S36–44.

31. Reiter MJ. Cardiovascular drug class specificity: beta-blockers. Prog Cardiovasc Dis 2004;47:11–33.

32. Lopez-Sendon J, Swedberg K, McMurray J, et al. Expert consensus document on beta-adrenergic receptor blockers. Eur Heart J 2004;25:1341–62.

33. McMurray J, Cohen-Solal A, Dietz R, et al. Practical recommendations for the use of ACE inhibitors, beta-blockers, aldosterone antagonists and angiotensin receptor blockers in heart failure: putting guidelines into practice. Eur J Heart Fail 2005;7:710–21.

34. Marchlinski FE, Jessup M. Timing the implantation of cardioverter-defibrillators in patients with non-ischemic cardiomyopathy. J Am Coll Cardiol 2006;47:2483–5.

35. Bardy GH, Lee KL, Mark DB, et al. Amiodarone or an implantable cardioverter-defibrillator for congestive heart failure. N Engl J Med 2005;352:225–37.

36. Boehmer JP. Device therapy for heart failure. Am J Cardiol 2003;91(6A):53D–59D.

37. Stevenson WG, Stevenson LW. Prevention of sudden death in heart failure. J Cardiovasc Electrophysiol 2001;12:112–14.

38. Demers C, McKelvie RS, Negassa A, Yusuf S, Investigators RPS. Reliability, validity, and responsiveness of the six-minute walk test in patients with heart failure. Am Heart J 2001;142:698–703.

39. Alla F, Briancon S, Guillemin F, et al. Self-rating of quality of life provides additional prognostic information in heart failure. Insights into the EPICAL study. Eur J Heart Fail 2002;4:337–43.

40. Rector T, Cohn J. Assessment of patient outcome with the Minnesota Living with Heart Failure Questionnaire: reliability and validity during a randomized, double-blind,

placebo-controlled trial of pimobendan. Am Heart J 1992;124:1017.

41. Uretsky BF, Thygesen K, Armstrong PW, et al. Acute coronary findings at autopsy in heart failure patients with sudden death: results from the Assessment of Treatment with Lisinopril and Survival (ATLAS) trial. Circulation 2000;102:611–16.

42. Bradley TD, Floras JS. Sleep apnea and heart failure: Part II: Central sleep apnea. Circulation 2003;107:1822–6.

43. Javaheri S. Heart failure and sleep apnea: emphasis on practical therapeutic options. Clin Chest Med 2003;24:207–22.

44. MacMahon KM, Lip GY. Psychological factors in heart failure: a review of the literature. Arch Intern Med 2002;162:509–16.

45. Vaccarino V, Kasl SV, Abramson J, Krumholz HM. Depressive symptoms and risk of functional decline and death in patients with heart failure. J Am Coll Cardiol 2001;38:199–205.

46. Opasich C, Rapezzi C, Lucci D, et al. Precipitating factors and decision-making processes of short-term worsening heart failure despite 'optimal' treatment (from the IN-CHF Registry). Am J Cardiol 2001;88:382–7.

47. Quaglietti SE, Atwood JE, Ackerman L, Froelicher V. Management of the patient with congestive heart failure using outpatient, home, and palliative care. Prog Cardiovasc Dis 2000;43:259–74.

48. Cohn JN, Tognoni G, Valsartan Heart Failure Trial I. A randomized trial of the angiotensin-receptor blocker valsartan in chronic heart failure. N Engl J Med 2001;345:1667–75.

49. Solomon SD, Wang D, Finn P, et al. Effect of candesartan on cause-specific mortality in heart failure patients: the Candesartan in Heart failure Assessment of Reduction in Mortality and morbidity (CHARM) program. Circulation 2004;110:2180–3.

50. Jessup M. Aldosterone blockade and heart failure. N Engl J Med 2003;348:1380–2.

51. Pitt B, Remme W, Zannad F, et al. Eplerenone, an aldosterone-receptor blocker, in patients with left ventricular dysfunction after myocardial infarction. N Engl J Med 2003;348:1309–21 [Erratum 2271].

52. Pitt B, Zannad F, Remme W, et al. The effect of spironolactone on morbidity and mortality in patients with severe heart failure. N Engl J Med 1999;341:709–17.

53. Steimle AE, Stevenson LW, Chelimsky-Fallick C, et al. Sustained hemodynamic efficacy of therapy tailored to reduce filling pressures in survivors with advanced heart failure. Circulation 1997;96:1165–72.

54. Taylor AL, Ziesche S, Yancy C, et al. Combination of isosorbide dinitrate and hydralazine in blacks with heart failure. N Engl J Med 2004;351:2049–57.

55. Rahimtoola SH. Digitalis therapy for patients in clinical heart failure. Circulation 2004;109:2942–6.

56. Rathore S, Wang Y, Krumholz HM. Sex-based differences in the effect of digoxin for the treatment of heart failure. N Engl J Med 2002;2002:1403–11.

57. The Digitalis Investigators Group. The effect of digoxin on mortality and morbidity in patients with heart failure. N Engl J Med 1997;336:525–33.

58. Cleland JG, Daubert JC, Erdmann E, et al. The effect of cardiac resynchronization on morbidity and mortality in heart failure. N Engl J Med 2005;352:1539–49.

59. Bristow MR, Saxon LA, Boehmer J, et al. Cardiac-resynchronization therapy with or without an implantable defibrillator in advanced chronic heart failure. N Engl J Med 2004;350:2140–50.

60. Goldberg LR, Jessup M. Stage B heart failure: management of asymptomatic left ventricular systolic dysfunction. Circulation 2006;113:2851–60.

4

Determinants of remodeling in systolic heart failure

John Harding and Thomas Cappola

Introduction • Clinical importance of remodeling • Pathophysiology of remodeling • Future directions

INTRODUCTION

Cardiac remodeling is a broad term that describes the change in size, shape, and function of the left ventricle (LV) that occurs in response to pathologic stress. The LV exhibits two classic patterns of remodeling, depending on the nature and duration of stress (Figure 4.1). Concentric remodeling, characterized by an increase in LV wall thickness and mass in the absence of chamber dilation, occurs in the early phases of pressure overload. Eccentric remodeling, characterized by chamber dilation and a decline in function, occurs in response to myocardial infarction, volume load, aortic or mitral regurgitation, and idiopathic dilated cardiomyopathy. There is substantial evidence in animal models that concentric remodeling often progresses to an eccentric phenotype in the situation of continued pathologic stress, but data in human subjects are less consistent.[1,2] Once initiated, remodeling progresses over time and ultimately results in symptomatic heart failure (Figure 4.2).

As reviewed elsewhere in this text, the use of cardiac resynchronization therapy (CRT) can induce a slowing or even reversal of remodeling in appropriately selected patients with eccentric remodeling, dyssynchrony, and systolic heart failure. However, remodeling is an extremely complex process, and it is important to appreciate the role of CRT in the larger context of factors that promote remodeling. This point is illustrated in Figure 4.3, which demonstrates the effect of CRT on serial changes in LV volume over 6 months of therapy. Although the efficacy of CRT is apparent, there is substantial variation in the progression or regression of remodeling in both the CRT and the placebo groups, indicating that factors other than conduction delay are playing a major role. The purpose of this chapter is to provide a brief overview of these determinants of remodeling in patients with systolic heart failure.

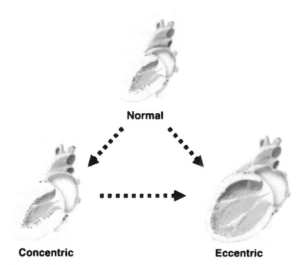

Figure 4.1 Overview of cardiac remodeling. (Adapted with permission from Jessup M, Brozena S. N Engl J Med 2003; 348:2007–18.[62] Copyright © 2003, Massachusetts Medical Society. All rights reserved)

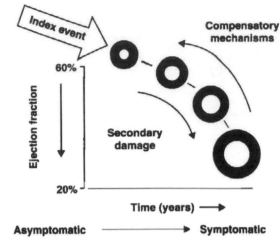

Figure 4.2 Progressive nature of cardiac remodeling and clinical heart failure. (Adapted with permission from Mann DL, Bristow MR. Mechanisms and models in heart failure: the biomedical model and beyond. Circulation 2005;111:2837–49.[19])

CLINICAL IMPORTANCE OF REMODELING

Two decades ago, White et al[3] first demonstrated the link between ventricular dilation after myocardial infarction and subsequent mortality. They followed 605 patients after myocardial infarction for a mean of 78 months and found that the post-infarction end-systolic volume had the greatest predictive value for mortality and was a more specific parameter than ejection fraction or end-diastolic volume alone. This important observation was extended to patients with idiopathic dilated cardiomyopathy by Douglas et al[4] Interestingly, patients with a more spherical LV and larger end-diastolic volumes had poorer survival compared with patients with a more ellipsoid LV, suggesting that ventricular size and geometry independently influence outcomes in systolic heart failure.

St John Sutton et al[5–7] extended these initial observations in what are now classic substudies of the Survival and Ventricular Enlargement (SAVE) clinical trial. After myocardial infarction, participants who experienced progressive ventricular dilation had increased mortality, progressive decline in ejection fraction, and greater risk for cardiac arrhythmias. Vasan et al[8] expanded these findings to the general population in a recent analysis of the Framingham Heart Study cohort. Participants in the general

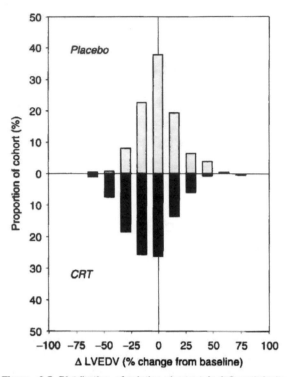

Figure 4.3 Distribution of relative changes in left ventricular end-diastolic volume (ΔLVEDV) over 6 months in 776 patients who participated in the MIRACLE and MIRACLE-ICD clinical trials. The CRT group (black) shows a leftward shift in the distribution of ΔLVEDV compared with the placebo group (gray), illustrating the therapeutic effect of CRT in promoting reverse remodeling. However, both groups show substantial variation in the degree of increase or decrease in LVEDV, as indicated by the widths of the distributions, and many patients experience large increases or decrease in LVEDV (>25%), even in the placebo group. Hence, factors other than CRT must have a strong influence on the progression of remodeling. Reprinted with permission from Journal of Cardiac Failure, Vol 12(3): Cappola TP, Harsch MR, Jessup M, et al. Predictors of Remodeling in CRT Era: Influence of Mitral Regurgitation, BNP and Gender. 182-8. 2006. With permission from Elsevier.

community whose LV end-diastolic dimensions were more than one standard deviation above average were more likely to develop congestive heart failure in the future. These and other studies demonstrate that cardiac remodeling is directly related to cardiovascular mortality in a broad range of patient populations. Moreover, virtually all lifesaving therapies in heart failure exert their clinical effects in association with slowing or reversal of remodeling.[5,6,9] As a result, the underlying mechanisms of cardiac remodeling have become a major focus of cardiovascular research over the past two decades.

PATHOPHYSIOLOGY OF REMODELING

Remodeling is a complex process mediated by pathogenetic factors at the cellular, whole-organ, and systemic levels (Figure 4.4), all of which interact to cause progressive LV dilation and failure. We briefly review each of these below, recognizing that many relevant factors remain undiscovered.

Cellular basis

Myocyte hypertrophy

Cardiac myocyte hypertrophy is one of the central pathologic features of remodeling, and has been the subject of intense research. Biomechanical stresses such as increased load, oxidative stress, inflammation, and neurohormonal activation activate a complex network of signaling pathways within cardiac myocytes that induce characteristic post-translational modifications, changes in gene expression, and changes in rates of protein synthesis (reviewed in references 10 and 11). Together, these result in a shift in contractile isoform expression, generation of new sarcomeres, an increase in myocyte size, and a shift in substrate preference away from fatty acids and toward glucose. The resulting myocyte phenotype is similar to that observed during fetal cardiac development, and, as such, the process of hypertrophy is often described as reactivation of a 'fetal program'. Patients with pressure overload typically add sarcomeres in parallel in response to stress (i.e., concentric

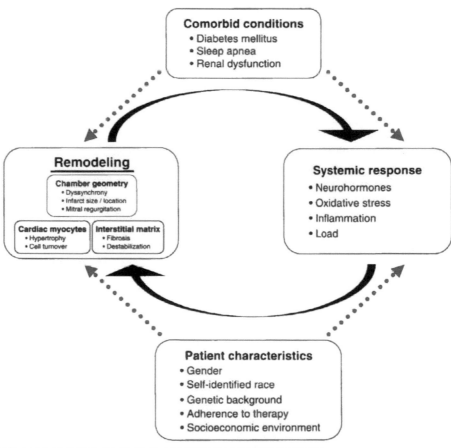

Figure 4.4 Overview of factors that contribute to remodeling in systolic heart failure.

hypertrophy), while patients with volume overload add sarcomeres in series (i.e., eccentric hypertrophy).[11] Initially, hypertrophy is an adaptive response to injury that minimizes ventricular wall stress, but over time it contributes to contractile dysfunction and progressive LV dilation.

Myocyte turnover: apoptosis and regeneration

In addition to hypertrophy, remodeling is associated with changes in myocyte turnover. Although this is a subject of considerable debate, many authors have suggested that apoptosis plays a significant role in the progression to symptomatic heart failure.[12] The same stressors that induce myocyte hypertrophy can also trigger myocyte apoptosis, contributing to loss of functional myocytes and progressive dilatation. It is difficult, however, to delineate how important the process of apoptosis is to ventricular remodeling, as the reported rate of apoptosis in patients with heart failure has a wide range in the literature.[12,13]

While apoptosis may play a central or perfunctory role in remodeling, novel therapeutic strategies have been developed that focus on negating cellular turnover with the introduction of stem cells or other myocardial progenitor cells that, in turn, differentiate into functioning cardiac myocytes. Although cell preparations and the methods of delivery vary greatly in the literature, pilot studies in patients have shown that progenitor cells may reduce LV volumes and increase ejection fraction in patients with acute and chronic ischemic heart failure.[14,15] Despite these early findings, randomized controlled clinical trials of cell-based therapies for ischemic heart failure have shown mixed results,[16-18] and larger trials are warranted to properly test the clinical efficacy and safety of such therapies.

Matrix remodeling/fibrosis

In addition to changes in cardiac myocytes, the interstitial matrix undergoes substantial pathologic change in association with cardiac remodeling,[19,20] including an increase in interstitial fibrosis and alteration in content of specific collagen isoforms.[21] The matrix is a highly dynamic tissue compartment regulated by a large family of proteases (matrix metalloproteinases, MMPs) and their endogenous inhibitors (tissue inhibitors of metalloproteinases, TIMPS). A growing literature suggests that changes in MMP activity, mediated by increases in MMP expression and/or decreased inhibition by TIMPs, destabilize the interstitial matrix and thereby promote ventricular dilation in the setting of pressure or volume load.[22] Accordingly, MMP inhibitors are being explored as a novel therapeutic strategy to attenuate post-infarction remodeling.[23,24]

Chamber geometry

Beyond changes at the cellular level, alterations in ventricular chamber geometry at the organ level can have a profound impact on the remodeling process.

Mitral regurgitation

As the ventricle dilates, it loses its normal ellipsoidal shape and becomes more spherical.[5] Sphericity contributes to increased wall stress via Laplace's law and causes mitral regurgitation by dilating the mitral valve annulus and stretching the papillary muscles, resulting in poor leaflet coaptation. Mitral regurgitation, in turn, exacerbates volume overload and begets further chamber dilation. Thus, it is no surprise that mitral regurgitation is common in patients with progressive remodeling, and the degree of regurgitation is often moderate to severe.[25,26] Trichon et al[26] prospectively analyzed over 2000 patients who presented for cardiac catheterization at their institution and found that 56% of patients with cardiomyopathy (ejection fraction <40%) had mitral regurgitation. Of these, almost 30% were graded moderate to severe (3+ to 4+). Importantly, survival at 1, 3, and 5 years was significantly lower in patients with moderate to severe mitral regurgitation, regardless of the etiology of heart failure. In addition, a substudy from the MIRACLE and MIRACLE-ICD clinical trials demonstrated that baseline mitral regurgitation is a significant risk factor for progressive ventricular dilation in patients with ischemic or non-ischemic cardiomyopathies.[27]

Myocardial infarction

The remodeling that occurs after myocardial infarction deserves special mention, because the extent and location of infarction can have a major impact on chamber geometry. For the first 48–72 hours after the initial injury, the primary means of acute remodeling occurs with infarct extension in the border zone between healthy and necrotic myocardium. Accordingly, strategies to improve perfusion either with thrombolytic therapy or primary coronary intervention have been employed to restore blood flow to the infarcted territory in order to limit infarct size.[28] Alterations in wall stress also play a role in infarct expansion in the acute setting and provide the rationale for using afterload reducing agents in the early post-infarct period. Pfeffer et al[29] demonstrated that a reduction in afterload within 30 days after myocardial infarction with the angiotensin-converting enzyme inhibitor (ACEI) captopril reduced wall stress and had a favorable impact both on long-term exercise capacity and on LV cavity dimension.

Dyssynchrony

As described elsewhere in this book, it has become clear that electrical and mechanical dyssynchrony contribute substantially to remodeling (Figure 4.4), and that resynchronization therapy induces reverse remodeling. The reader is referred to Chapter 2 for a detailed discussion of these mechanisms.

Neurohormonal activation

A variety of neurohormonal systems become activated at the systemic level in response to abnormal cardiac function. These responses serve to maintain vital organ perfusion in the acute setting, yet chronically they contribute to progressive remodeling and heart failure.

Sympathetic activation

Cohn et al[30] demonstrated the link between sympathetic activation and heart failure in their classic study showing that baseline plasma norepinephrine (noradrenaline) levels predict mortality in patient with heart failure. Moreover, plasma catecholamines have also been shown to associate with progressive ventricular dilation.[31] These are but two examples from an extensive body of evidence verifying a strong association between sympathetic activation and heart failure progression (reviewed in reference 19).

Elevated levels of catecholamines increase peripheral vasoconstriction, leading to increased mechanical load on the failing myocardium. Additionally, sympathetic stimulation directly promotes cardiac myocyte hypertrophy via adrenergic receptors on cardiac myocytes. Chronic adrenergic stimulation eventually leads to a downregulation of myocardial adrenergic receptor density and function, resulting in a diminished response to appropriate adrenergic surges in times of stress.[32] All of these mechanisms contribute to progressive remodeling and worse outcome.

Renin–angiotensin–aldosterone system

Activation of the renin–angiotensin–aldosterone system (RAAS) is one of the hallmarks of congestive heart failure, and has been the subject of intense research for more than two decades (reviewed in reference 11). In response to renal hypoperfusion and sympathetic stimulation, renin is released from the juxtaglomerular apparatus of the nephron into the circulation, where it converts the propeptide angiotensinogen to angiotensin I. In turn, angiotensin I is cleaved by angiotensin-converting enzyme (ACE) into the bioactive peptide angiotensin II (AII). AII is a potent vasoconstrictor that exacerbates remodeling via a number of mechanisms. These include increasing ventricular load and direct stimulation of pro-hypertrophic and pro-apoptotic signaling pathways in cardiac myocytes via specific AII receptors. In addition, AII stimulates aldosterone release by the adrenals, resulting in renal sodium and water retention, and remodeling of the myocardial matrix via a direct profibrotic effect of aldosterone on the myocardium.[33]

The most compelling evidence supporting the role of RAAS activation in promoting remodeling in humans comes from the results of large clinical trials demonstrating that RAAS inhibition improves clinical outcome and attenuates cardiac remodeling. These findings have been consistent in numerous trials using different strategies to blunt RAAS activation, including ACEIs,[29] AII receptor blockers,[34] and aldosterone antagonists.[35,36] Indeed, RAAS antagonists and beta-blockers form the cornerstone of modern heart failure pharmacotherapy and are reviewed in detail in Chapter 3.

Natriuretic peptides

To counterbalance the effects of systemic neurohormonal activation, the heart has evolved an 'endogenous hormonal system' composed mainly of natriuretic peptides. Most important among these is brain natriuretic peptide (BNP), which is synthesized and released by cardiac myocytes in response to biomechanical stressors. BNP is released as a prohormone and cleaved by the enzyme corin into a biologically inactive N-terminal fragment (NT-BNP) and a bioactive C-terminal fragment (CT-BNP). Acting through the specific cell-surface receptors, BNP causes vasodilation, natriuresis, and attenuation of hypertrophic signaling pathways in cardiac myocytes. As such, BNP can be regarded as an endogenous 'anti-remodeling' hormone. These findings have clinical importance, as elevated BNP in the peripheral circulation can aid in establishing the diagnosis and prognosis of heart failure patients.[37,38] Currently, infusion of recombinant CT-BNP is used clinically to treat decompensated heart failure by inducing vasodilation and natriuresis.[39] Whether chronic stimulation of natriuretic peptide receptors attenuates cardiac remodeling awaits the development of orally active BNP analogues.

Other neurohormones

Additional neurohormones are activated in association with heart failure, including endothelin,[40,41] apelin,[42] adrenomedullin,[43] and urocortin,[44] among others. As research continues, it seems likely that additional neurohormones will be discovered. In general, these neurohormones modulate vascular tone, renal sodium and water retention, and hypertrophic signaling pathways within myocytes. However, inhibitors of several of these neurohormones have failed to change the course of remodeling in clinical trials beyond the treatment effect caused by adrenergic receptor blockers and RAAS inhibitors. These findings suggest that our ability to treat heart failure via antagonism of additional neurohormones is beginning to plateau.

Inflammation and oxidative stress

Much as in the progression of atherosclerotic coronary vascular disease, inflammation plays a key role in ventricular remodeling. Inflammatory cytokines such as tumor necrosis factor α (TNF-α) and interleukin-6 (IL-6) are elevated in heart failure patients and promote hypertrophy and matrix remodeling in animal models. Inflammation also results in downstream elaboration of reactive oxygen species (ROS) that may directly damage cellular components and interfere with endogenous nitric oxide signaling (reviewed in reference 45). This has stimulated clinical research utilizing cytokine inhibitors and inhibitors of reactive species production.[46] Although preclinical data are compelling, these interventions have thus far shown no clinically meaningful effect on remodeling or outcome in clinical trials.[47]

Comorbid conditions

Obstructive sleep apnea

Recent evidence suggests that a large number of patients with heart failure have sleep-disordered breathing attributable to obstructive sleep apnea (OSA) and/or central sleep apnea (CSA), and that reduction of apneic events with continuous positive airway pressure (CPAP) can have favorable effects on ventricular remodeling.[48,49] Kaneko et al[48] demonstrated that 1 month of CPAP therapy significantly reduced hypopneic or apneic events and improved LV function when compared with patients on optimal medical therapy. Other studies have also shown CPAP to reduce LV afterload, which directly affects LV wall stress.[49]

Diabetes mellitus

Evidence from the SAVE trial revealed that in a well-described cohort, diabetic patients were more prone to develop heart failure after myocardial infarction. Despite a higher incidence of heart failure, diabetic patients exhibited less LV cavity dilation compared with non-diabetic controls.[50] This is consistent with a more concentric pattern of remodeling in diabetic patients, which may be attributable to increased large-artery stiffness and/or formation of advanced glycation end-products (AGE) within the cardiac interstitium in the setting of hyperglycemia.[51] While further research is necessary to define these mechanisms, diabetes should be viewed as an important clinical modifier of the remodeling process.

Renal insufficiency

Renal insufficiency is common in subjects with cardiac disease, and is associated with an acceleration in cardiac remodeling. Shlipak et al[52] illustrated the magnitude of this association in a population-based study of almost 6000 subjects. Renal insufficiency was associated with pathologic ventricular hypertrophy and with higher cardiovascular morbidity and mortality. A variety of mechanisms for this association have been postulated, including increased hypertension and vascular stiffness, and increased levels of neurohormones and other metabolites associated with poor renal function.

Patient characteristics

Gender

Several studies have demonstrated gender-specific features of cardiac remodeling. In response to pressure load or myocardial infarction, women tend to exhibit less ventricular dilation than men and are more likely to experience a phenotype of concentric remodeling.[53,54] This holds true even in more advanced stages of systolic heart failure, where women tend to dilate more slowly than men.[27] The mechanisms underlying these observations are poorly understood, but they are postulated to be due to differences in application of heart failure pharmacotherapies and/or to underlying biologic differences (e.g., differences in endogenous sex steroids) that may directly influence the remodeling response.

Self-identified race

Self-identified race has been associated with differences in cardiac remodeling in several observational studies.[55] In a substudy of the SOLVD clinical trial cohort, Dries et al[56] determined that self-identified African–Americans had higher risk of heart failure progression and higher mortality than self-identified Caucasians. There is now substantial debate regarding the meaning of self-identified race and the extent to which disease risk associated with race is due to inherited genetic predisposition or to different social, economic, and environmental factors that are associated with racial/ethnic groups. Properly studying the complexity of race and its influence on remodeling will require collaborative studies among cardiovascular researchers, geneticists, epidemiologists, and social scientists.

Genetic variation

The Framingham Offspring Study quantified cardiac hypertrophy in the general population using echocardiography in a large cohort of families, and found substantial heritability in LV mass.[57] This finding, which has since been validated in other cohorts,[58] strongly suggests than genetic variation passed within families predisposes patients to undergo different degrees of remodeling. At the same time, systolic heart failure cohorts in which patients have been rigorously phenotyped demonstrate substantial variation in the progression of remodeling.[27] This variation cannot be explained by clinical factors, and again suggests that genetic background of individual patients influences the clinical course of remodeling and heart failure. Defining these variants using modern genomic approaches has now become a major focus of heart failure research.

Adherence to therapy and socioeconomic environment

Although well beyond the scope of this text, it is important to recognize that patient behavior, adherence to prescribed therapy, and socioeconomic environment play substantial roles in determining the course and outcome of heart failure.[59]

As such, these factors will assuredly modify the course of cardiac remodeling. These observations are intuitive to practicing clinicians, and any complete treatment strategy or research effort in human subjects needs to address these components of heart failure progression.

FUTURE DIRECTIONS

As summarized in this chapter, ventricular remodeling is determined by complex interactions among numerous factors. CRT can induce a potent anti-remodeling effect by correcting electrical and mechanical dyssynchrony, but the role of resynchronization must be understood within this broader context (Figure 4.4). Although the future of heart failure therapeutics is impossible to predict, it is fair to assume that new treatments will build on at least three major themes. First, aspects of remodeling that are not directly addressed by any current treatments will hold promise as new therapeutic targets. Current examples under development include agents that directly target hypertrophic signaling in cardiac myocytes (e.g., histone deacetylase inhibitors[60] and type 5 phosphodiesterase inhibitors[61]) and cell-based therapies that aim to promote myocardial regeneration. Second, more effort will be spent focusing existing therapies on the subgroups of patients most likely to derive clinical benefit and least likely to experience toxicity. This 'personalized' approach will be accomplished using techniques ranging from more precise clinical guidelines for the use of drugs and devices to sophisticated pharmacogenomic profiling. Third, and perhaps most important, early recognition of risk factors for maladaptive remodeling may provide a remarkable opportunity to address remodeling in its early stages before a patient develops symptomatic heart failure.

REFERENCES

1. Berenji K, Drazner MH, Rothermel BA, Hill JA. Does load-induced ventricular hypertrophy progress to systolic heart failure? Am J Physiol Heart Circ Physiol 2005;289:H8–16.

2. Drazner MH. The transition from hypertrophy to failure: how certain are we? Circulation 2005 Aug 16;112:936–8.

3. White HD, Norris RM, Brown MA, et al. Left ventricular end-systolic volume as the major determinant of survival after recovery from myocardial infarction. Circulation 1987;76:44–51.

4. Douglas PS, Morrow R, Ioli A, Reichek N. Left ventricular shape, afterload and survival in idiopathic dilated cardiomyopathy. J Am Coll Cardiol 1989;13:311–15.

5. St John Sutton M, Pfeffer MA, Moye L, et al. Cardiovascular death and left ventricular remodeling two years after myocardial infarction: baseline predictors and impact of long-term use of captopril: information from the Survival and Ventricular Enlargement (SAVE) trial. Circulation 1997;96:3294–9.

6. St John Sutton M, Pfeffer MA. Prevention of post-infarction left ventricular remodeling by ACE-inhibitors. Cardiologia 1994;39(12 Suppl 1):27–30.

7. St John Sutton M, Lee D, Rouleau JL, et al. Left ventricular remodeling and ventricular arrhythmias after myocardial infarction. Circulation 2003;107:2577–82.

8. Vasan RS, Larson MG, Benjamin EJ, Evans JC, Levy D. Left ventricular dilatation and the risk of congestive heart failure in people without myocardial infarction. N Engl J Med 1997;336:1350–5.

9. Eichhorn EJ, Bristow MR. Medical therapy can improve the biological properties of the chronically failing heart. A new era in the treatment of heart failure. Circulation 1996;94:2285–96.

10. Frey N, Olson EN. Cardiac hypertrophy: the good, the bad, and the ugly. Annu Rev Physiol 2003;65:45–79.

11. Opie LH, Commerford PJ, Gersh BJ, Pfeffer MA. Controversies in ventricular remodelling. Lancet 2006; 367:356–67.

12. Narula J, Hajjar RJ, Dec GW. Apoptosis in the failing heart. Cardiol Clin 1998;16:691–710, ix.

13. Kitsis RN, Mann DL. Apoptosis and the heart: a decade of progress. J Mol Cell Cardiol 2005;38:1–2.

14. Perin EC, Dohmann HF, Borojevic R, et al. Transendocardial, autologous bone marrow cell transplantation for severe, chronic ischemic heart failure. Circulation 2003;107:2294–302.

15. Strauer BE, Brehm M, Zeus T, et al. Repair of infarcted myocardium by autologous intracoronary mononuclear bone marrow cell transplantation in humans. Circulation 2002;106:1913–18.

16. Assmus B, Honold J, Schachinger V, et al. Transcoronary transplantation of progenitor cells after myocardial infarction. N Engl J Med 2006;355:1222–32.

17. Schachinger V, Erbs S, Elsasser A, et al. Intracoronary bone marrow-derived progenitor cells in acute myocardial infarction. N Engl J Med 2006;355:1210–21.

18. Lunde K, Solheim S, Aakhus S, et al. Intracoronary injection of mononuclear bone marrow cells in acute myocardial infarction. N Engl J Med 2006;355: 1199–209.

19. Mann DL, Bristow MR. Mechanisms and models in heart failure: the biomechanical model and beyond. Circulation 2005;111:2837–49.

20. Hein S, Arnon E, Kostin S, et al. Progression from compensated hypertrophy to failure in the pressure-overloaded human heart: structural deterioration and compensatory mechanisms. Circulation 2003;107:984–91.

21. Polyakova V, Hein S, Kostin S, Ziegelhoeffer T, Schaper J. Matrix metalloproteinases and their tissue inhibitors in pressure-overloaded human myocardium during heart failure progression. J Am Coll Cardiol 2004;44:1609–18.

22. Thomas CV, Coker ML, Zellner JL, et al. Increased matrix metalloproteinase activity and selective upregulation in LV myocardium from patients with end-stage dilated cardiomyopathy. Circulation 1998;97:1708–15.

23. Ikonomidis JS, Hendrick JW, Parkhurst AM, et al. Accelerated LV remodeling after myocardial infarction in TIMP-1-deficient mice: effects of exogenous MMP inhibition. Am J Physiol Heart Circ Physiol 2005;288:H149–58.

24. Chapman RE, Scott AA, Deschamps AM, et al. Matrix metalloproteinase abundance in human myocardial fibroblasts: effects of sustained pharmacologic matrix metalloproteinase inhibition. J Mol Cell Cardiol 2003;35:539–48.

25. Mehra MR, Griffith BP. Is mitral regurgitation a viable treatment target in heart failure? The plot just thickened. J Am Coll Cardiol 2005;45:388–90.

26. Trichon BH, Felker GM, Shaw LK, Cabell CH, O'Connor CM. Relation of frequency and severity of mitral regurgitation to survival among patients with left ventricular systolic dysfunction and heart failure. Am J Cardiol 2003;91:538–43.

27. Cappola TP, Harsch MR, Jessup M, et al. Predictors of remodeling in the CRT era: influence of mitral regurgitation, BNP, and gender. J Card Fail 2006;12:182–8. Reprinted with permission from Elsevier.

28. Pfeffer MA, Braunwald E. Ventricular remodeling after myocardial infarction. Experimental observations and clinical implications. Circulation 1990;81:1161–72.

29. Pfeffer MA, Lamas GA, Vaughan DE, Parisi AF, Braunwald E. Effect of captopril on progressive ventricular dilatation after anterior myocardial infarction. N Engl J Med 1988;319:80–6.

30. Cohn JN, Levine TB, Olivari MT, et al. Plasma norepinephrine as a guide to prognosis in patients with chronic congestive heart failure. N Engl J Med 1984;311:819–23.

31. Cohn JN. Structural basis for heart failure. Ventricular remodeling and its pharmacological inhibition. Circulation 1995;91:2504–7.

32. Rockman HA, Koch WJ, Lefkowitz RJ. Seven-transmembrane-spanning receptors and heart function. Nature 2002;415:206–12.

33. Lijnen P, Petrov V. Induction of cardiac fibrosis by aldosterone. J Mol Cell Cardiol 2000;32:865–79.

34. Pitt B, Poole-Wilson PA, Segal R, et al. Effect of losartan compared with captopril on mortality in patients with symptomatic heart failure: randomised trial – the Losartan Heart Failure Survival Study ELITE II. Lancet 2000;355:1582–7.

35. Pitt B, Zannad F, Remme WJ, et al. The effect of spironolactone on morbidity and mortality in patients with severe heart failure. Randomized Aldactone Evaluation Study Investigators. N Engl J Med 1999;341:709–17.

36. Pitt B, Remme W, Zannad F, et al. Eplerenone, a selective aldosterone blocker, in patients with left ventricular dysfunction after myocardial infarction. N Engl J Med 2003;348:1309–21.

37. Maisel AS, Krishnaswamy P, Nowak RM, et al. Rapid measurement of B-type natriuretic peptide in the emergency diagnosis of heart failure. N Engl J Med 2002;347:161–7.

38. Omland T, Aakvaag A, Bonarjee VV, et al. Plasma brain natriuretic peptide as an indicator of left ventricular systolic function and long-term survival after acute myocardial infarction. Comparison with plasma atrial natriuretic peptide and N-terminal proatrial natriuretic peptide. Circulation 1996;93:1963–9.

39. Colucci WS, Elkayam U, Horton DP, et al. Intravenous nesiritide, a natriuretic peptide, in the treatment of decompensated congestive heart failure. Nesiritide Study Group. N Engl J Med 2000;343:246–53.

40. Fraccarollo D, Hu K, Galuppo P, Gaudron P, Ertl G. Chronic endothelin receptor blockade attenuates progressive ventricular dilation and improves cardiac function in rats with myocardial infarction: possible involvement of myocardial endothelin system in ventricular remodeling. Circulation 1997;96:3963–73.

41. Konstam MA, DeNofrio D. Endothelin expression and the progression of heart failure: exemplifying the vagaries of therapeutic development. Circulation 2004;109:143–5.

42. Chen MM, Ashley EA, Deng DX, et al. Novel role for the potent endogenous inotrope apelin in human cardiac dysfunction. Circulation 2003;108:1432–9.

43. Jougasaki M, Wei CM, McKinley LJ, Burnett JC Jr. Elevation of circulating and ventricular adrenomedullin in human congestive heart failure. Circulation 1995;92:286–9.

44. Rademaker MT, Cameron VA, Charles CJ, Richards AM. Integrated hemodynamic, hormonal, and renal actions of urocortin 2 in normal and paced sheep: beneficial effects in heart failure. Circulation 2005;112:3624–32.

45. Sawyer DB, Siwik DA, Xiao L, et al. Role of oxidative stress in myocardial hypertrophy and failure. J Mol Cell Cardiol 2002;34:379–88.

46. Hajjar RJ, Leopold JA. Xanthine oxidase inhibition and heart failure: novel therapeutic strategy for ventricular dysfunction? Circ Res 2006;98:169–71.

47. Mann DL, McMurray JJ, Packer M, et al. Targeted anticytokine therapy in patients with chronic heart failure: results of the Randomized Etanercept Worldwide Evaluation (RENEWAL). Circulation 2004;109:1594–602.

48. Kaneko Y, Floras JS, Usui K, et al. Cardiovascular effects of continuous positive airway pressure in patients with heart failure and obstructive sleep apnea. N Engl J Med 2003;348:1233–41.

49. Tkacova R, Rankin F, Fitzgerald FS, Floras JS, Bradley TD. Effects of continuous positive airway pressure on obstructive sleep apnea and left ventricular afterload in patients with heart failure. Circulation 1998;98:2269–75.

50. Solomon SD, St John SM, Lamas GA, et al. Ventricular remodeling does not accompany the development of heart failure in diabetic patients after myocardial infarction. Circulation 2002;106:1251–5.

51. Aronson D. Cross-linking of glycated collagen in the pathogenesis of arterial and myocardial stiffening of aging and diabetes. J Hypertens 2003;21:3–12.

52. Shlipak MG, Fried LF, Cushman M, et al. Cardiovascular mortality risk in chronic kidney disease: comparison of traditional and novel risk factors. JAMA 2005;293:1737–45.

53. Douglas PS, Katz SE, Weinberg EO, et al. Hypertrophic remodeling: gender differences in the early response to left ventricular pressure overload. J Am Coll Cardiol 1998;32:1118–25.

54. Crabbe DL, Dipla K, Ambati S, et al. Gender differences in post-infarction hypertrophy in end-stage failing hearts. J Am Coll Cardiol 2003;41:300–6.

55. East MA, Jollis JG, Nelson CL, Marks D, Peterson ED. The influence of left ventricular hypertrophy on survival in patients with coronary artery disease: Do race and gender matter? J Am Coll Cardiol 2003;41:949–54.

56. Dries DL, Exner DV, Gersh BJ, et al. Racial differences in the outcome of left ventricular dysfunction. N Engl J Med 1999;340:609–16.

57. Post WS, Larson MG, Myers RH, Galderisi M, Levy D. Heritability of left ventricular mass: the Framingham Heart Study. Hypertension 1997;30:1025–8.

58. Skelton TN, Andrew ME, Arnett DK, et al. Echocardiographic left ventricular mass in African–Americans: the Jackson cohort of the Atherosclerosis Risk in Communities Study. Echocardiography 2003; 20:111–20.

59. Ingelsson E, Lind L, Arnlov J, Sundstrom J. Socioeconomic factors as predictors of incident heart failure. J Card Fail 2006;12:540–5.

60. Kee HJ, Sohn IS, Nam KI, et al. Inhibition of histone deacetylation blocks cardiac hypertrophy induced by angiotensin II infusion and aortic banding. Circulation 2006;113:51–9.

61. Takimoto E, Champion HC, Li M, et al. Chronic inhibition of cyclic GMP phosphodiesterase 5A prevents and reverses cardiac hypertrophy. Nat Med 2005;11:214–22.

62. Jessup M, Brozena S. Heart failure. N Engl J Med 2003;348:2007–18.

5

Summary of all large randomized trials

Rajkumar K Sugumaran, Garrie J Haas, and William T Abraham

Introduction • **PATH-CHF** • **MUSTIC** • **MIRACLE** • **CONTAK-CD** • **MIRACLE ICD** • **COMPANION** • **CARE-HF** • **Conclusions**

INTRODUCTION

Over the past decade, cardiac resynchronization therapy (CRT) has evolved as an important treatment option for many patients with chronic heart failure who have remained symptomatic despite optimization of pharmacologic therapy. More than 10 years ago, observational studies provided the feasibility and acute hemodynamic data necessary to support proof of concept for CRT (Table 5.1). Over the past 5 years, more than 4000 patients have participated in randomized clinical trials that have validated the effectiveness of CRT in present-day clinical practice. These trials have evolved from relatively small studies utilizing a crossover design to assess various measures of functional status to larger trials with parallel control groups and composite endpoints including outcomes such as cardiac mortality, all-cause mortality, and heart failure hospitalizations. Completed clinical trials to date have provided convincing data supporting the efficacy of CRT in patients meeting a relatively narrow set of inclusion criteria including optimal medical therapy for heart failure, New York Heart Association (NYHA) classes III and IV, decreased left ventricular ejection fraction (LVEF) ≤35%, increased QRS duration, sinus rhythm, and biventricular pacing configuration. When patients have met these criteria, randomized clinical trials have consistently shown that CRT improves such functional endpoints as the 6-minute walk test (6MWT), NYHA class,

and quality-of-life (QOL) scores assessed with the Minnesota Living With Heart Failure Questionnaire (MLHFQ).[10,11] Importantly, a recently reported large clinical trial has shown that CRT, when combined with evidence-based medical therapies, not only improves clinical symptoms, exercise tolerance, and the frequency of hospitalizations, but also reduces mortality.[12] This chapter will summarize several of the important cardiac resynchronization clinical trials that have impacted clinical practice. An overview of the specific indications for CRT and the expected clinical outcome when utilized in the appropriate HF patient will be provided. Tables 5.2 and 5.3 summarize the clinical trials describing their design, the number of patients included, endpoints, and results.

PATH-CHF: PACING THERAPIES IN CONGESTIVE HEART FAILURE

The PATH-CHF trial was a single-blind, randomized, crossover, controlled trial designed to evaluate the clinical efficacy of hemodynamically optimized univentricular (right ventricular (RV) or left ventricular (LV)) or biventricular (BiV) pacing compared with no pacing in patients with advanced HF[13]. Inclusion criteria were a history of heart failure and LV systolic dysfunction of either ischemic or non-ischemic etiology, NYHA class III or IV, sinus rhythm >55 bpm, QRS duration >120 ms in at least two

Table 5.1 Observational trials of cardiac resynchronization therapy in heart failure[a]

Authors	Patients	Improvements
Cazeau et al (1994)[1]	Six-week technical feasibility study of four-chamber pacing in a 54-year-old with NYHA class IV heart failure, LBBB, 200 ms PR interval, and interatrial conduction delay	Clinical status
Foster et al (1995)[2]	Acute study of biventricular pacing in 18 postoperative coronary revascularization patients	Hemodynamics
Cazeau et al (1996)[3]	Eight patients with wide QRS and end-stage heart failure; comparing the effect of various ventricular pacing sites (RV apex, RVOT, RV apex–LV pacing); follow-up period 3–17 months	Hemodynamics and functional status in patients with LV or biventricular pacing only
Blanc et al (1997)[4]	Acute hemodynamic study comparing the effect of various ventricular pacing sites (RV apex, RVOT, LV, or biventricular pacing) in 27 patients with severe heart failure with first-degree AV block and/or IVCD	Hemodynamics in patients with LV or biventricular pacing only
Kass et al (1999)[5]	Acute hemodynamic study comparing various ventricular pacing modes (RV apex, RV septal, LV free wall, or biventricular pacing) in 18 patients with advanced heart failure	Hemodynamics in patients with LV or biventricular pacing only
Saxon et al (1998)[6]	Study of biventricular pacing in 11 postoperative cardiac surgery patients with depressed LV function	Hemodynamics
Gras et al (1998)[7]	(InSync Study, interim results, 3-month follow-up) European and Canadian multicenter trial of biventricular pacing in 68 patients with dilated cardiomyopathy, IVCD, and NYHA class III or IV heart failure	Quality of life, NYHA class, 6-minute walk distance
Leclercq et al (1998)[8]	Acute hemodynamic study comparing single-site RV DDD pacing with biventricular pacing in 18 patients with NYHA class III or IV heart failure	Hemodynamics for biventricular pacing only
Gras et al (2002)[9]	(InSync Study, final analysis, long-term follow-up) 117 patients (103 were successfully implanted with a CRT device) with idiopathic or ischemic dilated cardiomyopathy, NYHA class III or IV heart failure, LV dysfunction, and an IVCD	Quality of life, NYHA class. 6-minute walk distance

AV, atrioventricular; CRT, cardiac resynchronization therapy; IVCD, intraventricular conduction delay; LBBB, left bundle branch block; LV, left ventricular; NYHA, New York Heart Association; RV, right ventricular; RVOT, RV outflow tract.
[a]Modified from Hayes DL, Abraham WT. Cardiac Resynchronization Therapy. Blackwell: Malden, 2006:239–56.[14]

surface electrocardiograph (ECG) leads, and PR interval >150 ms. Patients were paced followed by no pacing (control phase), and crossed over to the other modality of pacing. The effects of pacing on peak oxygen consumption (VO_2) and anaerobic threshold during cardiopulmonary exercise testing (CPX) and on 6MWT were selected as primary endpoints. Secondary endpoints were NYHA class, QOL using the MLHFQ scale, and hospitalization frequency.

Acutely, BiV and LV pacing significantly improved hemodynamic parameters, aortic pulse pressure and LV contractility (dP/dt), compared with RV pacing ($p<0.01$). Statistically significant reductions in LV end-diastolic diameter (LVEDD) and end-systolic diameter (LVESD) were seen during chronic pacing ($p=0.007$). LV end-diastolic and end-systolic volumes (LVEDV and LVESV, respectively) were also decreased. Those patients who did not experience LV volume reduction (non-responders) had significantly higher baseline LVEDVs compared with those who did.[13,14] PATH-CHF also provided important information regarding

Table 5.2 Patient enrollment criteria for completed trials of cardiac resynchronization therapy[a]

| Study | No. of patients | Patient characteristics | | |
		NYHA class	QRS width (ms)	ICD indication
MUSTIC-SR[16]	58	III	>150	No
MUSTIC-AF[19]	43	III	>200	No
PATH-CHF[13]	41	III, IV	≥120	No
MIRACLE[21]	453	III, IV	≥130	No
CONTAK-CD[22]	490	II, III, IV	≥120	Yes
MIRACLE-ICD[23]	369	III, IV	≥130	Yes
COMPANION[27]	1520	III, IV	≥120	No
PATH-CHF II[15]	86	III, IV	≥120	Both
MIRACLE-ICD II[25]	186	II	≥130	Yes
CARE-HF[30]	813	III, IV	≥120	No

ICD, implantable cardioverter defibrillator; NYHA, New York Heart Association.

[a]Modified from Hayes DL, Abraham WT. Cardiac Resynchronization Therapy. Blackwell: Malden, 2006: 239–56.[14]

the optimal site for LV lead placement, which was observed with midlateral epicardial LV pacing. Although PATH-CHF had limitations, such as the small sample size, selected population, and short duration of control phase, it clearly identified a favorable response to CRT, including potential anti-remodeling effects (Figures 5.1 and 5.2).

PATH-CHF II was a prospective, single-blind, randomized, controlled, crossover study designed to assess the clinical efficacy of single-site LV pacing and degree of baseline conduction delay on the magnitude of clinical benefit.[15] This trial enrolled 86 patients with symptomatic HF (NYHA class II–IV), LV systolic dysfunction, sinus rhythm, and QRS duration >120 ms. Patients were randomized equally into long-QRS (baseline QRS >150 ms) and short-QRS (baseline QRS 120–150 ms) groups. The groups were compared during a 3-month period of active (univentricular pacing) and 3 months of inactive (ventricular inhibited) pacing. Results from CPX, 6MWT, and QOL scores were primary endpoints. Interestingly, only patients in the long-baseline-QRS group had a statistically significant improvement in the primary endpoints during univentricular pacing. It was therefore concluded from PATH-CHF II that in symptomatic heart failure patients with LV systolic dysfunction and long QRS (>150 ms), LV pacing significantly improves exercise tolerance

and QOL. This trial was the first to identify a potential differential response to CRT based on the baseline QRS duration.

MUSTIC: MULTISITE STIMULATION IN CARDIOMYOPATHIES STUDY

Similar to PATH-CHF, the MUSTIC trial was also a single-blind, randomized, crossover evaluation of CRT in patients with symptomatic heart failure and QRS prolongation. Entry criteria included NYHA class III heart failure on stable medical therapy, LVEF ≤35%, LVEDD >60 mm, sinus rhythm with a QRS duration >150 ms, and 6MWT distance <450 m.[16] Patients were randomized to BiV or no pacing, and then crossed over to the alternative pacing strategy; patients were blinded to their pacing mode.

Patients who were actively paced showed significant improvements in all primary and secondary endpoints.[16,17] The results also provided important physiologic, structural, and functional data illustrating that BiV pacing shortens total isovolumic time, reduces LV cavity size, and increases exercise tolerance in patients with dilated non-ischemic cardiomyopathy and ventricular conduction delay. While patients with an ischemic etiology for their heart failure also realized an improvement in exercise capacity with CRT, the degree of reverse remodeling in this group was less pronounced.[18,19] The MUSTIC trial

Table 5.3 CRT in randomized clinical trials[a]

Trials	Design	No. of patients	Endpoints Primary	Endpoints Secondary	Results summary
PATH-CHF	Crossover	41	• 6MWT • Peak VO$_2$	• NYHA functional class • QOL • Hospitalizations	• Improvement in: –6MWT –NYHA functional class –QOL • Less hospitalization
MUSTIC-SR	Crossover	58	• 6MWT	• NYHA functional class • QOL • Peak VO$_2$ • LV volumes • MR • Hospitalizations • Total mortality	• Improvement in –6MWT –NYHA functional class –QOL –Peak VO$_2$ –LV volumes –MR • Less hospitalization
MIRACLE	Parallel arms	453	• 6MWT • NYHA functional class • QOL	• Peak VO$_2$ • LVEF • LVEDD • MR • Clinical composite response	• Improvement in: –6MWT –NYHA functional class –QOL –LVEF –LVEDD –MR
MIRACLE-ICD	Parallel arms	555	• 6MWT • NYHA functional class • QOL	• Peak VO$_2$ • LVEF • LV volumes • MR • Clinical composite response	• Improvement in: –NYHA functional class –QOL
COMPANION	Parallel arms	1520	• All-cause mortality or hospitalization	• All-cause mortality and cardiac morbidity	• Reduced all-cause mortality/hospitalization
CARE-HF	Open label, randomized	814	• All-cause mortality	• NYHA functional class • QOL • LVEF • LVESV • Hospitalization for heart failure	• Reduced all-cause mortality/morbidity • Improvement in: –NYHA functional class –QOL –LVEF –LVESV
PATH-CHF	Crossover (no pacing vs LV pacing)	86	• 6MWT • Peak VO$_2$	• NYHA functional class	• Improvement in: –6MWT –QOL –Peak VO$_2$
CONTAK-CD	Crossover, parallel controlled	490	• 6MWT • NYHA functional class • QOL	• LVEF • LV volume • Composite of mortality hospitalization, and VT/VF	• Improvement in: –6MWT –NYHA functional class –QOL –LVEF –LV volume

CARE-HF, Cardiac Resynchronization–Heart Failure; CONTAK-CD, CONTAK–Cardiac Defibrillator; COMPANION, Comparison of Medical Therapy, Pacing and Defibrillation in Heart Failure; CRT, Cardiac Resynchronization Therapy; LV, left ventricular; LVEDD, LV end-diastolic dimension; LVEF, LV ejection fraction; LVESV, LV end-systolic volume; MIRACLE, Multicenter InSync Randomized Clinical Evaluation; MIRACLE-ICD, MIRACLE–implantable cardioverter defibrillator trial; MR, mitral regurgitation; MUSTIC, Multisite Simulation in Cardiomyopathies; NYHA, New York Heart Association; PATH-CHF, Pacing Therapies in Congestive Heart Failure trial; QOL, quality-of-life score; VF, ventricular fibrillation; VO$_2$, volume of oxygen; VT, ventricular tachycardia; 6MWT, 6-minute walk test.
[a]Reproduced from Ellenbogen KA, Wood MA, Klein HU. Why should we care about CARE-HF? J Am Coll Cardiol 2005;46:2199–203.[30]

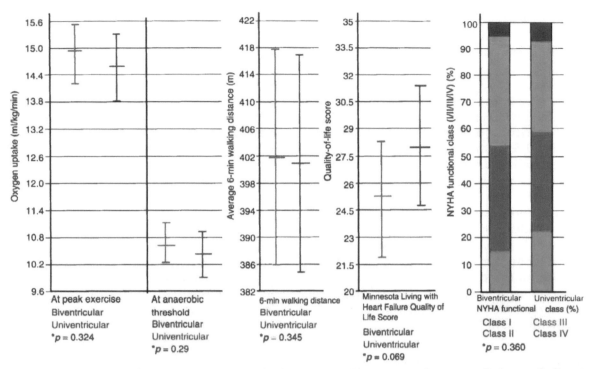

Figure 5.1 PATH-CHF. Biventricular pacing versus optimal univentricular pacing: oxygen uptake, average 6-minute walk distance, quality-of-life score (lower score better), and NYHA functional class. *36 LV patients, 4 RV patients.

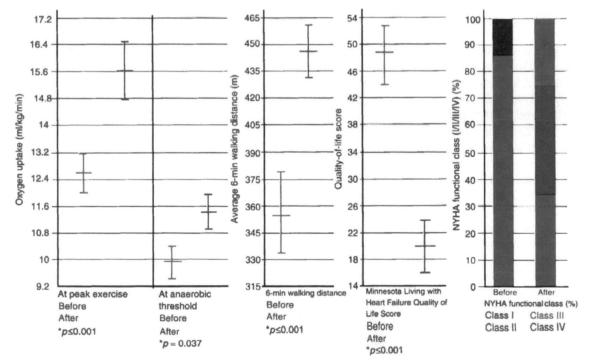

Figure 5.2 PATH-CHF. Clinical changes after 12 months of therapy: oxygen uptake, average 6-minute walk distance, quality-of-life score (lower score better), and NYHA functional class. *12 biventricular, 13 univentricular – LV, 4 univentricular – RV.

disclosed that placement of BiV pacing systems are superior to no pacing when assessed by such functional measurements as 6MWT, peak VO_2, and QOL.

A second MUSTIC trial (MUSTIC-AF) evaluated a similar set of endpoints in symptomatic heart failure patients with atrial fibrillation (AF) and ventricular dyssynchrony secondary to a paced QRS duration >200 ms.[19] BiV pacing evoked statistically significant improvements in several endpoints, including 6MWT distance, peak VO_2, and number of hospitalizations. These results suggest that BiV pacing is a reasonable consideration in AF patients who are bradycardic and pacer-dependent either because of native conduction disease or following AV node ablation for rate control. Therefore, MUSTIC-AF supports consideration of BiV pacing in patients undergoing AV node ablation who have a baseline reduction in LVEF.

MIRACLE: MULTICENTER INSYNC RANDOMIZED CLINICAL EVALUATION

The MIRACLE trial compared the effect of CRT on QOL and functional capacity in patients with heart failure and ventricular dysynchrony (QRS >130 ms).[20] A secondary objective was to assess the safety of CRT using the Medtronic InSync system. This was the first prospective, randomized, double-blind, parallel-controlled CRT trial designed to validate results from prior CRT studies and further evaluate the clinical efficacy and mechanisms of benefit of CRT. The inclusion criteria were NYHA class III or IV heart failure, QRS prolongation $\geqslant 130$ ms (mean 165 ms), LV systolic dysfunction with an LVEF $\leqslant 35\%$, LVEDD >55 mm (mean 69 mm), and 6MWT distance $\leqslant 450$ m.

Patients underwent a pre-discharge randomization to the control group (no CRT, $n = 225$) or CRT group ($n = 228$). Compared with the control group, CRT was associated with a significantly improved 6MWT distance (+39 m vs + 10 m; $p = 0.005$), improved NYHA class by at least one class (−1 vs 0; p <0.001), QOL (−18.0 points vs −9.0 points; $p = 0.001$), treadmill exercise time (+81 s vs +19 s; $p = 0.001$), and LVEF (+4.6% vs −0.2%; p <0.001). CRT was also associated with a modest but statistically significant improvement

in peak VO_2 (+1.1 ml/kg/min vs + 0.2 ml/kg/min; $p = 0.009$). The need for hospital admission (8% vs 15%; $p = 0.02$) and treatment with intravenous medication (7% vs 15%; $p = 0.004$) was lower in CRT patients compared with controls. Using a Heart Failure Clinical Composite Outcome Measure, a significantly higher percentage of CRT patients were classified as improved (67% vs 39%; p <0.001) and fewer CRT patients were classified as worsened (16% vs 27%). Death or worsening heart failure requiring hospitalization occurred less frequently in the CRT arm (28% vs 44%; hazard ratio (HR) 0.60; 95% confidence interval (CI) 0.37–0.96; $p = 0.03$).[20]

Thus, among patients with symptomatic heart failure and ventricular dyssynchrony as predicted by intraventricular conduction delay, BiV pacing was associated with improved functional class, increased 6MWT distance and peak VO_2, and improved QOL scores. These results provided the most encouraging and robust data to date, with 67% of CRT patients showing improvement in the clinical composite endpoint that included NYHA functional class and global assessment compared with 39% of placebo patients. The MIRACLE data suggest that CRT is safe and well tolerated, and improves QOL, functional class, exercise capacity, and heart failure composite response, thus suggesting an overall improvement in heart failure clinical status with CRT.

CONTAK-CD: CARDIAC RESYNCHRONIZATION THERAPY FOR THE TREATMENT OF HEART FAILURE IN PATIENTS WITH INTRAVENTRICULAR CONDUCTION DELAY AND MALIGNANT VENTRICULAR TACHYARRHYTHMIAS

The aim of CONTAK-CD was to assess the safety and effectiveness of CRT when combined with an implantable cardioverter defibrillator (ICD).[21] This study was the first to describe the results of CRT in a double-blind, randomized controlled fashion in patients with both symptomatic heart failure and ventricular tachyarrhythmias (VT). Prior CRT studies had restricted enrollment to patients with heart failure but without conventional indications for ICD therapy. Inclusion criteria for CONTAK-CD were NYHA class II–IV, LVEF $\leqslant$ 35%, QRS interval $\geqslant$ 120 ms, and conventional indications of an ICD. Patients ($n = 490$) were implanted with a device capable of providing both CRT and ICD therapy and randomized to CRT ($n = 245$) or control (no CRT, $n = 245$) for up to 6 months. The primary endpoint, namely progression of heart failure, was measured by the composite of all-cause mortality, hospitalization for heart failure, and VT/ventricular fibrillation (VF) requiring device intervention. Secondary endpoints included peak VO_2, 6MWT, NYHA, QOL, and echocardiographic analysis of LV structure and function. Results showed a 15% reduction in the primary endpoint of heart failure progression, which was not statistically significant ($p = 0.35$). CRT did, however, improve peak VO_2 ($p = 0.030$), 6MWT ($p = 0.043$), and LVEF ($p = 0.020$) in the NYHA class III/IV patients. In NYHA class II patients, the functional changes were less impressive and not significant. In addition to the favorable anti-remodeling effects (reductions in LVEDD and LVESD) observed in NYHA class III/IV patients treated with CRT, significant reductions in both parameters were also noted with CRT (vs control) in class II patients ($p = 0.024$ and $p = 0.014$, respectively).

MIRACLE ICD: MULTICENTER INSYNC IMPLANTABLE CARDIOVERSION DEFIBRILLATION RANDOMIZED CLINICAL EVALUATION

The purpose of the MIRACLE ICD trial was to compare the effect of CRT plus ICD (CRT-D) versus ICD alone on the QOL, functional capacity, and safety in patients with heart failure and ventricular dyssynchrony.[22,23] Patients with aged 18 years or more, with a history of cardiac arrest due to ventricular arrhythmia, inducible VF, or sustained VT, and with NYHA functional class III or IV heart failure, LVEF ⩽35%, QRS duration ⩾130 ms, LVEDD ⩾55 mm, and a stable heart failure drug regimen for 1 month or more were included.

Patients underwent a pre-discharge randomization to the control arm (ICD on, CRT off, $n = 182$) or control group (both ICD and CRT on, $n = 187$). Compared with the control arm, CRT was associated with a significantly improved NYHA class (−1 vs 0; $p = 0.007$) and QOL (−17.5 points

vs −11 points; $p = 0.02$), but no difference was observed in 6MWT (+55 m vs +53 m; $p = 0.36$). Many of the secondary endpoints were also improved in the CRT arm, including exercise treadmill time (+55.5 s vs −11 s; $p < 0.001$) and peak VO_2 (+1.1 ml/kg/min vs +0.1 ml/kg/min; $p = 0.04$). These observations suggested that heart failure patients, with an indication for an ICD, could benefit as much, if not more, from CRT than those patients without an ICD indication[22,23] (Figure 5.3).

A substudy, MIRACLE ICD II, was a randomized, double-blind, parallel, controlled trial of CRT in NYHA class II patients on optimal medical therapy, with LVEF ⩽35%, QRS ⩾130 ms, and an ICD indication.[24] The study randomized 186 patients implanted with a combined CRT-D device to CRT on ($n = 85$) or CRT off (ICD only ($n = 101$) served as the control). A total of 98 control and 82 CRT patients completed the study. After 6 months of follow-up, patients who received CRT demonstrated improvements in exercise time, 6MWT, and peak VO_2, although none of these differences reached statistical significance. The CRT group did have statistically significant improvements in the ventilatory response to exercise (VE/VCO_2; $p = 0.01$), NYHA class ($p = 0.05$), percentage of patients with improved overall clinical status ($p = 0.01$), and several echocardiographic parameters, including LVEDV ($p = 0.04$), LVESV ($p = 0.01$), and LVEF ($p = 0.02$).[24]

COMPANION: COMPARISON OF MEDICAL THERAPY, PACING, AND DEFIBRILLATION IN HEART FAILURE

The COMPANION trial was a multicenter, prospective, randomized controlled clinical trial designed to compare optimal medical therapy (OMT) with CRT or CRT-D in patients with advanced heart failure with an ischemic or non-ischemic etiology and no baseline indication for either a pacemaker or ICD.[25,26] Patients were selected based on the following inclusion criteria: NYHA III or IV with a prior heart failure hospitalization within the year prior to randomization, LVEF ⩽35%, LVEDD >55 mm, and QRS interval >120 ms. Subjects were randomized to OMT, CRT + OMT, and CRT-D + OMT. The primary endpoint was a combination of all-cause

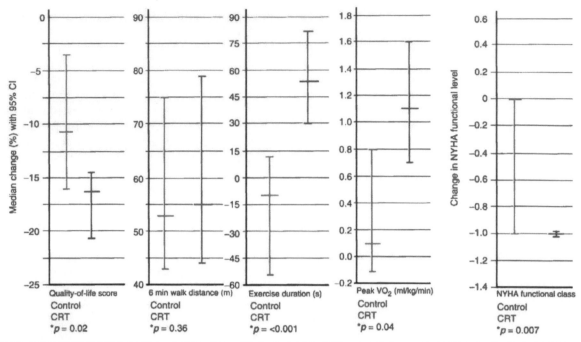

Figure 5.3 MIRACLE ICD. Primary and secondary outcomes: quality-of-life score (lower score better), 6-minute walk distance, exercise duration, peak VO₂, and NYHA functional class. CI, confidence interval.

mortality and all-cause hospitalization; secondary endpoints were all-cause mortality, cardiac morbidity, and exercise performance. While previous studies had not focused on a potential mortality benefit offered from CRT, COMPANION was the first trial powered to evaluate this endpoint in a prospective manner.[25,26]

The primary composite endpoint of all-cause mortality and all-cause hospitalization was reduced by approximately 19% in the CRT and CRT-D arms. Mortality through 1 year was reduced with CRT (HR 0.76; $p = 0.06$) and CRT-D (HR 0.64; $p = 0.003$) compared with medical therapy. Importantly, total mortality was reduced by 40% (from 19% to 11%) in patients implanted with CRT-D, while CRT alone resulted in a mortality reduction of 15% ($p = 0.06$). The time to death or heart failure hospitalization was significantly reduced with CRT (HR 0.75; $p = 0.002$) and with CRT-D (HR 0.72; $p < 0.001$) compared with control[26,27] (Figure 5.4).

An analysis examining the mode of death in COMPANION patients concluded that progressive heart failure was predominant in patients with advanced heart failure and was modestly reduced by both CRT and CRT-D. Only CRT-D reduced sudden cardiac death, resulting in a favorable and statistically significant effect of CRT-D on overall mortality.[28] COMPANION was the first large randomized trial to show an improvement in the composite endpoint of all-cause mortality and hospitalizations with CRT and CRT-D use in severe heart failure patients. Based on these results, the US Food and Drug Administration (FDA) approved the combined CRT-D device for those patients who are candidates for CRT therapy[28] (Figure 5.4).

CARE-HF: CARDIAC RESYNCHRONIZATION HEART FAILURE

The Cardiac Resynchronization Heart Failure Trial (CARE-HF) was a large, multicenter European study designed to evaluate the effect of CRT on long-term morbidity and mortality in a cohort of patients with advanced heart failure and cardiac dyssynchrony despite OMT.[29] The patient population consisted of age 18 years or more (mean 67 years), LVEF ≤35%; cardiac dyssynchrony as indicated by QRS duration > 120 ms

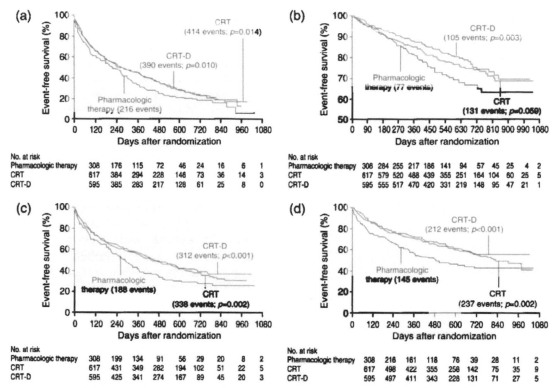

Figure 5.4 COMPANION. Survival curves: Kaplan–Meier estimates of (a) time to the primary endpoint of death from or hospitalization from any cause, (b) time to the secondary endpoint of death from any cause, (c) time to death from or hospitalization for cardiovascular causes, and (c) time to death from or hospitalization for heart failure. CRT, cardiac resynchronization therapy; CRT-D, cardiac resynchronization therapy – Defibrillator. (Reproduced from Bristow MR, Saxon LA, Boehmer J, et al. Cardiac-resynchronization therapy with or without an implantable defibrillator in advanced chronic heart failure. N Engl J Med 2004;350:2140–50.[26])

(median 160 ms), and sinus rhythm with NYHA class III or IV heart failure. Patients with a mildly increased QRS duration (120–149 ms) required evidence of ventricular dyssynchrony with echocardiography. Patients were randomized in an open-label manner to continued OMT alone ($n = 404$) or OMT combined with CRT ($n = 409$). The primary endpoint was all-cause mortality or unplanned hospitalization for a cardiovascular event, and the principal secondary endpoint was all-cause mortality alone.

Patients in the CRT group demonstrated a greater relative risk reduction of death and cardiovascular hospitalization ($p < 0.001$) and of all-cause mortality alone ($p < 0.002$) than the control group. Furthermore, the CRT group exhibited an improvement in symptoms, LVEF, functional

class, and QOL, as well as other echocardiographic and hemodynamic parameters ($p < 0.001$); death or hospitalization for worsening heart failure were also significantly reduced in the CRT group[29] (Figure 5.5).

Among patients with advanced heart failure and cardiac dyssynchrony despite OMT, treatment with CRT was associated with a reduction in the primary endpoint of all-cause mortality and hospitalization for major cardiovascular events compared with standard pharmacologic therapy. The results of CARE-HF accomplished the following: (i) first to show a benefit for CRT alone with respect to survival as a single endpoint; (ii) first to show a benefit for CRT for up to 18 months and continued improvement over time; (iii) first to show that neurohormonal measures

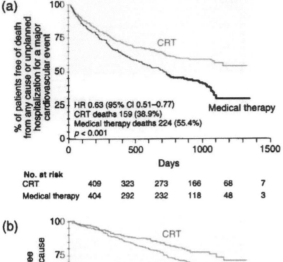

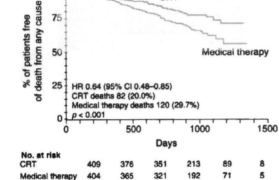

Figure 5.5 CARE-HF. Kaplan–Meier estimates of the time to the primary endpoint (a) and the principal secondary outcome (b). The primary outcome was death from any cause or an unplanned hospitalization for a major cardiovascular event. The principal secondary outcome was death from any cause. CRT, cardiac resynchronization therapy; HR, hazard ratio; CI, confidence interval. (Reproduced from Cleland JG, Daubert JC, Erdmann E, et al. The effect of cardiac resynchronization on morbidity and mortality in heart failure. N Engl J Med 2005;352:1539–49.[29])

(e.g., N-terminal pro-brain natriuretic peptide) improve dramatically with CRT; (iv) first to use direct measures of dyssynchrony as an inclusion criterion.[30] In patients with heart failure and cardiac dyssynchrony, CRT improved symptoms and QOL, and reduced complications and risk of death. These benefits are in addition to those afforded by standard pharmacologic therapy. CARE-HF supports the concept that CRT prolongs life in symptomatic heart failure patients, and ushers in a new era in the multimodality approach to heart failure therapeutics.[31,32]

CONCLUSIONS

A meta-analysis further illustrating the magnitude of benefit from CRT has been published by McAlister et al.[33] A total of 3216 patients from nine randomized controlled trials published prior to CARE-HF, but including COMPANION, identified multiple clinical benefits of CRT, including a consistent improvement in functional class, reduced HF hospitalizations, and an impressive reduction in all-cause mortality (HR 0.79; 95% CI 0.66–0.96) secondary primarily to fewer deaths from progressive heart failure.

While CRT is a relatively new treatment option for patients with heart failure, excellent clinical trial data as described in this chapter have resulted in the wide acceptance of CRT for patients meeting specific criteria. Current clinical guidelines recommend CRT for a highly selected patient population that generally includes NYHA class III or IV heart failure despite optimal medical therapy, sinus rhythm, intraventricular conduction delay, and LVEF less than 35% (Table 5.4). When treatment with CRT is targeted to this patient profile, clinical improvement may be expected in the majority of patients. Still, additional trials are needed to refine CRT patient selection and optimization. The prospective identification of those patients who do not respond favorably to CRT, despite meeting the basic selection criteria, has proven challenging and is a major area of investigation. Ongoing clinical trials are examining alternative and perhaps more sensitive methods to identify ventricular dyssynchrony rather than the traditional QRS prolongation. Given the potential for CRT to reverse or slow ventricular remodeling, studies designed to detect a benefit in less

---

Table 5.4 Current recommendations for CRT

- Symptomatic heart failure (NYHA class III–IV) on optimal medical therapy
- ≤ left ventricular ejection fraction (LVEF) ≤35%
- Intraventricular conduction delay (QRS duration ≥120 ms)
- Normal sinus rhythm.

NYHA, New York Heart Association.

symptomatic patients are underway. Whether BiV or LV-only pacing is the preferred method for CRT has yet to be determined. The common problem of atrial arrhythmia in heart failure has proven to be a major area of uncertainty when selecting patients for CRT. Studies to date have enrolled very few patients with atrial fibrillation – therefore the role of CRT in those with permanent or paroxysmal atrial arrhythmia remains in question. Despite the extensive CRT database that has been collected over the past few years and reviewed here, trials that are underway or planned should help to further refine the future utility of CRT.

ACKNOWLEDGMENTS

The authors would like to thank Ian for his assistance with the data representation.

REFERENCES

1. Cazeau S, Ritter P, Bakdach S, et al. Four chamber pacing in dilated caridomyopathy. Pacing Clin Electrophysiol 1994;17:1974–9.
2. Foster AH, Gold MR, McLaughlin JS. Acute hemodynamic effects of atrio–biventricular pacing in humans. Ann Thorac Surg 1995;59:294–300.
3. Cazeau S, Ritter P, Lazarus A et al. Multisite pacing for end-stage heart failure: early experience. Pacing Clin Electrophysiol 1996;19:1748–57.
4. Blanc JJ, Etienne Y, Gilard M, et al. Evaluation of different ventricular pacing sites in patients with severe heart failure: results of an acute hemodynamic study. Circulation 1997;96:3273–7.
5. Kass DA, Chen CH, Curry C, et al. Improved left ventricular mechanics from acute VDD pacing in patients with dilated cardiomyopathy and ventricular conduction delay. Circulation 1999;99:1567–73.
6. Saxon LA, Kerwin WF, Cahalan MK, et al. Acute effects of intraoperative multisite ventricular pacing on left ventricular function and activation/contraction sequence in patients with depressed ventricular function. J Cardiovasc Electrophysiol 1998;9:13–21.
7. Gras D, Mabo P, Tang T, et al. Multisite pacing as a supplemental treatment of congestive heart failure: preliminary results of the Medtronic Inc. InSync Study. Pacing Clin Electrophysiol 1998;21:2249–55.
8. Leclercq C, Cazeau S, Le Breton H, et al. Acute hemodynamic effects of biventricular DDD pacing in patients with end-stage heart failure. J Am Coll Cardiol 1998;21: 2249–55.
9. Gras D, Leclercq C, Tang AS, et al. Cardiac resynchronization therapy in advanced heart failure: the multisite InSync clinical study. Eur J Heart Fail 2002;4:311–20.
10. Williams L, Ellery S, Frenneaux M. The role of cardiac resynchronization therapy in heart failure. Minerva Cardioangiol 2005;53:249–63.
11. Israel CW, Butter C. Indication for cardiac resynchronization therapy: Consensus 2005. Herzschrittmacherther Elektrophysiol 2006;17:80–6.
12. Gotze S, Butter C, Fleck E. Cardiac resynchronization therapy for heart failure – from experimental pacing to evidence-based therapy. Clin Res Cardiol 2006;95: 18–35.
13. The PATH-CHF (PAcing THerapies in Congestive Heart Failure) Investigators; CPI Guidant Congestive Heart Failure Research Group. Impact of cardiac resynchronization therapy using hemodynamically optimized pacing on left ventricular remodeling in patients with congestive heart failure and ventricular conduction disturbances. J Am Coll Cardiol 2001;38:1957–65.
14. Hayes DL, Abraham WT. Cardiac Resynchronization Therapy. Blackwell: Malden, 2006:239–56.
15. Auricchio A, Stellbrink C, Butter C, et al., Clinical efficacy of cardiac resynchronization therapy using left ventricular pacing in heart failure patients stratified by severity of ventricular conduction delay. J Am Coll Cardiol 2003;42:2109–26.
16. Cazeau S, Leclercq C, Lavergne T, et al, for the Multisite Stimulation in Cardiomyopathies (MUSTIC) Study Investigators. Effects of multisite biventricular pacing in patients with heart failure and intraventricular conduction delay. N Engl J Med 2001;344:873–80.
17. Linde C, Braunschweig F, Gadler F, Bailleul C, Daubert JC. Long-term improvements in quality of life by biventricular pacing in patients with chronic heart failure: results from the Multisite Stimulation in Cardiomyopathy Study (MUSTIC). Am J Cardiol 2003;91:1090–5.
18. Duncan A, Wait D, Gibson D, Daubert JC;MUSTIC (Multisite Stimulation in Cardiomyopathies) Trial. Left ventricular remodelling and haemodynamic effects of multisite biventricular pacing in patients with left ventricular systolic dysfunction and activation disturbances in sinus rhythm: sub-study of the MUSTIC (Multisite Stimulation in Cardiomyopathies) trial. Eur Heart J 2003;24:430–41.
19. Linde C, Leclercq C, Rex S, et al. Long-term benefits of biventricular pacing in congestive heart failure: results from the MUltisite STimulation in cardiomyopathy (MUSTIC) study. J Am Coll Cardiol 2002;40:111–18.
20. Abraham WT. Rationale and design of a randomized clinical trial to assess the safety and efficacy of cardiac resynchronization therapy in patients with advanced heart failure: the Multicenter InSync Randomized

Clinical Evaluation (MIRACLE). J Card Fail 2000;
369–80.

21. Higgins SL, Hummel JD, Niazi IK, et al. Cardiac resynchronization therapy for the treatment of heart failure in patients with intraventricular conduction delay and malignant ventricular tachyarrythmias. J Am Coll Cardiol 2003;42:1454–9.

22. Young JB, Abraham WT, Smith AL, et al. Multicenter InSync ICD Randomized Clinical Evaluation (MIRACLE ICD) Trial Investigators. Combined cardiac resynchronization and implantable cardioversion defibrillation in advanced chronic heart failure: the MIRACLE ICD Trial. JAMA 2003;289:2685–94.

23. Pires LA, Abraham WT, Young JB, et al. MIRACLE and MIRACLE-ICD Investigators. Clinical predictors and timing of New York Heart Association class improvement with cardiac resynchronization therapy in patients with advanced chronic heart failure: results from the Multicenter InSync Randomized Clinical Evaluation (MIRACLE) and Multicenter InSync ICD Randomized Clinical Evaluation (MIRACLE-ICD) trials. Am Heart J 2006;151:837–43.

24. Abraham WT, Young JB, Leon AR, et al. Effects of cardiac resynchronization on disease progression in patients with left ventricular systolic dysfunction, an indication for an implantable cardioverter–defibrillator, and mildly symptomatic chronic heart failure. Circulation 2004;110:2864–8.

25. Morgan JM. The MADIT II and COMPANION studies: Will they affect uptake of device treatment? Heart 2004;90:243–5.

26. Bristow MR, Saxon LA, Boehmer J, et al. Cardiac-resynchronization therapy with or without an implantable defibrillator in advanced chronic heart failure. N Engl J Med 2004;350:2140–50.

27. Salukhe TV, Francis DP, Sutton R, Comparison of medical therapy, pacing and defibrillation in heart failure (COMPANION) trial terminated early;combined biventricular pacemaker–defibrillators reduce all-cause mortality and hospitalization. Int J Cardiol 2003;87:119–20.

28. Carson P, Anand I, O'Connor C, et al. Mode of death in advanced heart failure: the Comparison of Medical, Pacing, and Defibrillation Therapies in Heart Failure (COMPANION) trial. J Am Coll Cardiol 2005;46:2329–34.

29. Cleland JG, Daubert JC, Erdmann E, et al;Cardiac Resynchronization–Heart Failure (CARE-HF) Study Investigators. The effect of cardiac resynchronization on morbidity and mortality in heart failure. N Engl J Med 2005;352:1539–49.

30. Ellenbogen KA, Wood MA, Klein HU. Why should we care about CARE-HF? J Am Coll Cardiol 2005;46: 2199–203.

31. Cleland JG, Daubert JC, Erdmann E, et al. The effect of cardiac resynchronization on morbidity and mortality in heart failure. N Engl J Med 2005;352:1539–49.

32. Rivera DA, Bristow MR. Cardiac resynchronization – a heart failure perspective. Ann Noninvasive Electrocardiol 2005;10:16–23.

33. McAlister FA, Ezekowitz JA, Wiebe N, et al. Systematic review: Cardiac resynchronization in patients with symptomatic heart failure. Ann Intern Med 2004;141: 381–90.

6

Cardiac resynchronization therapy in special populations

Maria Rosa Costanzo and Mary Norine Walsh

Introduction • CRT in patients with ischemic versus non-ischemic cardiomyopathy • CRT in patients with mild heart failure symptoms • CRT in heart failure patients with normal QRS duration • CRT in heart failure patients with RBBB • Effects of CRT in heart failure patients with pacemakers 'upgraded' on biventricular pacing devices • CRT in heart failure patients with chronic AF • Conclusions

INTRODUCTION

In New York Heart Association (NYHA) class III–IV patients with left ventricular (LV) ejection fraction (LVEF) ≤35%, QRS duration ≥120 ms, and sinus rhythm, cardiac resynchronization therapy (CRT) consistently improves cardiac function, quality of life, functional capacity, and survival.[1-7] The effects of CRT, however, have not been thoroughly investigated in several patient populations that could potentially derive similar benefit. Early reports indicated that the benefit of CRT was greater in patients with non-ischemic than in those with ischemic cardiomyopathies. In more recent trials, however, CRT effects were independent of heart failure etiology.[8] The evidence that CRT can partially reverse myocardial remodeling mediating heart failure progression was largely obtained in NYHA class III patients.[1-7] It remains unknown if CRT can prevent heart failure progression in less symptomatic (NYHA class II) patients or meaningfully improve cardiac function in patients with advanced (NYHA class IV) heart failure. Enrollment in all major CRT trials required a QRS duration ≥120 ms.[1-7] Therefore, the effects of CRT in patients with a narrow QRS but with evidence of mechanical dyssynchrony have not been explored in depth. Similarly, the role of CRT in patients with atrial fibrillation (AF) remains largely unknown, because patients with this arrhythmia were excluded from most of the pivotal CRT studies.[1,3-5,7] The vast majority of CRT trial subjects had a left bundle branch block (LBBB) QRS configuration, and therefore scant data exist on the effects of CRT in patients with a prolonged QRS duration but a right bundle branch block (RBBB) QRS configuration.[1-7] Lastly, because right ventricular (RV) apical pacing produces a pattern of LV conduction similar to LBBB, the concern exists that persistent or even intermittent RV pacing may produce functional abnormalities similar to those induced by intrinsic LBBB.[9,10] Few data exist on whether the addition of a LV pacing lead will negate the deleterious effects of apical RV pacing in implantable cardioverter–defibrillator (ICD) recipients with underlying LV dysfunction.[11] This chapter will discuss the available data on heart failure patient populations who were absent from or poorly represented in CRT trials.

CRT IN PATIENTS WITH ISCHEMIC VERSUS NON-ISCHEMIC CARDIOMYOPATHY

The large randomized controlled clinical trials of CRT included patients with cardiomyopathy of both ischemic and non-ischemic causes[1-7] (Table 6.1). In most of these trials, patients were designated as having an ischemic etiology of heart failure on the basis of a history of prior myocardial infarction with electrocardographically evident infarct location, prior percutaneous coronary intervention, or prior coronary bypass surgery. Only one study – the PATH CHF (Pacing Therapies in Congestive Heart Failure) study – required coronary angiography for patient enrollment, but did not provide details of the angiographic findings.[1] The lack of coronary angiography as a prerequisite for assignment of a diagnosis of ischemic cardiomyopathy limits the analysis of differential effects of CRT according to the etiology of heart failure. Most CRT trials did not report their results according to the cause of heart disease. Notable exceptions

are MIRACLE ICD (Multicenter In Synch ICD Randomized Clinical Evaluation), COMPANION (Comparison of Medical Therapy, Pacing and Defibrillation in Heart Failure), and CARE-HF (Cardiac Resynchronization in Heart Failure).[4,5,7] In MIRACLE ICD, CRT effects on quality-of-life scores and NYHA class were not influenced by the etiology of heart failure.[4] According to a prespecified subgroup analysis performed in the CARE-HF trial, the benefits of CRT were similar in patients with ischemic and non-ischemic heart disease.[7] In the COMPANION trial, CRT – with or without the addition of an ICD – reduced the risk of the primary endpoint (all-cause death or hospitalization) to a similar extent in patients with and without ischemic heart disease.[5] In this study, however, there was a significant difference in the effect of CRT on the secondary

Table 6.1 Studies of resynchronization: representation of patients with ischemic heart failure etiology, atrial fibrillation (AF) and right bundle branch block (RBBB)

Study	Duration of treatment (months)	Sample size	Ischemic cause (%)	Mean LVEF ± SD (%)	NYHA class III or IV symptoms (%)	AF (%)	RBBB (%)
Crossover trials							
MUSTIC-SR [2]	3	58	37	23 ± 7	100	0	13
MUSTIC-AF [63]	3	43	43	26 ±10	100	100	NR
PATH-HF [1]	1	41	29	21 ± 7	100	0	7
CONTAK-CD [70]	3	490	69	22 ± 7	68	0	NR
Parallel-Arm Trials							
MIRACLE [3]	6	453	54	22 ± 6	100	0	NR
MIRACLE ICD [4]	6	555	35	21 ± 7	65	14	25
COMPANION [5]	12	1520	55	23	100	0	11
CARE-HF [7]	24.9	813	38	25	100	0	NR
Cohort studies							
Cazeau et al [71]	12	8	50	22 ±8	100	38	NR
InSynch Italian Registry [72]	12	117	48	22 ± 6	100	0	NR
Krahn et al [73]	6	45	69	19 ± 5	94	33	NR
Kuhlkamp et al [74]	3	84	NR	25 ± 7	68	12	NR
Leclercq et al [75]	6	37	38	23 ± 5	100	28	NR
Leon et al [60]	NR	20	55	22 ± 7	100	100	NR
Mortensen et al [76]	3	189	42	24 ± 7	83	0	NR
Molhoek et al [77]	6	40	48	24 ±9	NR	10	NR

COMPANION, Comparison of Medical Therapy, Pacing, and Defibrillation in Chronic Heart Failure; CONTAK-CD, Guidant CONTAK-CD CRT-D System trial; LVEF, left ventricular ejection fraction; MIRACLE, Multicenter InSynch Randomized Clinical Evaluation; MIRACLE ICD, Multicenter InSynch Implantable Cardioverter Defibrillator Randomized Clinical Evaluation; MUSTIC-AF, Multisite Stimulation in Cardiomyopathies – Atrial Fibrillation; MUSTIC-SR, MUSTIC – Sinus Rhythm; NR, not reported; NYHA, New York Heart Association; PATH-CHF, Pacing Therapies for Congestive Heart Failure.

endpoint of all-cause mortality between patients with and those without ischemic heart disease. Compared with optimal medical therapy, combined CRT–ICD therapy lowered all-cause mortality to a significantly greater degree in non-ischemic than in ischemic patients (50% vs 27%). In contrast, CRT alone produced a greater benefit in ischemic than in non-ischemic patients (28% vs 9%).[5]

The differential effects of CRT in ischemic versus non-ischemic cardiomyopathy may be due to the manner in which CRT influences myocardial oxygen consumption (MVO_2) and myocardial blood flow (MBF).[12] In 31 non-ischemic and 11 ischemic CRT responders, MVO_2 and MBF were evaluated by [^{11}C] acetate positron emission tomography (PET) before and 4 months after initiation of CRT.[12] The results of this study show that CRT improved ventricular efficiency and rendered more uniform the blood flow distribution between myocardial walls in patients with non-ischemic cardiomyopathy, but not in those with ischemic cardiomyopathy. Reverse ventricular remodeling, as measured by changes in LV end-diastolic dimension, was also greater in the non-ischemic than in the ischemic patients.[12] The strength of these results, however, is tempered by the fact that the patients with ischemic heart failure were only one-third of the study population.

An echocardiographic analysis from the MIRACLE (Multicenter InSynch Randomized Clinical Evaluation) study demonstrated that significant reverse remodeling and improvement in ejection fraction occurred in heart failure patients with both ischemic and non-ischemic LV dysfunction.[13] Although at 6 months after initiation of CRT, changes in LV volumes and LVEF were greater in patients with non-ischemic LV dysfunction than in patients with equivalent LV dysfunction due to ischemic heart disease, NYHA class, exercise capacity, and quality of life improved to a similar extent in the two heart failure etiology groups (Figure 6.1). A longer follow-up of MIRACLE study subjects revealed that the differences in reverse myocardial remodeling between ischemic and non-ischemic patients persisted.[14] In non-ischemic patients, LV volume reduction, which at 6 months was more than three-fold greater than that of ischemic patients, was sustained at 12 months.[14] In contrast, in the ischemic patients, the reduction in LV volume detected at 6 months was no longer present at 12 months. Despite these differences in measures of reverse myocardial remodeling, ischemic and non-ischemic patients continued to demonstrate similar improvements in clinical endpoints up to 18 months after CRT initiation. The results of other studies support the findings of the MIRACLE trial. A study of 34 patients with heart failure due to ischemic heart disease (defined as ≥50% stenosis in one of the major epicardial coronary arteries by angiography) and 40 patients with dilated cardiomyopathy revealed that after

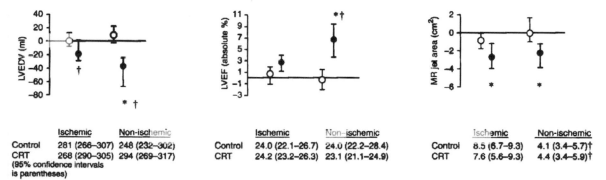

Figure 6.1 Median change from baseline in left ventricular end diastolic volume (LVEDV), left ventricular ejection fraction (LVEF), and mitral regurgitation (MR) jet area with two-sided 95% confidence intervals by heart failure etiology (open circles, control group; diamonds, cardiac resynchronization therapy (CRT) group); ≥*p<0.05, CRT vs control within subgroups; †p<0.05, treatment vs treatment between subgroup. (Reproduced with permission from St John Sutton MG et al. Circulation 2003;107: 1985–90.[13])

6 months of CRT, the two groups had similar improvements in QRS duration, NYHA class, quality-of-life scores, LVEF, mitral regurgitation, and annual hospitalizations. Furthermore, the percentage of responders to CRT, defined as patients who improved by at least one NYHA class after 6 months of CRT, was similar in the ischemic and non-ischemic group (65% vs 71%).[8]

CRT IN PATIENTS WITH MILD HEART FAILURE SYMPTOMS

The overwhelming majority of subjects in the large CRT trials were patients with NYHA class III heart failure symptoms.[1-7] Therefore, the effects of CRT in patients with cardiac dyssynchrony and milder heart failure symptoms are largely unknown. MIRACLE ICD II was a randomized, double-blind, parallel-controlled clinical trial of CRT in NYHA class II heart failure patients on optimal medical therapy with LVEF $\leq$35%, QRS $\geq$130 ms, and a class I ICD indication.[15] One hundred and one patients were randomized to the control group (ICD activated, CRT off) and 85 to the CRT group (ICD activated, CRT on). Compared with the control group at 6 months, the CRT group had greater improvement in ventricular remodeling indices, including LV diastolic and systolic volumes and LVEF, in ventilatory response to exercise, and in NYHA class. The CRT group had higher rates of clinical improvement than the control group (58% vs 36%; $p = 0.01$). Improvement of peak oxygen consumption (VO_{2max}), 6-minute walk distance (6MWD) and quality-of-life scores were similar in the control and CRT groups. The results of this study indicate that in mildly symptomatic, optimally treated heart failure patients with a wide QRS complex and an ICD indication, CRT did not alter exercise capacity, but was associated with improvement in cardiac structure and function and composite clinical response over 6 months.[15] These observations on the ability of CRT to limit heart failure progression must be confirmed in large, randomized, prospective trials of mildly symptomatic heart failure patients before a recommendation for CRT is extended to this population. Fortunately, two controlled clinical trials have been launched to determine if CRT, in combination with optimal medical therapy, can prevent or slow disease progression and reverse LV remodeling in patients with QRS duration $\geq$120 ms and milder than NYHA class III heart failure symptoms. MADIT-CRT (Multicenter Automatic Defibrillator Implantation Trial With Cardiac Resynchronization Therapy) is a randomized, open-label, active control, parallel assignment trial designed to determine if, compared with ICD therapy alone, combined ICD–CRT will reduce the risk of mortality and heart failure events by approximately 25% in subjects who are in NYHA class II with non-ischemic or ischemic cardiomyopathy and in subjects who are in NYHA class I with ischemic cardiomyopathy, LV systolic dysfunction (LVEF $\leq$30%), and prolonged intraventricular conduction (QRS duration $\geq$130 ms).[16]

REVERSE (REsynchronization reVErse Remodeling in Systolic left vEntricular dysfunction) is a prospective, multicenter, randomized, double-blind, parallel, controlled clinical trial designed to establish whether CRT, combined with optimal medical treatment, can attenuate heart failure disease progression compared with optimal medical treatment alone in patients with asymptomatic LV dysfunction with or without NYHA class I American College of Cardiology/American Heart Association (ACC/AHA) stage C or NYHA class II heart failure, QRS duration $\geq$120 ms, LVEF $\leq$40%, and LV end-diastolic diameter $\geq$55 mm.[17] It is anticipated that this study will include approximately 500 patients from 100 centers in the USA, Canada, and Europe, that enrollment will be completed by the end of 2006, and that follow-up will last for 5 years. Several aspects of this study deserve mention. The primary endpoint is a recently proposed heart failure clinical composite response, which may be more sensitive than any of its individual components in the detection of a treatment difference between CRT plus optimal medical treatment and pharmacological therapy alone.[18] Optimization of atrioventricular (AV) delay by echocardiogram is required in both active treatment and control groups to eliminate the possibility that inadequate LV diastolic filling might influence results. Finally decrease in LV end-systolic volume index is chosen as the principal secondary endpoint because a strong relationship has been demonstrated between this variable and clinical outcome.[17]

CRT IN HEART FAILURE PATIENTS WITH NORMAL QRS DURATION

Duration of QRS is an inadequate indicator of mechanical dyssynchrony. The use of QRS duration has been generally regarded as a surrogate of mechanical dyssynchrony, and its value resides in the simplicity and widespread use of the electrocardiogram (ECG).[19] Results of acute CRT studies indicate that improvement in contractility and stroke volume with CRT is smaller in patients with a QRS duration of 120–150 ms than in those with a QRS duration >150 ms. In addition, short-term (3 months) results suggested little or no improvements in exercise capacity and quality of life in patients with QRS duration of 120–150 ms.[20] In contrast, 1-year data have surprisingly showed a significant increase and near-comparable treatment effect in this patient population, compared with patients with QRS duration >150 ms.[21] Two additional observations have raised concerns about the ability of the QRS duration to predict mechanical dyssynchrony: (i) during atrial sensed sequential LV pacing alone, LV contractility and stroke volume significantly improve despite a QRS duration longer than that of intrinsic LBBB; (ii) QRS shortening during simultaneous RV and LV pacing is poorly correlated with clinical efficacy of CRT.[19,22] Taken together, these findings question the extent to which QRS duration is a valid measure of mechanical dyssynchrony. Notably, recent animal studies using tagged magnetic resonance imaging (MRI) have shown the dissociation that exists between electrical delay times and mechanical dyssynchrony.[22] However, this apparent dissociation may have other causes. The cut-off for defining abnormal QRS duration may be arbitrary, and perhaps vectocardiography or signal-averaging ECG should be used to provide a more precise definition of QRS duration. Furthermore, QRS duration should be adjusted for the degree of ventricular dilation. It is important to remember that the QRS complex results from the vectorial sum of electrical phenomena generated by myocardial masses over time. Thus, a myocardial mass whose contractility is temporally delayed can influence the QRS morphology and duration only if it has substantial volume. Minor regional and local changes in mass, represented electrically by a small vector, may not be adequately displayed in the standard ECG. However, such small masses may have enough volume or abnormal motion to be detected by imaging techniques.[19]

Mechanical dyssynchrony can be defined as mechanical dispersion of motion within the LV. This mechanical abnormality is caused by hidden electrical abnormalities.[19] Myocardial Purkinje cells form a diffuse network and propagate electrical impulses at high velocity in a uniform manner from the endocardium to the epicardium. In a region of myocardial disease, rearrangement of extracellular matrix and myocytes results in intramural disarray, which may influence the entry, the direction, and ultimately the velocity of propagation of electrical impulses within the diseased area. In an animal model of LBBB, regional differences have been demonstrated in the expression of genes and proteins mediating hypertrophy.[23] This indicates that, due to changes in activation sequence following the onset of LBBB, abnormal regional loading conditions are generated that induce variable degrees of hypertrophy. Recent electrophysiological mapping data have shown that with an abnormal activation sequence, the physiological endocardium-to-epicardium depolarization gradient is replaced by a diffuse activation wavefront traveling throughout the myocardial wall; the disorganized electrical depolarization creates abnormal local (endocardium, myocardium, and epicardium) loading conditions, leading to different degrees of transmural hypertrophy.[24] These intraventricular differences in hypertrophy and myocyte function can be detected with the appropriate imaging techniques. These methods, which include radionuclide imaging, MRI, echocardiography, and tissue Doppler imaging (TDI), are exhaustively discussed elsewhere in this textbook. The use of these imaging techniques has shown that the presence of mechanical dyssynchrony independently predicts prognosis in heart failure patients and that several measures of mechanical dyssynchrony predict response to CRT.[25-33]

Mechanical dyssynchrony has been measured in patients with intermediate (120–150 ms) and narrow (<120 ms) QRS duration. Mechanical systolic and diastolic dyssynchrony, as measured by echocardiography with TDI using a six basal, six mid-segmental model, were present, respectively, in 51% and 46% of 67 heart failure patients with QRS duration <120 ms[34] (Figure 6.2). In another echocardiographic and TDI study, inter- and intraventricular mechanical dyssynchrony were detected, respectively, in 12.5% and 29.5% of 61 patients with LVEF <35% and QRS duration <120 ms. Interestingly, there was no correlation between inter- and intraventricular dyssynchrony.[35] Similar results emerged

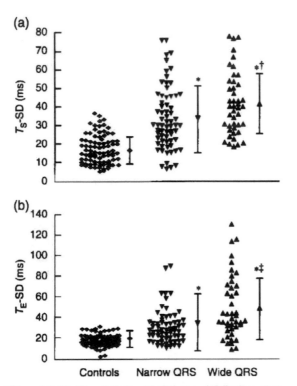

Figure 6.2 Scatter plot showing (a) the distribution of the standard deviation of the time to peak myocardial sustained systolic velocity T_S-SD and (b) early diastolic velocity T_E-SD of all 12 left ventricular segments in 88 normal controls, in 67 patients with heart failure and narrow QRS complexes (≤ 120 ms), and in 45 patients with heart failure and wide QRS complexes (> 120 ms). *p < 0.001 vs controls; †p = 0.009 vs normal-QRS group; ‡p = 0.002 vs normal-QRS group. (Reproduced with permission from Yu CM et al. Heart 2003; 89: 54–60.[34])

from another prospective TDI evaluation of the incidence of LV dyssynchrony in 64 heart failure patients with narrow QRS.[36] In this study, the correlation between QRS duration and severity of LV dyssynchrony was not significant ($r = 0.12$; $p > 0.05$). Among 106 patients with LVEF <35% and narrow QRS, a maximal temporal difference (T_S-diff) >91 ms from R wave to peak systolic point between eight myocardial segments was an independent risk factor for clinical events and mortality regardless of age, QRS duration, and use of β-blockers. The mean event-free survival was 16.3 months (95% confidence interval (CI) 11.9–20.7) in patients with T_S-diff >91 ms and 31.6 months (95% CI 28.0–35.1) in those with T_S-diff ≤ 91 ms ($p < 0.001$).[37] These results indicate that myocardial dyssynchrony assessed by TDI is a powerful predictor of clinical events in heart failure patients with normal QRS duration. The importance of these results is corroborated by the consistent finding that indices of mechanical dyssynchrony, not QRS duration, predict response to CRT. The presence and prognostic value of mechanical dyssynchrony in at least one-third of heart failure patients with QRS <120 ms beg the question of whether CRT improves the outcomes of heart failure patients with narrow QRS but evidence of mechanical dyssynchrony. In one study, CRT was performed in 52 patients with severe heart failure regardless of QRS duration, provided that there was evidence of inter- and intraventricular mechanical dyssynchrony.[38] In all patients, CRT produced significant improvement in cardiac function and exercise capacity. Comparison of the 14 patients with QRS duration ≤120 ms with the 38 patients with QRS duration >120 ms revealed similar improvement in LVEF, LV systolic and diastolic dimensions, mitral regurgitation area, interventricular delay, and posterolateral LV wall activation delay, LV filling time, deceleration time and 6MWD.[38] The major finding of this study is that CRT produces significant clinical and functional benefit in patients with QRS duration ≤120 ms who underwent biventricular (BiV) pacing because of documented mechanical dyssynchrony.[38] Importantly, the magnitude of improvement was similar to that achieved in patients with QRS duration >120 ms, who are the only patients with LV systolic dysfunction currently recognized as candidates for CRT by both practice guidelines and payers[39,40] (Table 6.2). The benefit of CRT in heart failure patients with mechanical dyssynchrony but narrow QRS and the findings that the degree of intraventricular dyssynchrony by TDI, and not the baseline QRS duration, predicts effectiveness of CRT argue in favor of using indices of mechanical dyssynchrony rather than QRS duration to identify optimal CRT candidates.[41] Admittedly, the data regarding the efficacy of CRT in patients with narrow QRS are derived from small, non-randomized studies using rather unsophisticated echocardiographic measurements.[42,43] However the results of these studies and the

growing body of evidence confirming the ability of indices of mechanical dyssynchrony to predict response to CRT underscore the need for larger randomized trials evaluating the effects of CRT in heart failure patients with proven mechanical dyssynchrony, regardless of their QRS duration.

CRT IN HEART FAILURE PATIENTS WITH RBBB

RBBB occurs less commonly than LBBB in patients with heart failure.[44-46] Although there has been a great deal of investigation on the efficacy of CRT in patients with prolonged QRS duration and a LBBB configuration, there is a

Table 6.2 Clinical, electrocardiographic, and echocardiographic characteristics before and after cardiac resynchronization therapy in patients with baseline QRS duration > 120 ms and in patients with QRS duration ≤120 ms[a,b]

Characteristics	QRS >120 ms (n = 38)	QRS ≤120 ms (n = 14)	p value[c]
QRS duration, baseline (ms)	168.2 ± 21.4	110.4 ± 10.9	< 0.001
QRS duration, follow-up (ms)	125.2 ± 9.1*	120.6 ± 13.1	0.453
NYHA, baseline	3.5 ± 0.5	3.3 ± 0.5	0.695
NYHA, follow-up	1.8 ± 0.5*	1.7 ± 0.6*	1.000
6MWD, baseline (m)	256.0 ± 65.4	276.4 ± 88.9	1.000
6MWD, follow-up (m)	394.2 ± 38.4*	369.9 ± 70.2†	0.362
Death	7 (18.4%)	3 (21.4%)	1.000[d]
LVEF, baseline (%)	22.6 ± 4.6	24.6 ± 5.0	0.591
LVEF, follow-up (%)	33.2 ± 5.4*	33.6 ±5.9*	1.000
LVEDD, baseline (mm)	77.4 ± 10.6	71.8 ± 9.2	0.490
LVEDD, follow-up (mm)	71.6 ± 10.7†	65.6 ± 8.5†	0.380
LVESD, baseline (mm)	64.8 ± 10.2	61.4 ± 8.4	0.839
LVESD, follow-up (mm)	57.9 ±11.0†	55.6 ± 8.2†	1.000
MR, baseline (cm²)	6.9 ±4.1	7.5 ± 4.7	1.000
MR, follow-up (cm²)	3.8 ± 2.9*	4.5 ± 3.5*	1.000
IVD, baseline (ms)	56.4 ± 31.1	42.5 ± 16.6	0.320
IVD, follow-up (ms)	15.9 ± 15.2*	6.4 ± 16.8*	0.178
Q-LW, baseline (ms)	421.8 ± 72.6	395.0 ± 53.9	0.987
Q-LW, follow-up (ms)	389.7 ± 55.3†	363.2 ± 47.3	0.472
E-A, baseline (ms)	425.3 ± 102.1	471.8 ± 166.3	0.687
E-A, follow-up (ms)	442.0 ± 120.8	437.5 ± 54.7	1.000
DT, baseline (ms)	121.5 ± 31.3	117.7 ± 25.8	1.000
DT, follow-up (ms)	157.2 ± 29.8*	148.5 ± 17.4†	0.223

[a] Adapted from Achilli A et al. J Am Coll Cardiol 2003;42:2117–24.[38]

[b] Data are presented as the mean value ±SD or percentage of patients.

[c] p-value based on analysis of variance or [d] Fisher exact test: * p <0.001; †p < 0.01; †p< 0.05 vs baseline.

NYHA, New York Heart Association; 6MWD, 6-minute walk distance; DT, deceleration time; E-A, left ventricular filling time; LVEF, left ventricular ejection fraction; IVD, interventricular delay; LVEDD, left ventricular end-diastolic diameter; LVESD, left ventricular end-systolic diameter; MR, mitral regurgitation area; Q-LW, posterolateral left ventricular wall delay.

shortage of data on the benefits of this therapy for patients with RBBB. All large randomized controlled clinical trials of CRT included patients with QRS duration of ≥120 ms.[1-7] Some (MIRACLE and MIRACLE ICD) enrolled only patients with QRS duration >130 ms[3,4] and one (MUSTIC: Multisite Stimulation in Cardiomyopathy) required an entry QRS duration >150 ms.[2] However, the average QRS duration of the enrolled patients was significantly longer.

As shown in Table 6.1, the numbers of patients with RBBB QRS configuration were not reported in all CRT trials, and, in the trials that did, RBBB patients comprised a small minority of enrolled subjects. Furthermore, most of the trials in which the number of patients with a RBBB QRS configuration was shown did not include prespecified analyses of CRT effects in this subgroup. Only MIRACLE ICD[4] and COMPANION[5] reported the effects of CRT in heart failure patients with RBBB. In MIRACLE ICD, the treatment effect of CRT on NYHA class and quality-of-life scores was not influenced by the morphology of the QRS complex. In COMPANION, all endpoints were met in the RBBB patient group, albeit with wider confidence intervals.

One study that focused exclusively on CRT in heart failure patients with complete RBBB demonstrated that this therapy resulted in an improvement in clinical status and exercise tolerance at 1 year.[47] Twelve patients with complete RBBB and QRS duration >140 ms, LVEF <35%, and LV end-diastolic diameter ≥60 mm underwent pacemaker implantation, and data were collected at 1, 6, and 12 months. Patients were considered responders to CRT if they experienced improvement in both NYHA class and exercise capacity. Although the LVEF was unchanged at 12 months, performance on maximal treadmill testing improved, as did NYHA class. In addition, at 12 months, QRS duration became shorter and there were significant reductions in mitral regurgitation, LV volumes, and electromechanical delay between LV free wall and septum, as measured by TDI. Compared with non-responders, the 75% of patients deemed to be responders had greater LV mechanical delay at baseline and greater reduction of intraventricular dyssynchrony after CRT. This improvement may be due to the fact that heart failure patients

with a RBBB QRS configuration have a concomitant left-sided intraventricular conduction delay. Regardless of the type of electrical delay, it appears that the patients most likely to benefit from CRT are those with echocardiographically detectable intraventricular mechanical dyssynchrony.

EFFECTS OF CRT IN HEART FAILURE PATIENTS WITH PACEMAKERS 'UPGRADED' TO BIVENTRICULAR PACING DEVICES

Similarly to intrinsic LBBB, RV-pacing-induced LBBB results in abnormal ventricular depolarization and worsening of mechanical dyssynchrony.[48] Experimental and clinical data suggest that, compared with atrial or no ventricular pacing, chronic RV pacing worsens systolic function and produces inter- and intraventricular dyssynchrony.[10] For heart failure patients with LBBB secondary to chronic RV pacing, the effects of CRT on QRS duration, ventricular synchrony, hemodynamics, and contractile function have not been extensively studied. Preliminary data suggest that upgrade to CRT in RV-paced heart failure patients improves functional capacity.[11] Placement of an LV lead in 15 NYHA class III–IV patients with QRS duration of 190 ± 27 ms and continuous RV pacing resulted in reductions in QRS duration (to 165 ± 18 ms; $p = 0.005$), LV electromechanical delay (calculated as the time from QRS initiation to onset of aortic flow: from 180 ± 33 ms to 161 ± 43 ms), LV end-diastolic volume (from 270 ± 70 ml to 254 ± 70 ml; $p = 0.0001$), and LV end-systolic volume (from 212 ± 61 ml to 192 ± 65 ml; $p = 0.001$), and improvements in LVEF (from 24 ± 6% to 31 ± 11%; $p = 0.02$), LV ejection time (from 252 ± 25 ms to 266 ± 21 ms; $p = 0.02$), and myocardial performance index (calculated as the sum of isovolumic contraction and relaxation divided by LV ejection time: from 0.90 ± 0.36 to 0.55 ± 0.20; $p = 0.01$)[49] (Figure 6.3). Diastolic function, as assessed by mitral valve deceleration time, was not affected by CRT. In this study, changes in QRS duration after CRT initiation were inversely correlated with increases in LVEF.[49] In contrast, among 16 RV-paced heart failure patients with a LVEF of 27 ± 5%, there was no correlation between QRS width and either inter- or intraventricular

(a)   Pre-'upgrade'   (b)   Post-'upgrade'

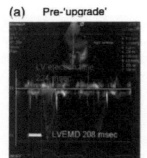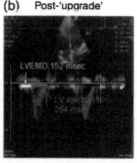

Figure 6.3 Left ventricular electromechanical delay (LVEMD), measured as the time from the beginning of the QRS interval to the onset of aortic outflow, is significantly shortened post 'upgrade' to cardiac resynchronization therapy (b) compared with pre 'upgrade' (right ventricular pacing) (a), indicating reduced interventricular dyssynchrony. Left ventricular ejection time, an index of systolic function, is lengthened post 'upgrade'. (Reproduced with permission from Horwich T et al. J Cardiovasc Electrophysiol 2004;15:1284–9.[49])

mechanical dyssynchrony.[50] Based upon this finding, the investigators recommended that mechanical dyssynchrony be documented before CRT is offered to RV-paced heart failure patients. Electrogram data in 18 ICD recipients upgraded to CRT–ICD revealed that, compared with the pre-CRT period, the rates of arrhythmias and appropriate ICD shocks significantly decreased during the first year after initiation of CRT.[51] Taken together, the data summarized above suggest that chronic RV pacing has detrimental clinical and hemodynamic effects, which may be attenuated by the addition of a LV-pacing lead for CRT. The data, however, come from small uncontrolled studies in which only some echocardiographic indices of mechanical dyssynchrony were examined and patients' follow-up was short. Prospective, randomized clinical trials are needed to confirm the long-term benefit of CRT in RV-paced heart failure patients.

CRT IN HEART FAILURE PATIENTS WITH CHRONIC AF

AF and heart failure are commonly encountered together, and either condition predisposes to the other.[52–54] Risk factors for both AF and heart failure include age, hypertension, valve disease, and myocardial infarction, as well as a variety of medical conditions and genetic variants. Heart failure and AF share common mechanisms, including myocardial fibrosis and dysregulation of intracellular calcium metabolism and neurohormonal function. It is not surprising, therefore, that the prevalence of chronic AF in the overall heart failure population is approximately 20%, and may be as high as 40% in patients with advanced heart failure.[52–54] Although the prognostic value of AF in heart failure patients remains controversial, in these patients AF often contributes to clinical deterioration because of loss of the contribution of atrial contraction to LV function, irregular heart rate, and frequently fast ventricular rates. Interestingly, one study showed that heart failure patients with both chronic AF and intraventricular conduction delay have a significantly higher 1-year mortality rate than heart failure patients in sinus rhythm (26.5% vs 14.5%; $p < 0.001$).[46] Importantly, data from a large UK District General Hospital indicate that as many as 40% of potential CRT candidates are in chronic AF.[55] It is now widely accepted that in heart failure patients with persistent AF and rapid ventricular response, rate control by atrioventricular node (AVN) ablation and permanent VVIR pacing produces, generally within 3 months, partial improvement of LV systolic dysfunction and its clinical consequences.[56] The data summarized above underscore the importance of the evaluation of the role of CRT in heart failure patients with chronic AF.

In one study, nine heart failure patients with LVEF $\leq 30\%$, AF, and AV block were evaluated by pressure–volume analysis. Ventricular stimulation was applied to the RV, LV free wall, and both RV and LV (BiV) at 80 and 120 bpm. At both heart rates, BiV pacing improved LV systolic function more than either site alone ($dP/dt_{max} = 810 \pm 83$, 924 ± 98, and 983 ± 102 mmHg/s for RV, LV, and BiV, respectively; $p < 0.05$), although LV pacing was significantly better than RV pacing. Diastolic function, as measured by isovolumic relaxation, was improved only by BiV pacing.[57] The results of this study indicate that in heart failure patients with AF and advanced AV block, CRT acutely enhances both systolic and diastolic LV function more than single-site RV or LV pacing. Another short-term study of 12 patients undergoing AVN ablation for drug-refractory AF confirmed that LV-based pacing is superior to RV apical pacing in terms of LV contractile function and diastolic filling.[58] In this study, in which 50% of the patients had preserved LVEF, BiV pacing did not improve diastolic function more than LV only pacing. OPSITE (Optimal Pacing SITE trial) was a prospective randomized, single-blind, 3-month crossover comparison of the effects of RV, LV, and BiV pacing on quality of life and exercise capacity of 56 patients with symptomatic chronic AF, uncontrolled ventricular rate, or heart failure.[59] Compared with RV pacing, after LV and BiV pacing, respectively, the Minnesota Living with Heart Failure Questionnaire (MLHFQ) score improved by 2% and 10%, the effort dyspnea item of the Specific Symptom Scale (SSS) changed by 0% and 2%, the Karolinska score by 6% and 14% (p <0.05 for BiV), the NYHA class by 5% and 11% (p <0.05 for BiV), the 6MWD by 12 m (+4%) and 4 m (+1%), and the LVEF by 5% and 5% (p <0.05 for both). Surprisingly, BiV pacing, but not LV pacing, was slightly better than RV pacing in the subgroup of patients with preserved LV systolic function and absence of native LBBB.[59] The results of this study indicate the improvement in quality of life and functional capacity is due predominantly to rhythm regularization resulting from AVN ablation. During the 3-month observation period, only modest or no additional favorable effects were provided by LV and BiV pacing compared with RV pacing.[59] As a result of these findings, the authors proposed that neither LV nor BiV pacing can be recommended as a first-line treatment for all patients with AF and should be reserved for patients who fail to improve with RV pacing alone or experience clinical deterioration late after AVN ablation. However, the results of this study should be interpreted with caution because of the heterogeneity of the patient population and the short follow-up period. The deleterious hemodynamic effects of apical RV pacing and the potential benefit of LV-based pacing therapy could have become apparent after a longer observation period.[10,48]

Indeed, in 20 NYHA class III–IV heart failure patients with LVEF ≤35% and prior (≥6 months)

AVN ablation and RV pacing for chronic AF, CRT produced significant improvement in LV function and symptoms of heart failure.[60] During a follow-up period of 17.3 ± 4.5 months, the NYHA class improved by 29% (p <0.001), the LVEF increased by 44% (p <0.001), the LV diastolic and end-systolic diameters decreased, respectively, by 6.5% (p <0.003) and 8.5% (p <0.01), hospitalizations were reduced by 81% (p <0.001), and the MLWHFQ scores improved by 33% (p <0.01).[60] Since the magnitude of improvement is similar to that produced by CRT in heart failure patients in sinus rhythm, the authors concluded that the benefits of BiV pacing in heart failure patients with AF are due more to the correction of cardiac dyssynchrony than to rhythm regularization resulting from AVN ablation. Similar improvement in LV performance and NYHA class, but no change in 6MWD or VO$_{2max}$, was observed 6 months after initiation of BiV pacing in 14 heart failure patients treated 20±19 months before study entry with AVN ablation for uncontrolled chronic AF.[61] Additional insights into the mechanisms of CRT-induced benefit in patients requiring AVN ablation for medically refractory AF are provided by the PAVE (Post AV Nodal Ablation Evaluation) study[62] (Figure 6.4). Of 184 patients with an LVEF of 46 ± 16% and NYHA class III or IV who required AVN ablation, 103 were randomized to receive a BiV pacing system and 81 an RV pacing system. At 6 months after AVN ablation, CRT-treated patients, compared with RV-paced patients, had a greater improvement above baseline in 6MWD (31% vs 24%; p = 0.04) without significant quality-of-life differences. At 6 months after AVN ablation LVEF was significantly higher in the BiV-than in the RV-paced group (46 ± 0.13% vs 41 ± 13%; p = 0.03). Patients with LVEF ≤45% or NYHA class II/III symptoms receiving a BiV pacemaker had greater improvement in 6MWD than those who were less symptomatic or had preserved LV systolic function.[62]

It is important to note, however, that the difference between the two pacing groups was due to a decline in 6MWD in the RV-paced group, rather than to an increase in 6MWD in the BiV group. A similar phenomenon was also noted with temporal changes in LVEF, which, over time, decreased in patients assigned to RV

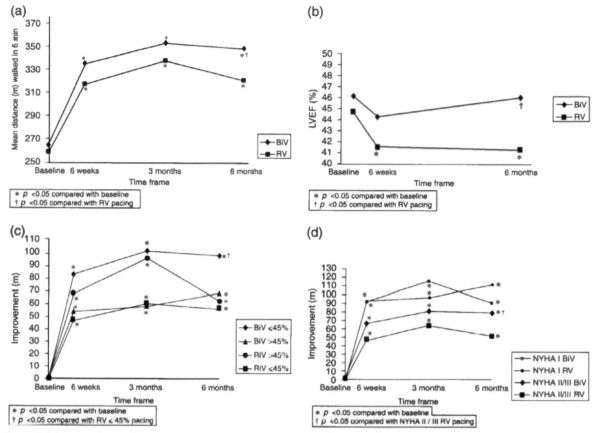

Figure 6.4 Results of the left ventricular-based cardiac stimulation PAVE (Post AV Nodal Ablation Evaluation) study. (a) Temporal changes in the 6-minute hallway walk test for patients randomized to biventricular (BiV) or right ventricular (RV) pacing. The baseline represents the 6-minute walk distance just prior to atrioventricular (AV) junction ablation. There is a significant improvement in the distance walked in both groups at 6 weeks postablation versus baseline, which remains at 3 months postablation. However, at 6 months postablation, the distance walked by patients randomized to RV pacing decreases, while that of the BiV group remains stable. (b) Temporal changes in the left ventricular ejection fraction (LVEF). Temporal changes in the 6-minute hallway walk test stratified by LVEF (>45% vs ≤45%) for patients randomized to BiV versus RV pacing. (d) Temporal changes in the 6-minute hallway walk test stratified by New York Heart Association (NYHA class I versus class II/III) for patients randomized to BiV versus RV pacing. (Reproduced with permission from Doshi RN et al. J Cardiovasc Electrophysiol 2005;16:1161–5.[62])

pacing, but remained stable in BiV recipients.[62] These findings imply that the clinical benefit of BiV pacing is attributable to the absence of the deleterious effects of chronic RV pacing.

This hypothesis is further supported by the results of the MUSTIC study.[63] In this single-blind, randomized, 6-month crossover comparison of BiV versus RV pacing in 59 NYHA class III patients with impaired systolic function and AF, the intention-to-treat analysis failed to reveal a significantly greater improvement in 6MWD in the BiV as compared with the RV group. The investigators attribute the inability to meet the study's primary endpoint to the 33% dropout rate in the RV-paced group, due to intolerance of the deleterious hemodynamic effects of RV pacing. Indeed, in the heart failure patients with AF who received effective BiV pacing, 6MWD and VO_{2max} increased, respectively, by 9.3% and 13%. In addition, the percentage of patients hospitalized during the 6-month crossover phase was 7% during BiV pacing and 23% during

RV pacing. In the MUSTIC study, 1-year follow-up of 42 patients in sinus rhythm and 33 patients with AF revealed similar increases in 6MWD (20% vs 17%), VO_{2max} (11% vs 9%), and LVEF (5% vs 4%), and similar decreases in mitral regurgitation area (45% vs 50%), NYHA class (25% vs 27%), and MLWHF score (36% vs 32%).[64] Only LV volumes were decreased to a greater extent in the sinus rhythm group than in the AF group. Although the results of this study must be interpreted with caution because the calculation of sample size was made only for the crossover phase and not for the 12-month follow-up time, the observed trends suggest that the benefits of BiV pacing in heart failure patients with AF are sustained at 1 year.[64]

It is difficult to reach definitive conclusions on the role of CRT in heart failure patients with chronic AF, because the studies performed in this population are for the most part small and not randomized. Furthermore, the severity of LV dysfunction, the measures of CRT effect, the types of pacing modes that are compared, the prevalence of AVN ablation, and the time from AVN ablation to CRT initiation, as well as the duration of follow-up, are highly variable[65–69] (Figure 6.5). Larger randomized clinical trials without these limitations are needed to clarify the role of CRT in heart failure patients with chronic AF.

CONCLUSIONS

The data summarized in this chapter suggest that CRT likely benefits patients with both ischemic

and non-ischemic etiologies of heart failure, but further confirmatory data are needed. In addition, CRT may benefit patient populations that are not specifically considered as appropriate candidates for BiV pacing by practice guidelines and healthcare payers. Preliminary studies suggest that CRT may prevent progression of heart failure in stage C patients with NYHA class I and II symptoms. Two ongoing controlled clinical trials, REVERSE and MADIT-CRT, will hopefully confirm the ability of CRT to attenuate or reverse myocardial remodeling in patients with mild heart failure symptoms. Larger prospective randomized trials are needed to confirm the benefits of CRT in patients with mechanical dyssynchrony despite normal QRS duration. The available data suggest that CRT is safe and effective in heart failure patients with chronic AF. Chronically RV paced patients may benefit from 'upgrade' to CRT because univentricular RV pacing results in alteration of the natural sequence of electrical activation and dyscoordinate mechanical contraction. In the future, rather than QRS duration, assessments of mechanical dyssynchrony by cardiac imaging may provide better criteria for the selection of CRT candidates.

REFERENCES

1. Auricchio A, Stellbrink C, Sack S, et al. Pacing Therapies in Congestive Heart Failure (PATH-CHF) Study Group. Long-term clinical effect of hemodynamically optimized cardiac resynchronization therapy in patients with heart failure and ventricular conduction delay. J Am Coll Cardiol 2002;39:2026–33.
2. Cazeau S, Leclercq C, Lavergne T, et al. Multisite Simulation in Cardiomyopathies (MUSTIC) Study Investigators. Effects of multisite biventricular pacing in patients with heart failure and intraventricular conduction delay. N Engl J Med 2001;344:873–80.
3. Abraham WT, Fisher WG, Smith AL, et al. MIRACLE Study Group. Multicenter InSync Randomized Clinical Evaluation. Cardiac resynchronization in chronic heart failure. N Engl J Med 2002;346:1845–53.
4. Young JB, Abraham WT, Smith AL, et al. Multicenter InSync ICD Randomized Clinical Evaluation (MIRACLE ICD) Trial Investigators. Combined cardiac resynchronization and implantable cardioversion defibrillation in advanced chronic heart failure: the MIRACLE ICD trial. JAMA 2003;289:2685–94.
5. Bristow MR, Saxon LA, Boehmer J, et al. Comparison of Medical Therapy, Pacing and Defibrillation in Heart

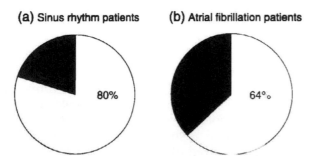

(a) Sinus rhythm patients   **(b)** Atrial fibrillation patients

80%   64%

Figure 6.5 Incidence of responders to cardiac resynchronization therapy in patients with sinus rhythm (a) is higher than in patients with atrial fibrillation (b). Black, non-responders; white, responders.[68]

Failure (COMPANION) Investigators. Cardiac resynchronization therapy with or without an implantable defibrillator in advanced chronic heart failure. N Engl J Med 2004;350:2140–50.

6. McAlister FA, Ezekowitz JA, Wiebe N, et al. Systematic Review: Cardiac resynchronization in patients with symptomatic heart failure. Ann Intern Med 2004; 141:381–90.

7. Cleland JGF, Daubert JC, Erdmann E, et al. The Cardiac Resynchronization–Heart Failure (CARE-HF) Study Investigators. The effect of cardiac resynchronization on morbidity and mortality in heart failure. N Engl J Med 2005;352:1539–49.

8. Molhoek SG, Bax JJ, van Erven L, et al. Comparison of benefits from cardiac resynchronization therapy in patients with ischemic cardiomyopathy versus idiopathic dilated cardiomyopathy. Am J Cardiol 2004;93:860–3.

9. Moss AJ, Zareba W, Hall WJ, et al. Prophylactic implantation of a defibrillator in patients with myocardial infarction and reduced ejection fraction. N Engl J Med 2002;346:877–83.

10. The DAVID Trial Investigators. Dual-chamber pacing or ventricular backup pacing in patients with an implantable defibrillator. The Dual Chamber and VVI Implantable Defibrillator (DAVID) trial. JAMA 2002; 288:3115–23.

11. Baker CM, Christopher TJ, Smith PF, et al. Addition of a left ventricular lead to conventional pacing systems in patients with congestive heart failure: early results in 60 consecutive patients. Pacing Clin Electrophysiol 2002;25:1166–71.

12. Linder O, Vogt J, Kammeier A, et al. Effect of cardiac resynchronization therapy on global and regional oxygen consumption and myocardial blood flow in patients with non-ischaemic and ischaemic cardiomyopathy. Eur Heart J 2005;26:70–6.

13. St John Sutton MG, Plappert T, Abraham WT, et al, for the Multicenter InSync Randomized Clinical Evaluation (MIRACLE) Study Group. Effect of cardiac resynchronization therapy on left ventricular size and function in chronic heart failure. Circulation 2003;107:1985–90.

14. St John Sutton MG, Plappert T, Hilpisch KE, et al. Sustained reverse left ventricular structural remodeling with cardiac resynchronization at one year is a function of etiology. Quantitative Doppler echocardiographic evidence from the Multicenter InSync Randomized Clinical Evaluation (MIRACLE). Circulation 2006;113:266–72.

15. Abraham WT, Young JB, Leon AR, et al, on behalf of the Multicenter InSynch ICD II Study Group. Effects of cardiac resynchronization on disease progression in patients with left ventricular systolic dysfunction, an indication for an implantable cardioverter-defibrillator, and mildly symptomatic chronic heart failure. Circulation 2004;110:2864–8.

16. Moss AJ, Brown MW, Cannom DS, et al. Multicenter Automatic Defibrillator Implanatation Trial – Cardiac Resynchronization Therapy (MADIT CRT): design and clinical protocol. Ann Nonivasive Electrocardiol 2005: 10:34–43.

17. Linde C, Gold M, Abraham WT, Daubert JC, for the REVERSE Study Group. Rationale and design of a randomized controlled trial to assess the safety and efficacy of cardiac resynchronization therapy in patients with asymptomatic left ventricular dysfunction with previous symptoms of heart failure or mild heart failure – the REsynchronization reVErses Remodeling in Systolic vEntricular dysfunction (REVERSE) study. Am Heart J 2006;151:288–94.

18. Packer M. Proposal for a new clinical end point to evaluate the efficacy of drugs and devices in the treatment of chronic heart failure. J Card Fail 2001;7:176–82.

19. Auricchio A, Yu CM. Beyond the measurement of QRS complex toward mechanical dyssynchrony: cardiac resynchronisation therapy in heart failure patients with a normal QRS duration. Heart 2004;90:479–81.

20. Auricchio A, Stellbrink C, Butter C, et al. Clinical efficacy of cardiac resynchronization therapy using left ventricular pacing in heart failure patients stratified by severity of ventricular conduction delay. J Am Coll Cardiol 2003;42:2109–16.

21. Butter C, Auricchio A, Stellbrink C, et al. Clinical efficacy of one year cardiac resynchronization therapy in heart failure patients stratified by QRS duration: results of the PATH-CHF II trial. Eur Heart J 2003; 24:363 (abst).

22. Leclercq C, Faris O, Tunin R, et al. Systolic improvement and mechanical resynchronization does not require electrical synchrony in the dilated failing heart with left bundle-branch block. Circulation 2002;106: 1760–3.

23. Spragg DD, Leclercq C, Loghmani M, et al. Regional alterations in protein expression in the dyssynchronous failing heart. Circulation 2003;108:929–32.

24. Auricchio A, Fantoni C, Regoli F, et al. Characterization of left ventricular activation in patients with heart failure and left bundle branch block. Circulation 2004; 109:1133–9.

25. Kerwin WF, Botvinick EH, O'Connell JW, et al. Ventricular contraction abnormalities in dilated cardiomyopathy: effect of biventricular pacing to correct interventricular dyssynchrony. J Am Coll Cardiol 2000; 35:1221–7.

26. Pitzalis MV, Iacoviello M, Romito R, et al. Cardiac resynchronization therapy tailored by echocardiographic evaluation of ventricular asynchrony. J Am Coll Cardiol 2002;40:1615–22.

27. Yu CM, Chau E, Sanderson JE, et al. Tissue Doppler echocardiographic evidence of reverse remodeling and

improved synchronicity by simultaneously delaying regional contraction after biventricular pacing therapy in heart failure. Circulation 2002;105:438–45.

28. Yu CM, Fung WH, Lin H, et al. Predictors of left ventricular reverse remodeling after cardiac resynchronization therapy for heart failure secondary to idiopathic dilated or ischemic cardiomyopathy. Am J Cardiol 2003;91:684–8.

29. Bax JJ, Molhoek SG, van Erven L, et al. Usefulness of myocardial tissue doppler echocardiography to evaluate left ventricular dyssynchrony before and after biventricular pacing in patients with idiopathic dilated cardiomyopathy. Am J Cardiol 2003;91:94–7.

30. Yu CM, Lin H, Fung WH, et al. Comparison of acute changes in left ventricular volume, systolic and diastolic functions, and intraventricular synchronicity after biventricular and right ventricular pacing for heart failure. Am Heart J 2003;145:846(G1–7).

31. Sogaard P, Egeblad H, Kim WY, et al. Tissue Doppler imaging predicts improved systolic performance and reversed left ventricular remodeling during long-term cardiac resynchronization therapy. J Am Coll Cardiol 2002;40:723–30.

32. Yu CM, Yip GWK, Zhang Q, et al. Tissue Doppler imaging is superior to delay longitudinal contraction or strain rate imaging on the prediction of reverse remodeling after cardiac resynchronization therapy for heart failure. Circulation 2004;110:66–73.

33. Yu CM, Zhang Q, Lin H, et al. Will cardiac resynchronization therapy reverse left ventricular remodeling in patients with mild prolongation of QRS complexes? J Am Coll Cardiol 2003;41:136A (abst).

34. Yu CM, Lin H, Zhang Q, et al. High prevalence of left ventricular systolic and diastolic asynchrony in patients with congestive heart failure and normal QRS duration. Heart 2003;89:54–60.

35. Ghio S, Constantin C, Klersy C, et al. Interventricular and intraventricular dyssynchrony are common in heart failure patients regardless of QRS duration. Eur Heart J 2004;25:571–8.

36. Bleeker GB, Schalij MJ, Molhoek SG, et al. Frequency of left ventricular dyssynchrony in patients with heart failure and a narrow QRS complex. Am J Cardiol 2005; 95:140–2.

37. Cho GY, Song JK, Park WJ, et al. Mechanical dyssynchrony assessed by tissue doppler imaging is a powerful predictor of mortality in congestive heart failure with normal QRS duration. J Am Coll Cardiol 2005;46:2237–43.

38. Achilli A, Sassara M, Ficili S, et al. Long-term effectiveness of cardiac resynchronization therapy in patients with refractory heart failure and 'narrow' QRS. J Am Coll Cardiol 2003;42:2117–24.

39. Hunt SA, Abraham WT, Chin MH, et al. ACC/AHA 2005 Guideline Update for the Diagnosis and Management of Chronic Heart Failure in the Adult: Summary Article:

a report of the American College of Cardiology/American Heart Association Task Force on Practice Guidelines (Writing Committee to Update the 2001 Guidelines for the Evaluation and Management of Heart Failure). Circulation 2005;112:1825–52.

40. Centers for Medicare and Medicaid Services. http://www.cms.hhs.gov/MLNMattersArticles/downloads/MM3604.pdf (Accessed August 5, 2006).

41. Yu CM, Fung JWH, Chan CK, et al. Comparison of the efficacy of reverse remodeling and clinical improvement for relatively narrow and wide QRS complexes after cardiac resynchronization therapy for heart failure. J Cardiovasc Electrophysiol 2004;15:1058–65.

42. Bleeker GB, Schalij MJ, Molhoek SG, et al. Relationship between QRS duration and left ventricular dyssynchrony in patients with end-stage heart failure. J Cardiovasc Electrophysiol 2004;15:544–9.

43. Kashani A, Barold SS. Significance of QRS complex duration in patients with heart failure. J Am Coll Cardiol 2005;46:2183–92.

44. Baldasseroni S, Gentile A, Gorini M, et al. Intraventricular conduction defects in patients with congestive heart failure: left but not right bundle branch block is an independent predictor of prognosis. A report from the Italian Network on Congestive Heart Failure (IN-CHF database). Ital Heart J 2003;4:607–13.

45. Wilensky RL, Yudelman P, Cohen AI, et al. Serial electrocardiographic changes in idiopathic dilated cardiomyopathy confirmed at necropsy. Am J Cardiol 1988; 62:276–83.

46. Baldasseroni S, Opasich C, Gorini M, et al. Left bundle-branch block is associated with increased 1-year sudden and total mortality rate in 5517 outpatients with congestive heart failure: a report from the Italian Network on Congestive Heart Failure. Am Heart J 2002;143:398–405.

47. Garrigue S, Reuter S, Labeque JN, et al. Usefulness of biventricular pacing in patients with congestive heart failure and right bundle branch block. Am J Cardiol 2001;88:1436–40.

48. Lee MA, Dae MW, Langberg JJ, et al. Effects of long term right ventricular apical pacing on left ventricular perfusion, innervation, function, and histology. J Am Coll Cardiol 1994;24:225–32.

49. Horwich T, Foster E, De Marco T, Tseng Z, Saxon L. Effects of resynchronization therapy on cardiac function in pacemaker patients 'upgraded' to biventricular devices. J Cardiovasc Electrophysiol 2004;15:1284–9.

50. Bordachar P, Garrigue S, Lafitte S, et al. Interventricular and intra-left ventricular electromechanical delays in right ventricular paced patients with heart failure: implications for upgrading to biventricular stimulation. Heart 2003;89:1401–5.

51. Ermis C, Seutter R, Zhu AX, et al. Impact of upgrade to cardiac resynchronization therapy on ventricular

arrhythmia frequency in patients with implantable cardioverter–defibrillators. J Am Coll Cardiol 2005; 46:2258–63.

52. Heist EK, Ruskin JN. Atrial fibrillation and congestive heart failure: risk factors, mechanisms, and treatment. Progr Cardiovasc Dis 2006;48:256–69.

53. Carson PE, Johnson GR, Dunkman WB, et al. The influence of atrial fibrillation on prognosis in mild to moderate heart failure. The V-HeFT studies. Circulation 1993;87(Suppl VI):VI-102–110.

54. Middlekauff HR, Stevenson WG, Stevenson LW. Prognostic significance of atrial fibrillation in advanced heart failure. A study of 390 patients. Circulation 1991; 84:40–8.

55. Farwell D, Patel NR, Hall A, et al. How many people with heart failure are appropriate candidates for biventricular resynchronization? Eur Heart J 2000;21: 1246–50.

56. Ozcan C, Jahangir A, Friedman PA, et al. Long-term survival after ablation of the atrioventricular node and implantation of a permanent pacemaker in patients with atrial fibrillation. N Engl J Med 2001;344: 1043–51.

57. Hay I, Melenovsky V, Fetics BJ, et al. Short-term effects of right–left heart sequential cardiac resynchronization in patients with heart failure, chronic atrial fibrillation, and atrioventricular nodal block. Circulation 2004;110: 3404–10.

58. Simantirakis EN, Vardakis KE, Kochiadakis GE, et al. Left ventricular mechanics during right ventricular apical or left ventricular-based pacing in patients with chronic atrial fibrillation after atrioventricular junction ablation. J Am Coll Cardiol 2004;43:1013–8.

59. Brignole M, Gammage M, Puggioni E, et al, on behalf of the Optimal Pacing SITE (OPSITE) Study Investigators. Comparative assessment of right, left, and biventricular pacing in patients with permanent atrial fibrillation. Eur Heart J 2005;26:712–22.

60. Leon AR, Greenberg JM, Kanuru N, et al. Cardiac resynchronization in patients with congestive heart failure and chronic atrial fibrillation: effect of upgrading to biventricular pacing after chronic right ventricular pacing. J Am Coll Cardiol 2002;39:1258–63.

61. Valls-Bertault V, Fatemi M, Gilard M, et al. Assessment of upgrading to biventricular pacing in patients with right ventricular pacing and congestive heart failure after atrioventricular junctional ablation for chronic atrial fibrillation. Europace 2004;6:438–43.

62. Doshi RN, Daoud EG, Fellows C, et al, for the PAVE Study Group. Left ventricular-based cardiac stimulation Post AV Nodal Ablation Evaluation (the PAVE study). J Cardiovasc Electrophysiol 2005;16:1161–5.

63. Leclercq C, Walker S, Linde C, et al. on behalf of the MUSTIC Study Group. Comparative effects of permanent biventricular and right-univentricular pacing in heart failure patients with chronic atrial fibrillation. Eur Heart J 2002;23:1780–7.

64. Linde C, Leclercq C, Rex S, et al, on behalf of the MUltisite STimulation In Cardiomyopathies (MUSTIC). Long-term benefits of biventricular pacing in congestive heart failure: results from the MUltisite STimulation In Cardiomyopathy (MUSTIC) Study. J Am Coll Cardiol 2002;40:111–18.

65. Puggioni E, Brignole M, Gammage M, et al. Acute comparative effect of right and left ventricular pacing in patients with permanent atrial fibrillation. J Am Coll Cardiol 2004;43:234–38.

66. Leclercq C, Alonso C, Pavin D, et al. Comparative effects of permanent biventricular pacing for refractory heart failure in patients with stable sinus rhythm or chronic atrial fibrillation. Am J Cardiol 2000;85:1154–6.

67. Garrigue S, Bordachar P, Reuter S, et al. Comparison of permanent left ventricular and biventricular pacing in patients with heart failure and chronic atrial fibrillation: prospective haemodynamic study. Heart 2002;87:529–34.

68. Molhoek SG, Bax JJ, Bleeker GB, et al. Comparison of response to cardiac resynchronization therapy in patients with sinus rhythm versus chronic atrial fibrillation. Am J Cardiol 2004:94:1506–9.

69. Kies P, Leclercq C, Crocq C, et al. Cardiac resynchronization therapy in chronic atrial fibrillation: impact on left atrial size and reversal to sinus rhythm. Heart 2006; 92:490–4.

70. Higgins SL, Hummel JD, Niazi IK, et al. Cardiac resynchronization therapy for the treatment of heart failure in patients with intraventricular conduction delay and malignant ventricular tachyarrhytmias. J Am Coll Cardiol 2003;42:1454–9.

71. Cazeau S, Ritter P, Lazarus A, et al. Multisite pacing for end-stage heart failure: early experience. Pacing Clin Electrophysiol 1996;19:1748–57.

72. Gras D, Leclercq C, Tang AS, et al. Cardiac resynchronization therapy in advanced heart failure: the multicenter InSynch clinical study. Eur J Heart Fail 2002;4:311–20.

73. Krahn AD, Snell L, Yee R, et al. Biventricular pacing improves quality of life and exercise tolerance in patients with heart failure and intraventricular conduction delay. Can J Cardiol 2002;18:380–7.

74. Kuhlkamp V. Initial experience with an implantable cardioverter defibrillator incorporating cardiac resynchronization therapy. J Am Coll Cardiol 2002;39:790–7.

75. Leclercq C, Cazeau S, Ritter P, et al. A pilot experience with permanent biventricular pacing to treat advanced heart failure. Am Heart J 2000;40:862–70.

76. Mortensen PT, Sogaard P, Mansour H, et al. Sequential biventricular pacing: evaluation of safety and efficacy. Pacing Clin Electrophysiol 2004;27:339–45.

77. Molhoek SG, Bax JJ, van Erven L, et al. Effects of resynchronization therapy in patients with end-stage heart failure. Am J Cardiol 2002;90:379–83.

7

Structural and functional left ventricular remodeling in heart failure with cardiac resynchronization therapy

Hind Rahmouni, Ted Plappert, and Martin St John Sutton

Introduction • Clinical trials of CRT • Conclusions

INTRODUCTION

Definition and prevalence of heart failure

Congestive heart failure (CHF) is a clinical symptom complex characterized by fatigue, dyspnea, reduced exercise tolerance, lower extremity and pulmonary edema associated with abnormal handling of sodium by the kidney. There are an estimated 25–30 million patients with heart failure worldwide. Heart failure may occur at any age, but has a predilection for the elderly, occurring in 6–10% of subjects over the age of 65 years. The prevalence of CHF increases with advancing age, and as the population ages, the management of heart failure will attain epidemic proportions. Currently, CHF is the most common hospital discharge diagnosis in patients aged over 65 years, and the costs for this diagnostic-related group (DRG) in the USA alone have already exceeded $28 billion per year.

Systolic versus diastolic heart failure

Between 30% and 50% of all patients presenting with heart failure have diastolic heart failure due to increased passive myocardial stiffness with preserved left ventricular (LV) function (LV ejection fraction (LVEF) ≥50%). Diastolic heart failure was initially believed to be a relatively benign condition, but the annual mortality from diastolic heart failure ranges between 5% and 15% and the readmission rate for new-onset heart failure approaches 50% within the first 6 months.[1–4] The remaining 50–70% of patients present with systolic heart failure, and are clinically indistinguishable from patients with diastolic heart failure. It is important to identify patients with systolic heart failure, as they are eligible for additional therapeutic options such as cardiac resynchronization therapy (CRT), which has never been tested in patients with primary diastolic heart failure.

Left ventricular remodeling

Systolic heart failure results from LV remodeling, which in 68% of patients is due to myocardial infarction and coronary artery disease. LV remodeling is a dynamic process of progressive LV dilation, distortion of LV cavity shape, and disruption of the mitral valve and subvalve geometry that results in mitral regurgitation, deterioration in LV contractile function, and development of heart failure. The occurrence of mitral regurgitation often escalates the remodeling process and hastens the onset of heart failure by further increasing the already-elevated LV loading conditions. The LV remodeling process is the final common pathway for most etiologies of heart failure, and portends a poor prognosis. The traditional treatment strategies in heart failure (Figure 7.1) include reduction of LV load (vasodilators), systemic blood pressure support for organ perfusion (intravenous ionotropes), and a combination of load reduction and neuro-hormonal blockade (angiotensin-converting enzyme inhibitors (ACEIs), angiotensin-receptor blockers (ARBs), and β-receptor blockers). These treatment strategies attenuate remodeling, but have had little effect on long-term survival. The aim of new therapeutic interventions is not only to attenuate progressive LV remodeling to heart failure, but also to reverse this remodeling process. 'Reverse remodeling' is a relatively new concept in heart failure, where progressive LV dilation and deterioration in contractile function in patients are not simply arrested, but are partially reversed. CRT is a relatively new form of therapy that has proved to be efficacious in a highly selected population of patients with systolic heart failure.

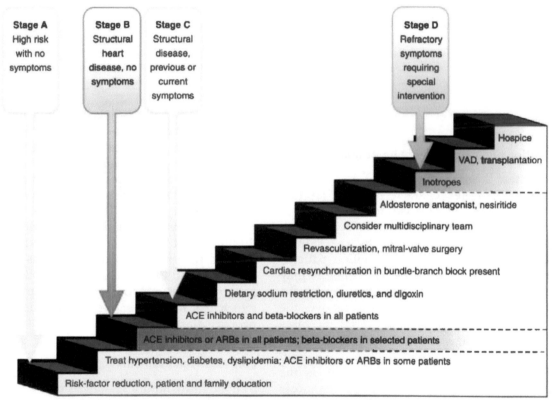

Figure 7.1 Patients with stage A heart failure are at high risk for heart failure but do not have structural heart disease or symptoms of heart failure. This group includes patients with hypertension, diabetes, coronary artery disease, previous exposure to cardiotoxic drugs, or a family history of cardiomyopathy. Patients with stage B heart failure have structural heart disease but have no symptoms of heart failure. This group includes patients with left ventricular (LV) hypertrophy, previous myocardial infarction, LV systolic dysfunction, or valvular heart disease, and all of whom would be considered to have New York Heart Association (NYHA) class I symptoms. Patients with stage C heart failure have known structural heart disease and current or previous symptoms of heart failure. Their symptoms may be classified as NYHA class I, II, III, or IV. Patients with stage D heart failure have refractory symptoms of heart failure at rest despite maximal medical therapy, are hospitalized, and require specialized interventions or hospice care. All such patients would be considered to have NYHA class IV symptoms. ACE, angiotensin-converting enzyme; ARB, angiotensin-receptor blocker; VAD, ventricular assist device. (Reproduced from Jessup M, Brozena S. Heart failure. N Engl J Med 2003;348:2007–18.)

Cardiac resynchronization therapy

CRT has become an established treatment for a population of patients with New York Heart Association (NYHA) symptom class III/IV heart failure refractory to optimal medical treatment and with evidence of LV dyssynchrony demonstrated by prolongation of the QRS duration >130 ms. The prevalence of electrocardiographic QRS duration (>130 ms) is reported to be between 33% and 50% of all patients with systolic heart failure, which is significantly higher than the estimated 1.5% prevalence in the general population.[5,6] The longer the QRS duration, the higher the mortality, independent of all other patient demographics. In the normal heart, the short QRS duration (<100 ms) reflects the rapid velocity of electrical activation of the ventricles from the atrioventricular (AV) node. Electrical impulse propagation in the normal heart occurs via the specialized conducting tissue of the His–Purkinje network. By contrast, in left bundle branch block (LBBB), QRS prolongation is mostly due to slow cell-to-cell conduction from the right ventricle (RV) that has a tenfold slower conduction velocity than the Purkinje system and therefore delays initiation of LV depolarization and contraction. LBBB results in abnormal septal motion (Figure 7.2) and also regional differences in the timing of onset and peak systolic myocardial contraction velocity. Recently, Doppler tissue imaging and tissue tracking techniques have been shown to be superior to QRS prolongation as a means of identifying non-uniformity of contraction and used as a surrogate for LV dyssynchrony.

Aims of CRT in advanced heart failure

The aims of CRT in heart failure patients are both acute and chronic. Acute aims are to optimize AV timing, prolong LV filling, and coordinate RV and LV contraction by minimizing inter- and intraventricular mechanical delay and facilitating ventricular interaction. The long-term goals are for the acute changes described above to translate into structural and functional reverse remodeling, alleviation of symptoms, and improved survival. A consistent finding in both small uncontrolled open-label studies and the eight large randomized clinical trials of CRT[7-14] (Table 7.1) has been the improvement in exercise capacity, NYHA symptom class, and quality of life in the majority (65–75%) of patients with systolic heart failure. These beneficial effects of CRT were achieved in patients already receiving optimal medical therapy with ACEIs or ARBs, β-receptor blocking agents, and diuretics. Only two of the eight large randomized CRT trials, COMPANION[11] ($n = 1520$) and CARE-HF[12] ($n = 814$), were statistically powered to assess all-cause mortality, and only five of the eight studies[8-10,12,14] had measurements of LV size and/or LVEF as secondary endpoints that

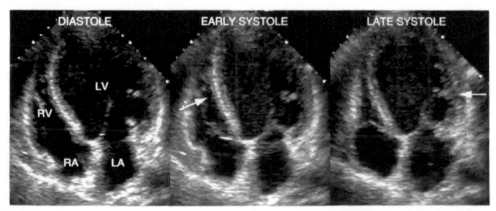

Figure 7.2 Transthoracic apical four-chamber view of a patient with dilated cardiomyopathy at end-diastole (right), early systole (central), and late systole (left), showing paradoxical ventricular septal wall contraction (central panel arrow) and late inward motion of the lateral wall (right panel arrow). LV, left ventricle; RV, right ventricle; RA, right atrium; LA, left atrium.

Table 7.1 CRT in randomized clinical trials

Trial	Design	No. of patients	Endpoints Primary	Endpoints Secondary	Results summary

PATH-CHF[7]	Crossover	41	6MWT
			Peak VO$_2$
				NYHA functional class
				QOL
				Hospitalizations
					Improvement in:
					  6MWT
					  NYHA functional class
					  QOL
					Less hospitalizations

MUSTIC-SR[8]	Crossover	58	6MWT	NYHA functional class
				QOL
				Peak VO$_2$
				LV volumes
				MR
				Hospitalizations
				Total mortality
					Improvement in:
					  6MWT
					  NYHA functional class
					  QOL
					  Peak VO$_2$
					  LV volumes
					  MR
					Less hospitalizations

MIRACLE[9]	Parallel arms	453	6MWT
			NYHA functional class
			QOL
				Peak VO$_2$
				LVEF
				LVEDD
				MR
				Clinical composite response
					Improvement in:
					  6MWT
					  NYHA functional class
					  QOL
					  LVEF
					  LVEDD
					  MR

MIRACLE ICD[10]	Parallel arms	555	6MWT
			NYHA functional class
			QOL
				Peak VO$_2$
				LVEF
				LV volumes
				MR
				Clinical composite response
					Improvement in:
					  NYHA functional class
					  QOL

COMPANION[11]	Parallel arms	1520	All-cause mortality or hospitalization	All-cause mortality and cardiac morbidity	Reduced all-cause mortality/ hospitalization

CARE-HF[12]	Open label, randomized	814	All-cause mortality	NYHA functional class
				QOL
				LVEF
				LVESV
				Hospitalization for heart failure
					Reduced mortality/ morbidity
					Improvement in:
					  NYHA functional class
					  QOL
					  LVEF
					  LVESV

PATH-CHF II[13]	Crossover (no pacing vs LV pacing)	86	6MWT
			Peak VO$_2$
				NYHA functional class
				QOL
					Improvement in:
					  6MWT
					  QOL
					  Peak VO$_2$

CONTAK CD[14]	Crossover, parallel controlled	490	6MWT
			NYHA functional class
			QOL
				LVEF
				LV volumes
				Composite of mortality, hospitalizations, VT/VF
					Improvement in:
					  6MWT
					  NYHA functional class
					  QOL
					  LVEF
					  LV volumes

CARE-HF, Cardiac Resynchronization – Heart Failure; CONTAK CD, CONTAK – Cardiac Defibrillator; COMPANION, Comparison of Medical Therapy, Pacing and Defibrillation in Heart Failure; CRT, cardiac resynchronization therapy; LV, left ventricular; LVEDD, LV end-diastolic dimension; LVEF, LV ejection fraction; LVESV, LV end-systolic volume; MIRACLE, Multicenter InSync Randomized Clinical Evaluation; MIRACLE ICD, MIRACLE Implantable Cardioverter Defibrillator; MR, mitral regurgitation; MUSTIC, Multisite Simulation in Cardiomyopathics; NYHA, New York Heart Association; PATH-CHF, Pacing Therapies in Congestive Heart Failure; QOL, quality-of-life score; VF, ventricular fibrillation; VO$_2$, volume of oxygen; VT, ventricular tachycardia; 6MWT, 6-minute walk test.

allowed quantification of structural and functional remodeling associated with CRT. In addition, serial changes in echocardiographic LV dimensions and volumes, LVEF, and severity of mitral regurgitation enabled examination of the relations between changes in LV volumes and exercise capacity and between structural changes (LV volumes and/or LVEF) and changes in quality of life and NYHA symptom class during remodeling.

The purpose of this chapter is to describe the structural and functional LV remodeling induced by CRT, determine whether the salutary effects on symptoms and remodeling are continued beyond 6 months, identify predictors of response to CRT (described in detail in Chapter 18), and mention briefly the subgroup of patients who fail to respond to CRT.

CLINICAL TRIALS OF CRT

In five randomized CRT trials involving approximately 4000 patients, echocardiographic images of the LV were obtained as part of the study protocol. This echocardiographic data has enabled exploration of the potential mechanisms of reverse remodeling with CRT, and the relationships between changes in LV architecture and function and improvement in symptoms. Enrollment criteria were concordant across most of the randomized trials and included severe

symptomatic systolic heart failure in NYHA symptom class III/IV, LV systolic dysfunction, LVEF ≤35%, and prolonged QRS duration ≥120/130 ms. Before randomization, patients were on stable optimal heart failure therapy for a minimum of 4 weeks for ACEIs or ARBs, and for a minimum of 3 months for β-adrenergic receptor blockade. The COMPANION[11] and CARE-HF[12] studies, which enrolled 1520 and 814 heart failure patients, respectively, demonstrated improvements in the combined endpoint of all-cause mortality and hospitalization (COMPANION) and the combined endpoint of reduced mortality and morbidity (CARE-HF). Clinical follow-up ranged from 1 month to 29 months, with a mean follow-up period of 3–6 months.

In these selected patients with heart failure, CRT results in significant reduction in LV size assessed either as linear M-mode echocardiographic measurements of cavity dimensions (Figure 7.3) or LV volume computations by transthoracic echocardiography (TTE) and modified Simpson's method of disks as recommended by the American Society of Echocardiography.[15] Changes in LV volumes occur early after initiation of CRT, and become statistically significant at 1 week compared with control patients.[16] There is further progressive reduction in end-diastolic and end-systolic LV diameters and LV volumes at 3 and 6 months compared with their baseline

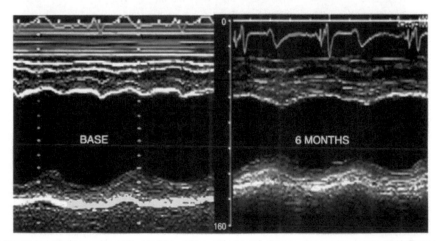

Figure 7.3 M-mode echocardiogram at baseline (left) and 6 months (right) after cardiac resynchronization therapy. Note the reduction in LV diameters and the synchronous contraction of the septal and posterior walls at 6 months compared with baseline.

values (Figures 7.4 and 7.5) in the majority of patients (65–75%), or compared with the control group who had the CRT device placed but with biventricular pacing turned off. In the control group, LV volumes either remained unchanged or increased. Concomitant with the reduction in LV cavity size/volume, LV mass decreased progressively with CRT at 3 and 6 months, but at a slower rate than the decrease in LV volumes. LV cavity shape assessed as a sphericity index changed from a globular to a more normal ellipsoidal configuration in the treatment group, while LV volumes, LV mass, and cavity shape did not improve in the control group over time.[17]

The changes in LV size and LV cavity shape with CRT were associated with an increase in ejection fraction at 3 months, with further incremental improvement at 6 months. Cardiac index increased with CRT at 6 months, but declined significantly in the control group over the same time period. This structural and functional reverse LV remodeling with CRT occurred independently of the use of β-adrenergic receptor blockers. Evidence for this observation is provided by the finding that there were no changes in LV volumes or ejection fraction in the control group compared with patients in the control group who were not on β-adrenergic receptor blockers.

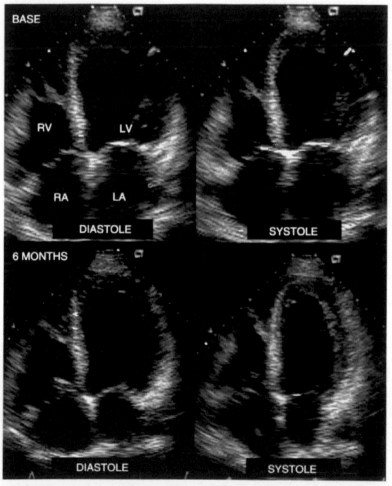

Figure 7.4 Transthoracic apical four-chamber view at baseline (top) and after cardiac resynchronization therapy (bottom). At 6 months, the end-diastolic and end-systolic volumes are reduced compared with baseline, and the left ventricle has a more elliptical shape, reflecting the reverse remodeling. LV, left ventricle; RV, right ventricle; RA, right atrium; LA, left atrium.

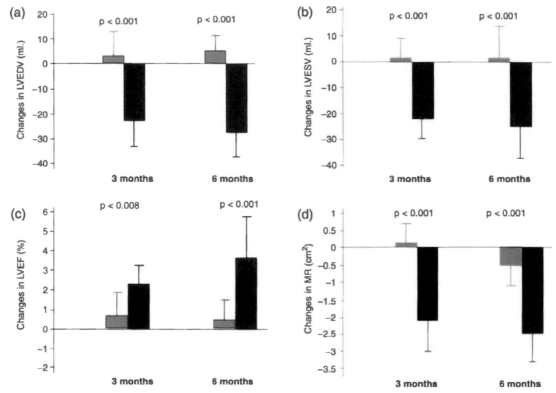

Figure 7.5 Median change (with 95% confidence intervals) in LVEDV (a), LVESV (b), LVEF (c), and MR (d) at 3 and 6 months after randomization in the control group (gray) and the CRT group (black). LVEDV, left ventricular end-diastolic volume; LVESV, left ventricular end-systolic volume; LVEF, left ventricular ejection fraction; MR, mitral regurgitation. (Reproduced with permission from St John Sutton MG, Plappert T, Abraham WT, et al. Multicenter InSync Randomized Clinical Evaluation (MIRACLE) Study Group. Effect of cardiac resynchronization therapy on left ventricular size and function in chronic heart failure. Circulation 2003;107:1985–90.[17])

By contrast, patients taking β-adrenergic receptor blockers on CRT exhibited a highly significant degree of reverse remodeling, indicating that CRT and β-blocker therapy are complementary.[17]

Mitral regurgitation and CRT

The severity of mitral regurgitation decreased with CRT by 3 months, and this change was sustained at 6 months (Figure 7.6). Two different potential mechanisms can be invoked for the decrease in mitral regurgitation induced by CRT. The first is that the coordination of the timing of contraction of the two papillary muscles allows synchronization of the initiation and completion of LV contraction[18] (Figure 6.7). The second is due to the structural and functional reverse remodeling that reduces the

diameter of the LV short axis, restores the mitral annular area and subvalve geometry to near normal, and approximates the papillary muscles that facilitate appropriate coaptation of the anterior and posterior mitral valve leaflets (Figure 7.8). Reduction in volumes with CRT was on a different temporal schedule from the regression of LV hypertrophy.

Effects of CRT on LV diastolic function

Hitherto, no CRT trials have been conducted on primary diastolic LV heart failure, but several studies have reported changes in diastolic function with CRT in patients with systolic heart failure. Optimization of AV timing with synchronized biventricular pacing resulted in prolonged LV diastolic filling time, separation of

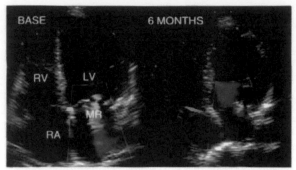

Figure 7.6 Color Doppler transthoracic apical four-chamber views: (a) before CRT, demonstrating regurgitant flow in the left atrium during systole, indicating severe mitral regurgitation; (b) 6 months after CRT, with a significant reduction in severity of mitral regurgitation.

the passive filling phase (E wave) from atriosystolic contraction (A wave) and activation of ventricular contraction at the end of atrial systolic contraction. Isovolumic relaxation time and peak velocities during E wave, A wave, and

E/A wave changed after CRT. However, the deceleration time of the E wave shortened at 3 and 6 months and the interventricular mechanical delay (IVMD) decreased significantly by 6 months compared with the controls, in whom none of these changes occurred. The myocardial performance index (MPI), also known as the Tei index,[19] represents combined diastolic and systolic myocardial function, and is calculated as the sum of the isovolumic relaxation time and isovolumic contraction time (ICT) divided by the ejection time (LVET):

$$\text{Tei index} = \frac{\text{IVRT} + \text{ICT}}{\text{LVET}}$$

This index improved with CRT at 6 months – largely due to shortening of the ICT.

Linear regression analysis of the combined populations of MIRACLE and MIRACLE ICD showed that two diastolic parameters – higher E/A velocity ratios and shorter E-wave deceleration

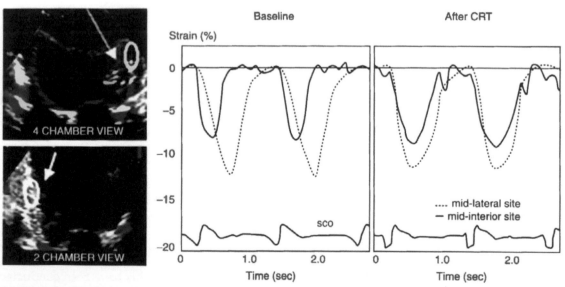

Figure 7.7 Echocardiographic strain images from the four- and two-chamber views, with corresponding time–strain plots from sites adjacent to papillary muscles before and after cardiac resynchronization therapy. Baseline plots demonstrate late peak strain occurring in the anterolateral papillary muscle site compared with the posteromedial papillary muscle site. Peak strain is aligned after cardiac resynchronization therapy in these sites. (From Kanzaki H, Bazaz R, Schwartzman D, et al. A mechanism for immediate reduction in mitral regurgitation after cardiac resynchronization therapy: insights from mechanical activation strain mapping. J Am Coll Cardiol 2004;44:1619–25.[18])

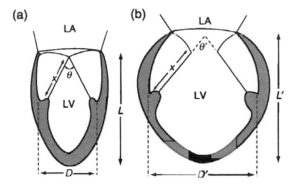

Figure 7.8 Schematic demonstrating the possible mechanism of mitral regurgitation. Left ventricular dilation due to volume overload (a) results in the left ventricle (LV) becoming more spherical compared to a normal heart (b): (a)→(b). There is an increase in the mitral valve ring circumference and the left ventricular diameter (D→D') and length (L→L'). The angle θ subtended by the papillary muscles to the mitral annulus increases (θ→θ'), but there is no elongation of the mitral valve leaflets or chordae (x→x), which results in incomplete cusp coaptation and mitral regurgitation. LA, left atrium.

time – correlated with the change in LV end-diastolic volume over time and that these factors predict LV remodeling.[20]

Need for continued CRT and reverse LV remodeling

In a novel open-label observational study of 25 patients with NYHA class III/IV heart failure and QRS duration $\geq$130 ms, the need for continuous CRT was clearly demonstrated.[16] CRT induced reductions in LV volume and severity of mitral regurgitation and an increase in LVEF over a 3-month period. After providing the above evidence for reverse LV remodeling with CRT, cessation of CRT resulted in recurrent LV dilation, acute deterioration in LVEF, and return of the severe mitral regurgitation present at baseline (Figure 7.9). Deterioration in clinical status has also been reported in individual patients who have been shown to have lost

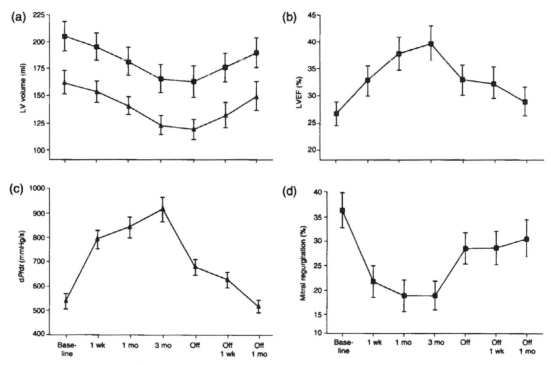

Figure 7.9 Changes in left ventricular end-diastolic (squares) and end-systolic (triangles) volumes (a), ejection fraction (b), dP/dT (c), and mitral regurgitation (d) before and after biventricular pacing, as well as when pacing was suspended for 1 month. (Reproduced with permission from Yu CM, Chau E, Sanderson JE, et al. Tissue Doppler echocardiographic evidence of reverse remodeling and improved synchronicity by simultaneously delaying regional contraction after biventricular pacing therapy in heart failure. Circulation 2002;105:438–45.[16])

the stimulus for reverse LV remodeling because of dislodgement or fracture of the coronary sinus LV electrode or a similar occurrence with the RV electrode and termination of synchronized biventricular pacing.

Durability of effect of CRT on LV remodeling

Heart failure has an inexorably progressive downhill course. The combination of ACEIs, ARBs, aldosterone antagonists, diuretics, and digoxin may attenuate and even slow the rate of the remodeling to end-stage LV dysfunction and demise, but with notable exceptions they do not reverse the remodeling process. CRT is unequivocally associated with reverse LV remodeling, but at present, CRT has only proven efficacy in patients with NYHA class III/IV, prolonged QRS duration, and systolic dysfunction, who comprise only one-third to one-half of the 50–70% of the patients overall presenting with systolic heart failure.

In addition to the relatively small target population (10–15% of the total number of heart failure patients), CRT appears to induce reverse LV remodeling consistently in only 65–75% of the selected patients (Figure 7.10). In current times of fiscal responsibility, the costs for the device and device placement, and a track record of 65–75% success rate for CRT, have to be offset

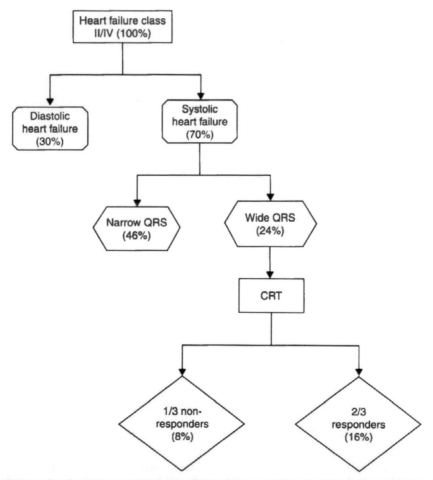

Figure 7.10 Flow diagram showing the target population of heart failure patients who benefit from CRT. Note that patients with heart failure class III/IV already represent only 30% of the whole population of heart failure patients.

by the combination of minimal device-related complications and continued subjective and objective effects at long-term follow-up.

Clinical information and serial echocardiographic data from MIRACLE, MUSTIC, and CARE-HF have shown that the symptomatic benefits in terms of NYHA class, exercise capacity (usually the 6-minute hall walk), and quality of life are sustained for at least 12–24 months, independently of the various etiologies of heart failure. The MIRACLE trial (Figure 7.11) provided an opportunity to quantify the magnitude and frequency of reverse remodeling – specifically LV volumes and LVEF – in more than 200 patients who were initially randomized to the active CRT arm and followed for a minimum of 1 year of continuous CRT.

LV end-diastolic volume (EDV) and end-systolic volume (ESV) were both decreased compared with baseline values at 12 months. However, the mean difference for both EDV and ESV between baseline and 6 months and between baseline and 12 months were greater at 6 months – which is consistent with a trend for LV volumes to return to baseline by 12 months. Furthermore, the proportions of patients who experienced a decrease in LVEDV and LVESV at 6 months were 71% and 74%; and at 12 months, they were 58% and 60%. LVEF, by contrast, increased progressively from a mean of 24% at baseline to 29% at 6 months and to 31% at 12 months.

Examination of the baseline demographics that correlated with structural remodeling (change in LVEDV) at 6 months were age ≥65 years, or more, female sex, QRS duration ≥170 ms and LVEF ≤ 25%, whereas at 12 months the only correlations were QRS duration ≥170 ms and LVEF ≤ 25%.[21] It is not clear from any other large randomized CRT trials whether this apparent trend for loss of efficacy is real or the result of different heart failure etiologies.

Impact of etiology of CHF on reverse remodeling with CRT

All eight large randomized CRT trials included heart failure patients with diverse etiologies, but the major representations were ischemic cardiomyopathy and idiopathic dilated cardiomyopathies. A number of small studies have indicated that reverse LV structural and functional remodeling differ according to etiology of heart failure in both magnitude and longevity, although in the more than 1000 patients in the MIRACLE program, NYHA symptom class, quality of life using the Minnesota Living with Heart Failure questionnaire, and 6-minute hall

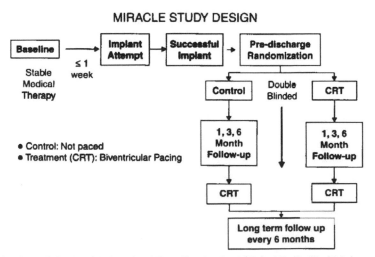

Figure 7.11 Study design of the MIRACLE (Multicenter InSync Randomized Clinical Evaluation) trial.

walk did not differ between patients with ischemic versus non-ischemic etiologies for heart failure at 6, 12, 18, and 24 months.[22]

Most heart failure trials in concordance with optimal clinical practice guidelines do not require every heart failure patient to undergo coronary arteriography to assign an ischemic versus a non-ischemic etiology. The diagnostic assignment to ischemic dilated cardiomyopathy is made by the referring physician on the basis of a clinical history of chest pain, prior myocardial infarction, or evidence of coronary artery disease by electrocardiography, echocardiography, or radionuclide myocardial perfusion scan, and is often (but not always) corroborated by cardiac catheterization. Therefore, there is potential for imprecision or misclassification and subsequent incorrect diagnostic assignment.

Reverse LV remodeling and increase in LVEF occurred in patients with heart failure of ischemic and non-ischemic etiologies.[23] The magnitude of

the reduction in LV end-diastolic volume and the increase in LVEF after 6 months of CRT was significantly greater (twofold) in the non-ischemics compared with the ischemics (Figure 7.12) – concordant with a prior observation.[24,25] These discrepancies between ischemics and non-ischemics in reverse remodeling profiles could not be ascribed either to differences in baseline demographics between the two etiologies or to the disparate use of β-adrenergic receptor blocking agents. Examination of changes in LV volumes between 6 and 12 months of continuous CRT showed that CRT had a persistent and consistently different effect on reverse remodeling in ischemic heart failure as compared with non-ischemic heart failure. When the time-dependent changes in LV volumes were assessed by cause of heart failure at 6 and 12 months using a random-effects statistical model adjusted for age, sex, and baseline heart rate, QRS duration, ejection fraction, and LV volumes because of

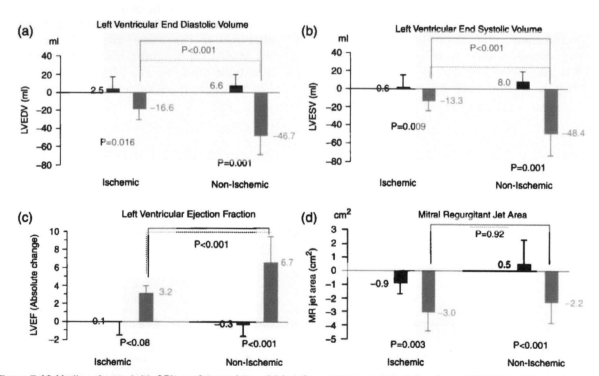

Figure 7.12 Median change (with 95% confidence intervals) in left ventricular end-diastolic volume (LVEDV) (a), left ventricular end-systolic volume (LVESV) (b), left ventricular ejection fraction (LVEF) (c), and mitral regurgitation (MR) jet area (d) at baseline and 6 months after biventricular pacing in the control group (circles) and the CRT group (diamonds) in ischemic versus non-ischemic patients.

differences between ischemic and non-ischemic patients. The difference in changes in LV end-diastolic volume by etiology of heart failure remained significant.[21] In the ischemic heart failure patients, the beneficial reduction in LV volumes achieved at 6 months had almost completely regressed by 12 months. In contrast, the reduction in LV volumes in the non-ischemic heart failure patients at 6 months was more than threefold greater than in the ischemic patients, and this difference was sustained at 12 months.

The late recurrence of LV dilatation in ischemic heart failure with CRT beyond 6 months may relate to the deterioration in LV function due to repetitive episodes of ischemia and the inexorable progressive loss of viable myocardium that typifies ischemic cardiomyopathy, rather than a loss of efficacy of cardiac resynchronization therapy. The determination of predictors of response to CRT before device implantation is the subject of intense investigation, as is a plausible explanation for the differential effect of CRT in ischemic versus non-ischemic causes of heart failure.

CONCLUSIONS

CRT is an important advance in the treatment of a selected population of advanced heart failure patients (NYHA class III/IV) whose 1-year mortality rate is 15–30%. CRT not only improves ventricular efficiency, but also reverses the process of geometrical and functional remodeling. CRT, in reducing LV size, interrupts the vicious cycle fueled by chronically increased wall stress that leads to progressive deterioration of LV function. The observed differences in response to CRT therapy between ischemic and nonischemic patients still need to be clarified. Future studies will hopefully identify predictors of a positive response to CRT before device implantation.

REFERENCES

1. Vasan RS, Larson MG, Benjamin EJ, et al. Congestive heart failure in subjects with normal versus reduced left ventricular ejection fraction: prevalence and mortality in a population-based cohort. J Am Coll Cardiol 1999; 33:1948–55.

2. Chen HH, Lainchbury JG, Senni M, Bailey KR, Redfield MM. Diastolic heart failure in the community: clinical profile, natural history, therapy, and impact of proposed diagnostic criteria. J Card Fail 2002;8:279–87.

3. Redfield MM, Jacobsen SJ, Burnett JC Jr, et al. Burden of systolic and diastolic ventricular dysfunction in the community: appreciating the scope of the heart failure epidemic. JAMA 2003;289:194–202.

4. Dauterman KW, Go AS, Rowell R, et al. Congestive heart failure with preserved systolic function in a statewide sample of community hospitals. J Card Fail 2001;7:221–228.

5. Baldasseroni S, Opasich C, Gorini M, et al. Italian Network on Congestive Heart Failure Investigators. Left bundle-branch block is associated with increased 1-year sudden and total mortality rate in 5517 outpatients with congestive heart failure: a report from the Italian Network on Congestive Heart Failure. Am Heart J 2002;143:398–405.

6. Eriksson P, Hansson PO, Eriksson H, Dellborg M. Bundle-branch block in a general male population: the study of men born 1913. Circulation 1998;98:2494–500.

7. Auricchio A, Stellbrink C, Sack S, et al. Pacing Therapies in Congestive Heart Failure (PATH-CHF) Study Group. Long-term clinical effect of hemodynamically optimized cardiac resynchronization therapy in patients with heart failure and ventricular conduction delay. J Am Coll Cardiol 2002;39:2026–33.

8. Cazeau S, Leclercq C, Lavergne T, et al. Multisite Stimulation in Cardiomyopathies (MUSTIC) Study Investigators. Effects of multisite biventricular pacing in patients with heart failure and intraventricular conduction delay. N Engl J Med 2001;344:873–80.

9. Abraham WT, Fisher WG, Smith AL, et al. MIRACLE Study Group. Multicenter InSync Randomized Clinical Evaluation. Cardiac resynchronization in chronic heart failure. N Engl J Med 2002;346:1845–53.

10. Young JB, Abraham WT, Smith AL, et al. Multicenter InSync ICD Randomized Clinical Evaluation (MIRACLE ICD) Trial Investigators. Combined cardiac resynchronization and implantable cardioversion defibrillation in advanced chronic heart failure: the MIRACLE ICD trial. JAMA 2003;289:2685–94.

11. Bristow MR, Saxon LA, Boehmer J, et al. Comparison of Medical Therapy, Pacing, and Defibrillation in Heart Failure (COMPANION) Investigators. Cardiac-resynchronization therapy with or without an implantable defibrillator in advanced chronic heart failure. N Engl J Med 2004;350:2140–50.

12. Cleland JG, Daubert JC, Erdmann E, et al. Cardiac Resynchronization-Heart Failure (CARE-HF) Study Investigators. The effect of cardiac resynchronization on morbidity and mortality in heart failure. N Engl J Med 2005;352:1539–49.

13. Auricchio A, Stellbrink C, Butter C, et al. Pacing Therapies in Congestive Heart Failure II Study Group, Guidant Heart Failure Research Group. Clinical efficacy of cardiac resynchronization therapy using left ventricular pacing in heart failure patients stratified by severity of ventricular conduction delay. J Am Coll Cardiol 2003;42:2109–16.

14. Lozano I, Bocchiardo M, Achtelik M, et al. VENTAK CHF/CONTAK CD Investigators Study Group. Impact of biventricular pacing on mortality in a randomized crossover study of patients with heart failure and ventricular arrhythmias. Pacing Clin Electrophysiol 2000;23:1711–12.

15. Lang RM, Bierig M, Devereux RB, et al. Chamber Quantification Writing Group, American Society of Echocardiography's Guidelines and Standards Committee, European Association of Echocardiography. Recommendations for chamber quantification: a report from the American Society of Echocardiography's Guidelines and Standards Committee and the Chamber Quantification Writing Group, developed in conjunction with the European Association of Echocardiography, a branch of the European Society of Cardiology. J Am Soc Echocardiogr 2005;18:1440–63.

16. Yu CM, Chau E, Sanderson JE, et al. Tissue Doppler echocardiographic evidence of reverse remodeling and improved synchronicity by simultaneously delaying regional contraction after biventricular pacing therapy in heart failure. Circulation 2002;105:438–45.

17. St John Sutton MG, Plappert T, Abraham WT, et al. Multicenter InSync Randomized Clinical Evaluation (MIRACLE) Study Group. Effect of cardiac resynchronization therapy on left ventricular size and function in chronic heart failure. Circulation 2003;107: 1985–90.

18. Kanzaki H, Bazaz R, Schwartzman D, et al. A mechanism for immediate reduction in mitral regurgitation after cardiac resynchronization therapy: insights from mechanical activation strain mapping. J Am Coll Cardiol 2004;44:1619–25.

19. Tei C, Ling LH, Hodge DO, et al. New index of combined systolic and diastolic myocardial performance: a simple and reproducible measure of cardiac function – a study in normals and dilated cardiomyopathy. J Cardiol 1995;26:357–66.

20. Cappola TP, Harsch MR, Jessup M, et al. Predictors of remodeling in the CRT era: influence of mitral regurgitation, BNP, and gender. J Card Fail 2006;12:182–8.

21. Sutton MG, Plappert T, Hilpisch KE, et al. Sustained reverse left ventricular structural remodeling with cardiac resynchronization at one year is a function of etiology: quantitative Doppler echocardiographic evidence from the Multicenter InSync Randomized Clinical Evaluation (MIRACLE). Circulation 2006;113:266–72.

22. Abraham WT, Leon AR, Young JB. Benefits of cardiac resynchronization therapy sustained for 18 months: results from the MIRACLE program. Circulation 2003; 108(Suppl IV): IV-629 (abst).

23. St John Sutton M, Lee D, Rouleau JL, et al. Left ventricular remodeling and ventricular arrhythmias after myocardial infarction. Circulation 2003;107:2577–82.

24. The RESOLVD Investigators. Effects of metoprolol CR in patients with ischemic and dilated cardiomyopathy: the Randomized Evaluation of Strategies for Left Ventricular Dysfunction Pilot Study. Circulation 2000;101:378–84.

25. Molhoek SG, Bax JJ, van Erven L, et al. Comparison of benefits from cardiac resynchronization therapy in patients with ischemic cardiomyopathy versus idiopathic dilated cardiomyopathy. Am J Cardiol 2004;93:860–3.

8

Selecting appropriate patients for cardiac resynchronization therapy: What can we learn from clinical trial evidence?

Philip B Adamson

Introduction • Definition of clinical response to CRT • Prospective randomized clinical trials • Patient selection: application to clinical practice • Summary

INTRODUCTION

Cardiac resynchronization therapy (CRT) can be achieved using biventricular pacing systems in patients with symptomatic chronic heart failure who have a comorbidity of intraventricular conduction delay (IVCD) and QRS duration >120 ms. Current evidence suggests that approximately 70% of patients with IVCD who experience persistent New York Heart Association (NYHA) class III or IV heart failure symptoms despite maximal benefits of medical therapy, including diuretics, angiotensin intervention, and beta-blockade, have measurable improvement in their heart failure syndromes with the addition of CRT to their complex medication and device options.[1-5] In a very short period of time, over 4000 patients have enrolled in randomized controlled trials to evaluate this intervention, leading to consensus agreement that CRT is a standard of care for appropriate patients.[6] This rapid accumulation of data creates challenges to integrate principles from prospective trials into daily clinical practice. The intention of this chapter is to highlight commonalities of patient selection criteria for clinical trials with the expressed goal of using the currently accepted indications for CRT therapy to identify patients more likely to respond to this invasive therapy option.

DEFINITION OF CLINICAL RESPONSE TO CRT

It is difficult to consistently define what represents a clinical response to CRT. Additionally, no other therapy in heart failure has had such attention paid to 'responder' rates, which may be due to the fact that the initial major clinical trials with CRT only assessed quality of life, 6-minute hall walk distance (6MWD), or NYHA functional classification, which led the US Food and Drug Administration (FDA) to grant regulatory approval for CRT with an indication only to reduce heart failure symptoms. The CARE-HF (Cardiac Resynchronization in Heart Failure) trial, then, was very important because it examined the effects of CRT, without an implantable cardioverter–defibrillator, on mortality – not just heart failure morbidity.[4] The 37% reduction in overall mortality observed in patients randomized to CRT in the CARE-HF trial changed the primary impact and indication of the therapy. However, it is still important to ensure that application of this therapy conforms to the inclusion and exclusion criteria of major clinical trials, which form the basis for consensus recommendations. Future clinical trial evidence will undoubtedly lead to revised patient selection criteria, but the intent of this chapter is to outline what currently describes patient populations most likely to benefit from CRT.

Seventy percent of patients enrolled in the MIRACLE (Multicenter InSync Randomized Clinical Evaluation) trial improved at least one NYHA symptom classification at 6 months,[2] but evidence from the MUSTIC (Multisite Stimulation in Cardiomyopathy) follow-up trial[7,8] and CARE-HF suggested that many patients continue to show clinical improvement even after 18 months of continued therapy. Since the long-term follow-up portion of the MUSTIC trial was uncontrolled, it is difficult to determine how much the CRT intervention was actually responsible for the continued clinical improvement, but the CARE-HF trial averaged 29 months of follow-up and confirmed a sustained effect of CRT on heart failure symptoms and reversal of adverse remodeling.[4] These data raise the important question of how long one must wait before labeling the patient a 'nonresponder'. It appears that some patients take longer than 6 months before having measurable changes in their heart failure symptoms. Therefore, patient and provider expectations about response to CRT should reflect the experience of randomized clinical trials and provide enough time for the intervention to impact heart failure symptoms.

Examining the long-term impact of CRT on heart failure symptoms reveals that only 24% of patients receiving CRT still had NYHA class III or IV symptoms after 18 months of continuous therapy in the CARE-HF trial, compared with 50% of those in the medication only arm of the trial.[4] On the other hand, findings from CARE-HF reiterated the important point that medical therapy offered to patients with heart failure is effective in reducing heart failure symptoms. In that trial, 50% of patients treated with medications alone improved to less severe symptom classes, and many would no longer qualify for device therapy after prolonged exposure to appropriate neurohormonal intervention. These findings justify the need to provide maximal medical therapy prior to referral for device implantation in order to increase the likelihood of an acceptable clinical outcome.

The magnitude of response to CRT in the CARE-HF trial, however, was profound, with 1 death and 3 hospitalizations prevented in the population studied for every 9 CRT implants. In contrast, 1 life was saved for about every 11 ICD implants in SCD-HeFT (Sudden Cardiac Death in Heart Failure Trial), with no reported impact on hospitalizations or quality of life.[9] This magnitude of effect suggests that the results of CARE-HF should de-emphasize the attention given to 'response rate'.

Other considerations in determining 'clinical response'

Heart failure syndromes have traditionally been considered to consist of progressive worsening of symptoms and pump function, so should those patients who remain the same NYHA class be considered responders? Indeed, many would consider prevention of clinical deterioration 'success' when considering heart failure populations. If prevention of deterioration is a positive 'response', then the overall response to CRT may be much higher than 70%. In the MIRACLE trial, the clinical composite was used as a secondary endpoint, and according to this marker only 16% of patients worsened.[2] With the clinical composite and considering patients who do not worsen over time as a successful intervention, CRT symptom response rates may be as high as 84%. If response is defined only as an improvement in NYHA symptom classification, however, then less than two-thirds of patients improved.[10] Therefore, improved predictors of response are needed, and a thoughtful definition of response is warranted to match outcomes with expectations.

Other surrogate endpoints, such as reversal of adverse myocardial remodeling, are also cited as evidence of a 'response' to heart failure therapies such as neurohormonal intervention or CRT.[11] For example, small studies of patients receiving CRT demonstrated that those with significant intraventricular mechanical delay measured by M-mode echocardiography prior to CRT device implantation were more likely to have a reduced left ventricular (LV) end-diastolic diameter at 3 months of follow-up.[12] This method was incorporated in the CARE-HF trial for inclusion of patients with QRS duration between 120 and 150 ms.[4] Those patients with QRS duration in this range, but without echocardiographic evidence of mechanical dyssynchrony, were excluded from the trial. No results are available comparing the response to CRT in the patients with echocardiographic evidence for intraventricular mechanical delay and QRS < 150 ms with the response in those with QRS > 150 ms. Tissue Doppler echocardiographic and other imaging modalities demonstrate improvement in LV and remodeling over time with CRT,[13–16] but prospective evaluation of these modalities as predictors of response is not yet available. Certainly data from small imaging studies are promising and suggest that QRS duration may not be the best means to identify potential intraventricular dyssynchrony,[17–21] but until prospective trial evidence using imaging as the basis for CRT prescription is available, traditional CRT indications should be used to apply therapy in a clinical setting. Additionally, evidence suggests that many patients with IVCD do not have corresponding mechanical dyssynchrony and some patients with normal QRS duration have significant mechanical dyssynchrony.[22,23] Future application of CRT will undoubtedly include inclusion criteria that are not solely based on electrocardiographic criteria, but results of randomized trials are not yet available.

Controversy about 'response' rates in patients receiving CRT led to concerns about selection criteria and raised many very important questions. Is improvement in NYHA classification the only outcome that should be considered a 'response' to CRT? Should CRT be offered to patients with less symptomatic heart failure, especially now that it is clear that the intervention decreases mortality? Should selection criteria change to reflect imaging evidence of ventricular dyssynchrony? It is helpful to clearly understand the populations studied in clinical trials and their characteristics to more effectively apply this technology in the therapy mix for patients with heart failure.

PROSPECTIVE RANDOMIZED CLINICAL TRIALS

Almost all clinical trial designs intend to apply CRT to patients with very symptomatic heart failure syndromes (NYHA class III or IV) who have interventricular dyssynchrony defined as prolonged interventricular conduction (QRS duration > 120 ms). One trial, CARE-HF, also incorporated echocardiographic evidence of ventricular dyssynchrony in patients with QRS duration 120–150 ms.[4] The echocardiogram method used, described by Pitzalis et al,[12] measures the time from maximal displacement of the interventricular septum to the maximum displacement of the posterior wall when interrogated in the parasternal window. Patients with prolongation of this echocardiogram interval (>130 ms) tend to have improved reverse remodeling after 6 months of CRT,[12] so it was part of the CARE-HF hypothesis that shorter QRS durations (i.e., 120–150 ms) may not indicate the presence of dyssynchrony and may include individuals into the trial with little likelihood of clinical improvement.

Overall, the intent of CRT trial designs should be carefully considered when prescribing this modality to patients with heart failure. Many factors influence trial design, such as costs, duration of follow-up, and choosing a population with the highest likelihood of successful investigation. Once major trials are positive, then, the inclusion and exclusion criteria used form the basis for consensus recommendations, regulatory approval, and reimbursement for the intervention. For example, choosing patients with NYHA class III and IV heart failure formulated the official indication for CRT use in heart failure patients, but, in reality, the vast majority of patients randomized in CRT trials reported symptoms consistent with NYHA class III heart failure (Figure 8.1). In fact, 85% or more of patients enrolled in all prospective clinical trials evaluating CRT had NYHA class III heart failure. Therefore, the vast majority of experience in clinical trials involves patients with less severe class III heart failure symptoms. A closer look at clinical experience suggests that CRT may be less effective in patients with more advanced heart failure symptoms, corresponding to unstable NYHA class IV.

A recent study of patients receiving CRT examined the prognostic value of long-term heart rate variability derived from an implanted CRT device. This study found that patients who reported NYHA class IV heart failure at implantation were more likely to require hospitalization in the follow-up period.[24] Detailed analysis of patients requiring hospitalization in the

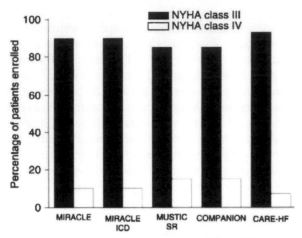

Figure 8.1 Percentage of patients enrolled in CRT clinical trials with NYHA class III or IV heart failure: MIRACLE;[2] MIRACLE ICD;[31] MUSTIC;[1] COMPANION;[3] CARE-HF.[4]

18 months following CRT implantation found that the group was characterized by very low long-term heart rate variability (<50 ms), inability to tolerate beta-blocker therapy at enrolment, and higher probability of NYHA class IV symptoms at baseline evaluation[24] (Figure 8.2). These data suggest that patients with unstable heart failure syndromes characterized by sympathetic activation (low heart rate variability), severe symptoms, and inability to tolerate beta-blockers are less likely to benefit from CRT – at least based on their need for hospitalization in the follow-up period.

The concept of applying CRT to less symptomatic patients was also supported by data from a clinical trial randomizing NYHA class II patients to receive CRT.[25] After 6 months of therapy, CRT patients had more evidence for LV reverse remodeling, including reduced LV end-systolic and diastolic volumes with improved ejection fractions.[25] Understandably, symptoms and distances walked in these relatively asymptomatic patients were not different between CRT and non-CRT groups. Nevertheless, improved reversal of the underlying heart failure pathophysiology is an important surrogate endpoint acceptable for evaluating the impact of an intervention over a short period of time.

In summary, clinical trials examining potential benefits of CRT in heart failure have focused on stable patients with NYHA class III heart

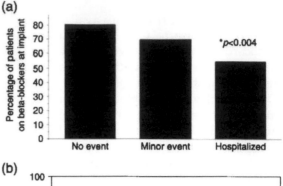

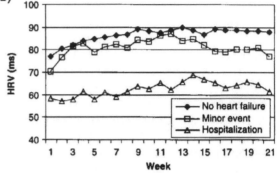

Figure 8.2 Percentage of patients using beta-blocker therapy at the time of CRT device implantation (a), with continuously measured heart rate variability (HRV) shown in (b). Patients experiencing a hospitalization in the follow-up period (18 months) were more likely to be NYHA class IV, not able to tolerate beta-blocker therapy, and characterized by sympathetic activation (very low heart rate variability). Minor events were classified as office visits requiring intravenous diuretics. All events were adjudicated by an independent panel. (Modified with permission from Adamson PB et al. Circulation 2004;110:2389–94.[24])

failure characterized by the ability to tolerate beta-blockers and other neurohormonal intervention. More symptomatic patients, especially those with American College of Cardiology (ACC) stage D persistently symptomatic heart failure,[6] seemed somewhat less likely to benefit from CRT. However, clinical trial evidence in class IV patients is less robust, as 15% or less of the patients enrolled in clinical trials were this symptomatic. Defining 'response', however, is a difficult task and depends on the duration of follow-up and which clinical characteristics are used to establish benefit. Emphasis on 'responder' rates, however, may be less important with the beneficial effects on mortality demonstrated by the CARE-HF trial.

PATIENT SELECTION: APPLICATION TO CLINICAL PRACTICE

It may not be reasonable to expect a 100% response to any therapy in a complex syndrome such as chronic heart failure. If the 84% response is accurate, then application of clinical trial inclusion and exclusion criteria in applying this therapy in 'real-world' experience would be reasonable. However, there are several suggestions for revising patient selection criteria for CRT beyond those used in initial clinical trials in an attempt to improve patient response to the therapy.

Most refinements in patient selection focus on redefining cardiac dyssynchrony using imaging techniques rather than relying on prolonged QRS duration. It is important to emphasize that the only randomized clinical trial that included echocardiographic evidence for dyssynchrony was CARE-HF, and this was only applied to those patients with QRS duration 120–150 ms. Other investigational methods for patient selection include tissue Doppler timing of regional mechanical activation, even in patients with normal QRS duration. This method of defining the underlying 'lesion' of dyssynchrony may improve outcomes and may include some patients who might benefit from CRT.[21-23]

Another group of patients who were systematically excluded from prospective clinical trials comprises patients with permanent atrial fibrillation at the time of CRT implantation. The MUSTIC trial enrolled patients with atrial fibrillation and IVCD and analyzed their experience separately from the normal-sinus-rhythm group.[1] However, since the atrial fibrillation group was so small, it is difficult to generalize conclusions from that experience to clinical practice. MUSTIC patients with atrial fibrillation preferred their experience with CRT to no therapy once they were crossed-over.[1] Subsequent small studies suggest that patients with atrioventricular (AV) nodal ablation for atrial fibrillation rate control improve with CRT ventricular rate support.[26] Although CRT did not prevent atrial fibrillation in the CARE-HF trial compared with maximal medical therapy, mortality was less in patients who developed atrial fibrillation after device implantation.[4] Small-study evidence, then, would suggest that patients with atrial fibrillation seem to improve with CRT therapy, especially if ventricular rate control is achieved with AV nodal ablation.

Another group of patients who may benefit from CRT are those with severely symptomatic LV dysfunction who have high-grade AV block and need ventricular rate support from permanent pacing. Experience from the DAVID (Dual Chamber and VVI Implantable Defibrillator) trial found that when prophylactic ICDs force right ventricular (RV) apical pacing at 70 bpm, patients decompensate and die more often than if the ICD is programmed as a back-up pacemaker (lower rate limit 40 bpm).[27] The risk for adverse outcomes was worse in those with an abnormal QRS complex on the surface electrocardiogram during non-paced activation.[28] This evidence is not conclusive, but certainly suggests that the ventricular dyssynchrony created by traditional RV pacemakers increases symptoms and, possibly, mortality in patients with LV dysfunction. Prospective clinical trials are now ongoing to evaluate the utility of CRT in patients with AV nodal disease and a need for ventricular rate support. Until those trials have been completed, special consideration should be given to apply CRT to symptomatic heart failure patients with LV systolic dysfunction who need ventricular pacing support due to high-grade AV block.

Finally, prospective clinical trials did not randomize patients in whom the LV lead was not placed transvenously. This excluded about 10% of patients in whom the complete system was not implanted at the first attempt. Common practice following CRT approval, however, relies on transthoracic epicardial lead placement, even though no prospective clinical trial data are available to justify this approach. Promising results available from small groups of patients do seem to justify epicardial lead placement when transvenous LV lead placement is not possible.[29]

SUMMARY

Clinical trial evidence supports the use of CRT in patients with persistent NYHA class III or IV heart failure in combination with maximally tolerated medical therapy if QRS duration is >120 ms. Long-term mortality is reduced and morbidity benefits are significant, with over 80% of patients either improving or not worsening after CRT devices are implanted. A closer look at clinical trial populations shows that most patients studied have NYHA class III stable heart failure without overt signs of sympathetic activation. This suggests that CRT should not be considered a 'bail-out' or 'last-resort' therapy, but should be considered in all appropriate patients, especially if their class III symptoms are stable.

Most patients studied in prospective clinical trials were in normal sinus rhythm, but limited clinical evidence in patients with atrial fibrillation suggests that this group may also improve with CRT, especially in the setting of AV nodal ablation. Finally, CRT should be considered in heart failure patients who need ventricular rate support from permanent pacing.

Several clinical considerations should be made in case properly selected patients do not respond to CRT after a reasonable waiting period. Proper device function, lead placement, and LV capture are essential parameters to examine. Further adjustment in medications, such as decreasing loop diuretic dosing, are also important clinical parameters that may provide

better outcomes in patients declared non-responders.[30] Overall, proper patient selection, education, and informed expectations are certain to maximize this lifesaving device intervention for patients with refractory heart failure syndromes (Figure 8.3).

REFERENCES

1. Cazeau S, Leclercq C, Lavergne T, et al, for the Multisite Stimulation in Cardiomyopathies Study Investigators. Effects of multisite bi-ventricular pacing in patients with heart failure and intra-ventricular conduction delay. N Engl J Med 2001;344:873–80.
2. Abraham WT, Fisher WG, Smith AL, et al, for the MIRACLE Study Group. Cardiac Resynchronization in Chronic Heart Failure. N Engl J Med 2002;346:1845–53.
3. Bristow MR, Saxon LA, Boehmer J, et al. Cardiac-resynchronization therapy with or without an implantable defibrillator in advanced chronic heart failure. N Engl J Med 2004;350:2140–50.
4. Cleland JG, Daubert JC, Erdmann E, et al. The effect of cardiac resynchronization on morbidity and mortality in heart failure. N Engl J Med 2005;352:1539–49.
5. Freemantle N, Tharmanathan P, Calvert MJ, et al. Cardiac resynchronisation for patients with heart failure due to left ventricular systolic dysfunction – a systematic review and meta-analysis. Eur J Heart Fail 2006;8:433–40.
6. Hunt SA, Abraham WT, Chin MH, et al. ACC/AHA 2005 Guideline Update for the Diagnosis and Management of Chronic Heart Failure in the Adult – Summary article. A report of the American College of Cardiology/American Heart Association Task Force on Practice Guidelines. J Am Coll Cardiol 2005;46:1116–43.
7. Linde C, Leclercq C, Rex S, et al. Long-term benefits of biventricular pacing in congestive heart failure: results from the MUltisite Stimulation In Cardiomyopathy (MUSTIC) study. J Am Coll Cardiol 2002;40:111–18.
8. Linde C, Braunschweig F, Gadler F, et al. Long-term improvements in quality of life by biventricular pacing in patients with chronic heart failure: results from the Multisite Stimulation in Cardiomyopathy study (MUSTIC). Am J Cardiol 2003;91:1090–95.
9. Bardy GH, Lee KL, Mark DB, et al. Sudden Cardiac Death in Heart Failure Trial (SCD-HeFT) Investigators. Amiodarone or an implantable cardioverter–defibrillator for congestive heart failure. N Engl J Med 2005; 352: 225–37.
10. Pires LA, Abraham WT, Young JB, et al. Clinical predictors and timing of New York Heart Association class improvement with cardiac resynchronization therapy in patients with advanced chronic heart failure: results from the Multicenter InSync Randomized Clinical

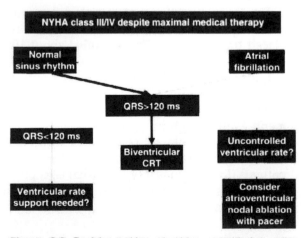

Figure 8.3 Decision-making algorithm considering most patients who may be candidates for cardiac resynchronization therapy (CRT). Thick lines denote the most evidence for use (i.e., normal sinus rhythm with refractory class III or IV heart failure and wide QRS complex).

Evaluation (MIRACLE) and Multicenter InSync ICD Randomized Clinical Evaluation (MIRACLE-ICD) trials. Am Heart J 2006;151:837–43.

11. Patten RD, Udelson JE, Konstam MA. Ventricular remodeling and its prevention in the treatment of heart failure. Curr Opin Cardiol 1998;13:162–7.

12. Pitzalis MV, Iacoviello M, Romito R, et al. Ventricular asynchrony predicts a better outcome in patients with chronic heart failure receiving cardiac resynchronization therapy. J Am Coll Cardiol 2005;45:65–9.

13. Saxon LA, De Marco T, Schafer J, et al. Effects of long-term biventricular stimulation for resynchronization on echocardiographic measures of remodeling. Circulation 2002;105:1304–10.

14. Yu CM, Chau E, Sanderson JE, et al. Tissue Doppler echocardiographic evidence of reverse remodeling and improved synchronicity by simultaneously delaying regional contraction after biventricular pacing therapy in heart failure. Circulation 2002;105:438–45.

15. St. John Sutton MG, Plappert T, Abraham WT, et al. Effect of cardiac resynchronization therapy on left ventricular size and function in chronic heart failure. Circulation 2003;107:1985–90.

16. Sutton MG, Plappert T, Hilpisch KE, et al. Sustained reverse left ventricular structural remodeling with cardiac resynchronization at one year is a function of etiology: quantitative Doppler echocardiographic evidence from the Multicenter InSync Randomized Clinical Evaluation (MIRACLE). Circulation 2006;113:266–72.

17. Stellbrink C, Breighardt OA, Franke A. Impact of cardiac resynchronization therapy using hemodynamically optimized pacing on left ventricular remodeling in patients with congestive heart failure and ventricular conduction disturbances. J Am Coll Cardiol 2001;38:1957–65.

18. Bax JJ, Ansalone G, Breithardt OA, et al. Echocardiographic evaluation of cardiac resynchronization therapy: ready for routine clinical use? A critical appraisal. J Am Coll Cardiol 2004;44:1–9.

19. Sogaard P, Egeblad H, Kim WY, et al. Tissue Doppler imaging predicts improved systolic performance and reversed left ventricular remodeling during long-term cardiac resynchronization therapy. J Am Coll Cardiol 2002;40:723–30.

20. Sogaard P, Hassager C. Tissue Doppler imaging as a guide to resynchronization therapy in patients with congestive heart failure. Curr Opin Cardiol 2004;19:447–51.

21. Westenberg JJ, Lamb JH, van der Geest RJ, et al. Assessment of left ventricular dyssynchrony in patients with conduction delay and idiopathic dilated cardiomyopathy: head-to-head comparison between tissue Doppler imaging and velocity-encoded magnetic resonance imaging. J Am Coll Cardiol 2006;2042–8.

22. Turner MS, Bleasdale RA, Vinereanu D, et al. Electrical and mechanical components of dyssynchrony in heart failure patients with normal QRS duration and left bundle-branch block: impact of left and biventricular pacing. Circulation 2004;109:2544–9.

23. Auricchio A, Yu CM. Beyond the measurement of QRS complex toward mechanical dyssynchrony: cardiac resynchronization therapy in heart failure patients with normal QRS duration. Heart 2004;90:479–81.

24. Adamson PB, Smith AL, Abraham WT, et al. Continuous autonomic assessment in patients with symptomatic heart failure: prognostic value of heart rate variability measured by an implanted cardiac resynchronization device. Circulation 2004;110:2389–94.

25. Abraham WT, Young JB, Leon A, et al. Effects of cardiac resynchronization on disease progression in patients with left ventricular systolic dysfunction, an indication for an implantable cardioverter–defibrillator, and mildly symptomatic chronic heart failure. Circulation 2004;110:2864–8.

26. Leon AR, Greenberg JM, Kanuru N, et al. Cardiac resynchronization in patients with congestive heart failure and chronic atrial fibrillation: effect of upgrading to biventricular pacing after chronic right ventricular pacing. J Am Coll Cardiol 2002;39:1258–63.

27. Wilkoff BL, Cook JR, Epstein AE, et al. Dual-chamber pacing or ventricular backup pacing in patients with an implantable defibrillator: the Dual Chamber and VVI Implantable Defibrillator (DAVID) trial. JAMA 2002;288:3115–23.

28. Hayes JJ, Sharma AD, Love JC, et al. Abnormal conduction increases risk of adverse outcomes from right ventricular pacing. J Am Coll Cardiol 2006;1628–33.

29. Mair H, Sachweh J, Meuris B, et al. Surgical epicardial left ventricular lead versus coronary sinus lead placement in biventricular pacing. Eur J Cardiothorac Surg 2005;27:235–42.

30. Aranda JM Jr, Woo GW, Schofield RS, et al. Management of heart failure after cardiac resynchronization therapy: integrating advanced heart failure treatment with optimal device function. J Am Coll Cardiol 2005;46:2193–8.

31. Young JB, Abraham WT, Smith AL, et al. Combined cardiac resynchronization and implantable cardioversion defibrillation in advanced chronic heart failure: the MIRACLE ICD trial. JAMA 2003;289:2685–94.

9

Anatomy of the coronary venous system

Monique RM Jongbloed, Martin J Schalij, and Adriana C Gittenberger-de Groot

Introduction • Embryonic development of the coronary venous system • Nomenclature of the adult coronary venous system • Anatomy of the coronary sinus and the major tributaries of the coronary venous system • Anatomical variations in the coronary venous system • Potential difficulties and hazards of CRT: case examples • Integration of anatomy with electrophysiology

INTRODUCTION

Implantation of a biventricular pacing device requires proper knowledge of the target veins for implantation of the left ventricular lead, and awareness of potential difficulties that may be encountered. In this chapter, the anatomy of the coronary sinus and the tributaries of the coronary venous system, as well as their variations, are discussed. First, a description of the embryonic development of the coronary veins draining the heart is provided. Thereafter, attention will focus on the adult anatomy, and on the consequences of variations in anatomy for clinical practice in relation to the implantation of devices for cardiac resynchronization therapy (CRT). These difficulties will be illustrated by several case examples.

EMBRYONIC DEVELOPMENT OF THE CORONARY VENOUS SYSTEM

In vertebrates, the heart is the first organ to be formed, and becomes functional during early embryogenesis. After fusion of the bilateral splanchic mesoderm in the embryo, the primitive myocardial heart tube is formed (Figure 9.1a, b). After looping, the heart tube consists of several segments: the sinus venosus or inflow region of the heart, the primitive atrium, the ventricular inlet segment, the ventricular outlet segment and the outflow tract.[1] The sinus venosus becomes incorporated into the atrium and receives the venous inflow of the cardiac veins.

The coronary sinus develops from this sinus venosus segment of the embryonic heart. The sinus venosus has a paired origin, and in the 4th week of development it consists of a left and right sinus horn connected by a small transverse part (Figure 9.1c). Each sinus horn receives blood from three significant embryonic veins: the *vena vitellinae* or *omphalomesenterica*, the *vena umbilicalis*, and the *vena cardinalis communis* (the future caval veins and coronary sinus) (Figure 9.1c). During the 4th and 5th weeks of development, left-to-right shunting of the blood flow causes growth in favour of the right sinus horn and shifting of the ostium of the sinus venosus to the right atrium. During further development in humans, the left umbilical vein and left vitellin vein obliterate, and eventually also the major part of the left common cardinal vein (Figure 9.1d). All that remains of the left sinus horn is the *coronary sinus*, and the *oblique vein of Marshall* (the embryological remnant of the left superior vena cava) (Figure 9.1e; see also Figure 9.2b, c). Due to the left-to-right shunting of the blood, the right sinus horn and concomitant veins enlarge, and eventually the caval veins will form.[2,3] The right sinus horn becomes incorporated into the atria, with the major part forming the smooth walled part of the right atrium, bordered by the left and right venous valves. Part of the right venous valve (the future crista terminalis), together with the venous sinus septum (a ridge present at the medial atrial wall), forms the *eustachian* valve, which covers

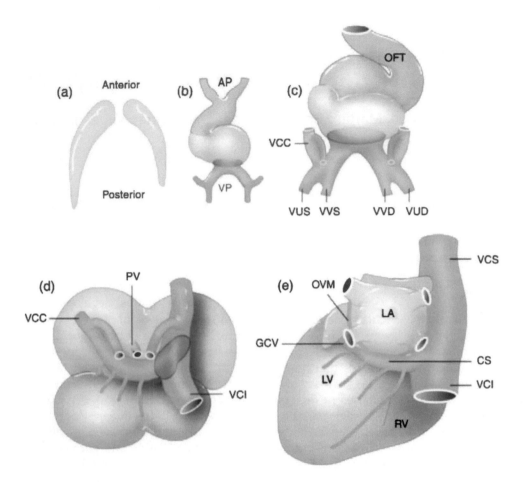

Figure 9.1 Embryology of the heart. The heart develops from two (asymmetrical) plates of bilateral splanchic mesoderm (a), which fuse to form a primitive linear heart tube (b). This heart tube already consists of an arterial pole (AP) and venous pole (VP). The venous pole of the tube is the site where the venous inflow part, or sinus venosus, of the heart will develop (depicted in dark blue). At the sinus venosus segment of the heart, two sinus horns can be observed: a right sinus horn and a left sinus horn (c). Each horn consists of three major veins: the vena cardinalis communis (VCC), the vena umbilicalis sinistra (VUS, for the left sinus horn) and dextra (VUD, for the right sinus horn), and the vena vitellinna sinistra (VVS) and dextra (VVD), respectively. The coronary sinus and the vein of Marshall develop from the left horn of the sinus venosus segment of the embryonic heart. Here the first anlage of a posterior coronary vascular network is found (future coronary veins that drain in the coronary sinus). Rapid growth in favor of the right sinus horn causes a left-to-right shunt of the blood flow, and the right sinus horn is incorporated into the right atrium and will form the smooth-walled part of the right atrium. The left sinus horn will mainly regress, and what remains are the coronary sinus and the vein of Marshall, which will often obliterate (d, e). CS, coronary sinus; GCV, great cardiac vein; LA, left atrium; LV, left ventricle; OFT, outflow tract; OVM, oblique vein of Marshall; PV, primitive pulmonary vein; RV, right ventricle; VCI, vena cava inferior; VCS, vena cava superior.

the inferior vena cava. The part of the right venous valve ventral to where it fuses with the venous sinus septum forms the *thebesian* valve, which covers the ostium of the coronary sinus[2] (Figure 9.2a). This valve can be variable in size and form – uni- or bicuspid; complete or incomplete; circular, cribiform, crescent-shaped, or threadlike – and may hamper access to the coronary sinus. Also, a thick smooth membrane may occlude the coronary sinus ostium (ostium atresia).[4] Inside the coronary sinus, the *valve of Vieussens* is present[4] (Figure 9.2b). The site of the

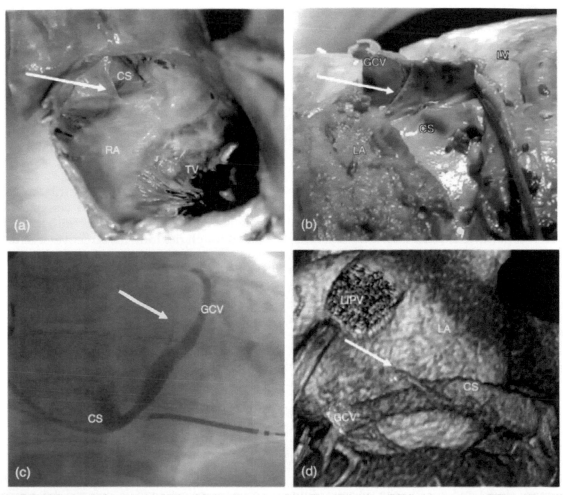

Figure 9.2 (a) Anatomical specimen obtained from a human cadaver. The right atrium (RA) has been opened. The ostium of the coronary sinus (CS) is bordered by the Thebesian valve (arrow). In the lower half of the picture, the tricuspid valve (TV) can be observed. (b) Specimen obtained from a human cadaver, demonstrating the valve of Vieussens (arrow) bordering the ostium of the great cardiac vein (GCV). This site corresponds (often within a few millimeters) to the site where the oblique vein of Marshall opens into the coronary venous system. (c) Venogram of the coronary sinus and great cardiac vein (right anterior oblique view). The oblique vein of Marshall (arrow) can be used to mark the anatomical border between the great cardiac vein and the coronary sinus. As this structure is often obliterated, it cannot be observed with venography in every individual. (d) Volume-rendered reconstruction obtained by multi–slice computed tomography, demonstrating the oblique vein of Marshall (arrow) as a border structure between the great cardiac vein and the coronary sinus. LA, left atrium; LIPV, left inferior pulmonary vein; LV, left ventricle.

valve of Vieussens is in close proximity to the insertion of the oblique vein of Marshall (Figure 9.2c, d), which can be used to mark the border between the coronary sinus and the great cardiac vein (see the section below on the anatomy of the coronary sinus). Uni- or bicuspid complete or incomplete valves may also be present at the ostia of each of the tributaries of the coronary venous system. The function of these valves is

believed to be the prevention of backflow of blood in the venous system during cardiac presystole.[4]

In 1–3% of subjects, an extensive network of threads and fibers is connected with the eustachian and thebesian valves – the so-called *Chiari network*. This network is considered to be a congenital remnant of the right venous valve and is probably of no clinical significance in the majority of cases, although it may cause entrapment of catheters and pacemaker leads.[5]

Several forms of an anomalous development of (one of the components of) the coronary venous system are known. When the left cardinal vein persists completely, it forms a left superior vena cava that usually drains into the coronary sinus. The coronary sinus is often enlarged in this situation, because it drains not only the cardiac veins, but also the blood flow of the persisting left superior vena cava. Other congenital anomalies that can be encountered in clinical practice (albeit relatively rarely) include the absence of a coronary sinus draining into the right atrium (cardiac veins may drain separately into the left and right atria – associated with a persistent left superior vena cava in the majority of cases). These include ostial atresia or an unroofed coronary sinus.[6] Total occlusion of the coronary sinus ostium by a pronounced Thebesian valve, and a double construct of the coronary sinus (sinus coronarius duplex) can also be encountered.[4]

Part of the *tributaries* of the coronary venous system are, from early onwards, always in contact with the coronary sinus. Differentiation of the coronary sinus and its tributaries in the embryo and fetus expands from proximal towards distal – in other words, it starts with connections to the left cardinal vein (the future coronary sinus) and runs in the subepicardium towards the apex of the heart. Only the ingrowth of the anterior veins into the right atrium is a separate event.[7] Initially, the primitive coronary vasculature connecting to the left cardinal vein of the sinus venosus is not yet differentiated into a proper cardiac vein. The coronary vessel network that grows out in the atrioventricular sulcus and as a ring around the arterial trunk still has to differentiate into coronary arteries and veins.[8] After connection of endothelial strands from this peritruncal ring to the aorta (the future coronary arteries) and simultaneously to the anterior part of the right atrium, arterial and venous differentiation takes place. Vessels that connect to the coronary sinus and right atrium will eventually form the coronary venous system.[9] Throughout development, there is a close anatomical association between the coronary arteries and the coronary veins.

Arteriovenous connections that are present proximally in the vascular tree gradually disappear, and a process of remodeling into a capillary network takes place, connecting the arterial and venous systems.[9] The different tributaries of the coronary venous system draining the myocardium are discussed below.

NOMENCLATURE OF THE ADULT CORONARY VENOUS SYSTEM

In the next section, the different tributaries that drain the myocardium via the coronary sinus into the right atrium are described. The posterolateral tributaries form the target vessels for percutaneous placement of the left ventricular lead in cardiac resynchronization therapy. As the nomenclature used in the literature varies, an overview of the main components of the coronary venous system and their synonyms is provided in Table 9.1. The nomenclature in the first column is the terminology used in this chapter.

ANATOMY OF THE CORONARY SINUS AND THE MAJOR TRIBUTARIES OF THE CORONARY VENOUS SYSTEM (Figure 9.3)

The *coronary sinus* runs at the dorsal side of the heart in the posterior atrioventricular groove or coronary sulcus, and is covered by muscular fibers of the left atrium.[10] There is a close anatomical association with the coronary arteries. The coronary sinus drains into the right atrium, through an oval ostium.[11] Distal from the coronary sinus, the first vein that drains into the coronary sinus is the *great cardiac vein*. This vein runs from anterior to posterior, together with the circumflex branch of the left coronary artery in the left coronary sulcus. The border between the coronary sinus and the great cardiac vein is marked by the *oblique vein of Marshall*. As explained above, this vein is a remnant of the left superior vena cava, which regresses in humans and persists as a small vessel that can sometimes be cannulated, but becomes fibrotic distally in the majority of cases.[12] The *oblique vein of Marshall* descends obliquely on the posterior surface of the left atrium near the site of the valve of Vieussens[4] (Figure 9.2b–d). More distally, the great cardiac

Table 9.1 Nomenclature of the adult coronary venous system

Terminology used in this chapter	Abbreviation	Synonyms		Association with coronary artery
		Latin name	Other	
Coronary sinus	CS			
Posterior interventricular vein	PIV	Vena cardiaca media/ vena interventricularis posterior	Middle cardiac vein	Right descending posterior branch of the RCA (or LCA if left-dominant system)
Posterior vein of LV	PVLV	Vena posterior ventriculi sinistri/vena ventriculi sinistri posterior	Left posterior ventricular vein	
Great cardiac vein	GCV	Vena cardiaca magna	Left coronary vein/ vena coronaria sinistra	Ramus circumflex of the LCA
Anterior interventricular vein	AIV	Vena interventricularis anterior		LAD artery from LCA
Left marginal vein	LMV	Vena marginalis sinistra		
Small cardiac vein	SCV	Vena cardiaca parva	Right coronary vein/ vena coronaria dextra	RCA (in the right coronary sulcus)
Right marginal vein	RMV	Vena marginalis dextra		
Anterior cardiac veins	ACV	Venae cardiacae anteriores		
Oblique vein of Marshall	OVM	Vena obliqua atrii sinistri	Oblique vein of the LA	
Thebesian vessels	ThV	Venae cardiacae cordis minimae	Smallest cardiac vessels	
Eustachian valve	EV	Valvula ostii venae cavae inferioris		
Thebesian valve	TV	Valvula ostii sinus coronarii		
Valve of Vieussens	VV	Valvula ostii venae cardiacae magnae	Valvula ostii venae coronariae sinistrae	

LA, left atrium; LAD, left anterior descending; LCA, left coronary artery; LV, left ventricle; RCA, right coronary artery.

vein is termed the *anterior interventricular vein.* This runs in an anterior position from the apex of the left ventricle in the anterior interventricular sulcus, together with the anterior descending branch from the left coronary artery. The anterior ventricular vein drains the apical region and anterior walls of both ventricles, part of the interventricular septum (via the anterior septal veins), and part of the left atrium.[4]

A variable number of posterolateral tributaries of the coronary venous system can be encountered, which are discussed below. With the ostium of the coronary sinus in the right atrium as a reference, from proximal to distal,

and towards the *left* side of the heart, the following vertical posterolateral tributaries draining into the coronary veins can be encountered.

The *posterior interventricular vein* ascends from the apex at the dorsal site of the heart in the posterior interventricular sulcus towards the crux cordis. This vein runs together with the descending posterior artery (the interventricular branch of the right coronary artery or the left coronary artery in the case of a right- or left-dominant system, respectively). It drains the apical region and the posterior walls of the right and left ventricles, as well as part of the posterior area of the interventricular septum (via the posterior

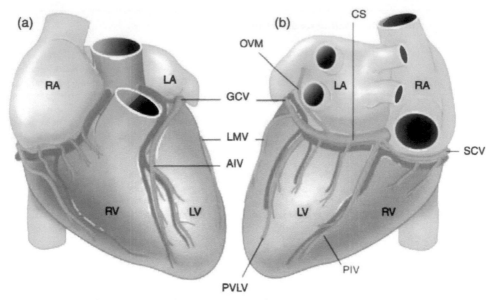

Figure 9.3 Anatomy of the adult coronary venous system: (a) anterior view; (b) posterior view. The coronary venous system is depicted in blue and the coronary arteries in red. For a description of the different components see the text. AIV, anterior interventricular vein; CS, coronary sinus; GCV, great cardiac vein; LA, left atrium; LMV, left marginal vein; LV, left ventricle; OVM, oblique vein of Marshall; PIV, posterior interventricular vein; PVLV, posterior vein of the left ventricle; RA, right atrium; RV, right ventricle; SCV, small cardiac vein.

septal veins).[4] The insertion of the posterior interventricular vein into the coronary sinus is close to its entrance into the right atrium in the majority of cases.

More distally, at the posterolateral wall of the left ventricle, the major branch draining into the coronary venous system is the *posterior vein of the left ventricle*, which drains the lateral and posterior walls of the left ventricle. There can be a variable number of additional posterior branches. The posterior vein of the left ventricle drains into either the coronary sinus or the great cardiac vein.[4] It is at this site, and more distally towards the left margin of the heart, that we often find the target vessel for placement of the left ventricular lead. The *left marginal vein* runs along the left margin of the heart and drains into the great cardiac vein in the majority of cases and into the coronary sinus in a minority of cases.

Towards the *right* side of the heart, the first component of the coronary venous system that runs in the coronary sulcus is the *small cardiac vein*. This vein runs in the posterior right coronary sulcus together with the right coronary artery. The small cardiac vein drains blood from the posterior and lateral walls of the right ventricle. In some patients, the small cardiac vein may drain directly into the coronary sinus.[4]

The *right marginal vein* runs along the right margin of the heart and either drains into the small cardiac vein or enters the right atrium independently.

The *venae cardiacae anteriores* consist of three or four small vessels that drain part of the anterior and anterolateral surface of the right ventricle and enter the right atrium independently in the majority of cases, either directly or by first fusing into a single vessel or sinus.

The *veins of Thebesius* are very small cardiac vessels, part of the so-called smaller cardiac venous system, that conduct blood directly from the coronary system into the heart chambers.[4] These veins do not drain into the coronary sinus. They do not belong to the anterior cardiac veins and open independently on the endocardial surfaces of the right and left cardiac chambers.[4]

Figure 9.4 depicts the coronary venous system as it can be seen using multislice computed tomography (CT) and fluoroscopy. The terminal part of the great cardiac vein often appears 'kinked' as it leaves the coronary sulcus and continues into the coronary sinus.[4] Although the presence of the ligament of Marshall is a more reliable feature, on angiography this kink can often be seen and used as a point of recognition for the transition of the great cardiac vein into the coronary sinus, the place where the valve of Vieussens can be present (see also the small arrow in Figure 9.10d). In patients with chronic congestive heart failure, enlargement of the various components of the coronary venous system can be observed[4] (probably as a result of a general enlargement of the heart).

Variable drainage patterns of the coronary venous system, as well as variations in the occurrence of its different components, may occur.

ANATOMICAL VARIATIONS IN THE CORONARY VENOUS SYSTEM

Anatomical studies describe large interindividual variations in the anatomy of the adult coronary venous system.[4,13] Based on the observations by von Lüdinghausen and at our center, we created three groups of anatomical variants.[4,11]

In the first variant (Figure 9.5a), there is continuity of the cardiac veins at the crux cordis; the small cardiac vein connects to the coronary sinus at the crux cordis. This variant is observed in 29–36% of subjects. The small cardiac vein may also enter the right atrium independently. In the second variant (Figure 9.5b), observed in the majority of subjects (approximately 60%), the small cardiac vein and anterior cardiac veins enter the right atrium separately from the coronary sinus. The posterior interventricular vein connects to the coronary sinus at the crux cordis.

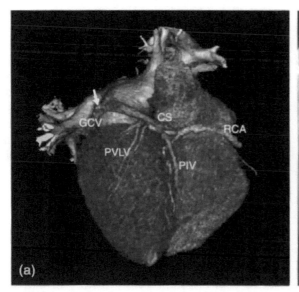
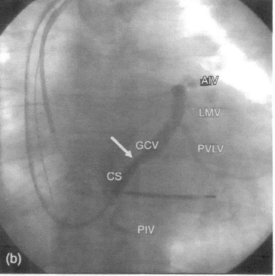

Figure 9.4 Dorsal view of a volume-rendered reconstruction of (a) multislice computed tomography and a venogram (b), demonstrating the coronary venous system. The border between the great cardiac vein and the coronary sinus can be recognized by the oblique vein of Marshall. However, as this structure may be obliterated, contrast filling is often not sufficient to recognize this structure on CT/angiography. Another way to recognize this transition is that the terminal part of the great cardiac vein often appears 'kinked' as it leaves the coronary sulcus and continues into the coronary sinus (arrow).[4] Although the presence of the vein of Marshall is a more reliable feature, this kink can often be seen on angiography and used as a point of recognition for the transition of the great cardiac vein into the coronary sinus, the place where the valve of Vieussens can be present (see also the small arrow in Figure 9.10d). AIV, anterior interventricular vein; CS, coronary sinus; GCV, great cardiac vein; LA, left atrium; LMV, left marginal vein; LV, left ventricle; OVM, oblique vein of Marshall; PIV, posterior interventricular vein; PVLV, posterior vein of the left ventricle; RA, right atrium; RCA, right coronary artery; RV, right ventricle.

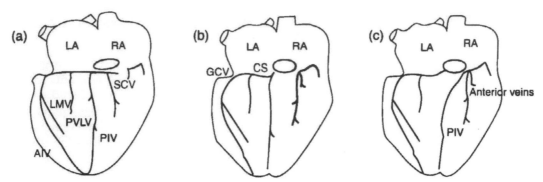

Figure 9.5 (a–c) Anatomical variants of the drainage pattern of the coronary venous system, modified after von Ludinghausen.[4] For explanation, see text. AIV, anterior interventricular vein; CS, coronary sinus; GCV, great cardiac vein; LA, left atrium; LMV, left marginal vein; PIV, posterior interventricular vein; PVLV, posterior vein of the left ventricle; RA, right atrium; SCV, small cardiac vein. (Reproduced with permission from Jongbloed MR et al. J Am Coll Cardiol 2005;45:749–53.[11])

Finally, in the third variant (Figure 9.5c), there is no connection between the coronary sinus and the posterior interventricular vein. The latter is connected to the small cardiac vein or enters the right atrium independently. This variant is the rarest, and is observed in 3–10% of subjects.[4,11] The different components of the coronary venous system may also not be connected at all, so that the coronary sinus, posterior veinous branches, and anterior veins all enter the right atrium independently (approximately 1% of cases).[4] As the more anterior branches are not usually selected for positioning of the left ventricular lead, the clinical consequences of these variations of insertion are limited; however, they may cause problems when advancing the catheter into the coronary venous system.

Of greater clinical significance are variations in the anatomy of the posterolateral branches of the cardiac venous system, as there is significant interindividual variation in the presence of the major branches draining the heart. As the posterior interventricular vein is encountered in practically all patients, the posterior vein of the left ventricle may be absent in 5% of patients and the left marginal vein may only be present in 73–88%, although reports on the presence of the veins vary.[4,13] Also, in our own studies using high-spatial-resolution multislice CT, only in limited percentages of patients were all tributaries observed.[11] Figure 9.6 shows examples of variable occurrence of posterolateral branches as observed with multislice CT. Furthermore, the diameter of

the ostia can be only a few millimeters, hampering correct positioning of the LV lead.[4]

The veins of the coronary venous system can both run under and cross over coronary arteries.[4,13] Compression of cardiac veins can be caused by crossing sclerosed or calcified segments of branches of coronary arteries (when the vein runs underneath the coronary artery – an example is shown in Figure 9.6a), which may also cause problems when advancing catheters. Furthermore, the presence of valves in the coronary venous system may cause problems in advancing catheters and achieving adequate lead positioning. In the next section, three case examples of problematic left ventricular lead placement are described.

POTENTIAL DIFFICULTIES AND HAZARDS OF CRT: CASE EXAMPLES

Case example 1

A 70-year-old man with a history of end-stage heart failure based on ischemic cardiomyopathy and mitral regurgitation grade II/III was referred for implantation of a CRT device with an implantable cardioverter–defibrillator (ICD) (because of non-sustained ventricular tachycardia). On the electrocardiogram (ECG) prior to implantation, there was sinus rhythm, a left deviation of the cardiac axis, and left bundle branch block (Figure 9.7a). Echocardiography demonstrated a dilated left ventricle (biplane left

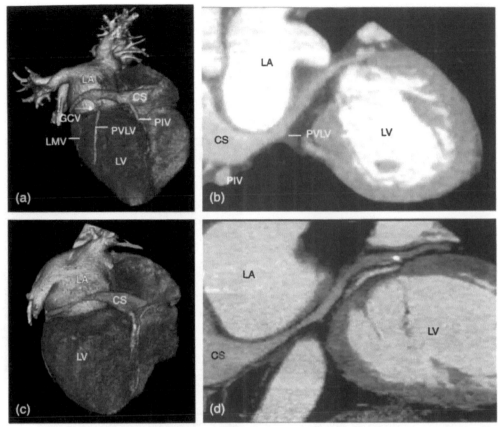

Figure 9.6 Volume-rendered reconstructions, dorsal views (a, c) and curved multiplanar reformats (b, d) of multislice CT scans, demonstrating variability in the cardiac venous system. In (a) and (b), several posterolateral side branches are present, whereas high-resolution imaging of the coronary venous system in the patient in (c) and (d) did not show significant side-branches. The veins of the coronary venous system can both run under or cross over coronary arteries. In (a), the posterior vein of the left ventricle (PVLV) runs under the circumflex branch of the left coronary artery and appears to be compressed by this branch (arrow). AIV, anterior interventricular vein; CS, coronary sinus; GCV, great cardiac vein; LA, left atrium; LMV, left marginal vein; LV, left ventricle; PIV, posterior interventricular vein. Reprinted and modified from J AM Coll Cardiol, Volume 45; Jongbloed M, Lamb H, Bax J. Noninvasive Visualization of the cardiac venous system using multislice computed tomography. Pages 749–753. American College of Cardiology Foundation (2005), with permission from Elsevier.

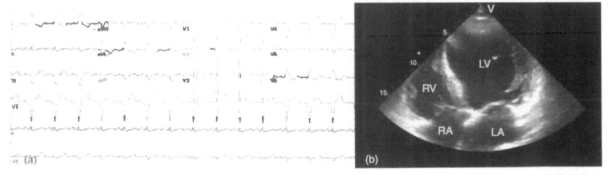

Figure 9.7 (a) ECG prior to implantation of the biventricular pacing device of the patient in Case example 1, demonstrating sinus rhythm with a left deviation of the cardiac axis and left bundle branch block. (b) A 4-chamber view with a marked dilated left ventricle (measured diameter 7.2 cm). LA, left atrium; LV, left ventricle; RA, right atrium; RV, right ventricle.

ventricular ejection fraction 29%) (Figure 9.7b) with significant septal-to-lateral delay (not shown). During the implantation procedure of the left ventricular lead, a block of contrast flow in the coronary sinus was observed during contrast injection, which limited visualization of the distal part of the coronary venous system, indicating obstruction (Figure 9.8a). The site of obstruction corresponds to the position of the valve of Vieussens (see Figure 9.2).

A guidewire was advanced in the coronary sinus (Figure 9.8b), but the left ventricular lead

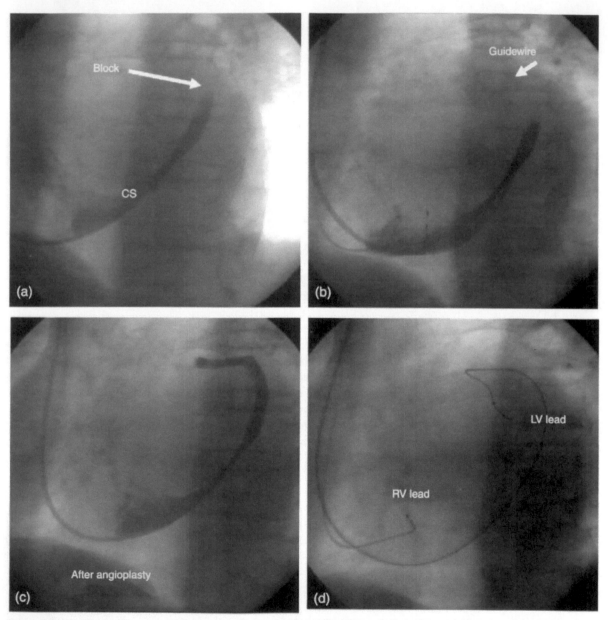

Figure 9.8 Venograms of the patient described in Case example 1: left oblique views. (a) After injection of contrast into the coronary sinus (CS), a block in contrast flow was observed, limiting imaging of the distal coronary venous system. (b) A guidewire was advanced and could be passed besides the obstructing valve. (c) After balloon angioplasty, imaging of the distal coronary venous system could be achieved. However, no suitable posterolateral branches were observed, nor were they seen after balloon occlusion (balloon not shown). (d) Final position of the pacemaker leads. LV, left ventricular; RV, right ventricular.

still could not be advanced through the obstructing valve. Balloon angioplasty was performed, after which the distal coronary venous system could be depicted and the lead further advanced in the coronary venous system. However, positioning of the lead was not feasible because of the lack of posterolateral tributaries (after balloon occlusion of the proximal venous system, no tributaries were visible on angiography) (Figure 9.8c). Eventually, a small anterolateral branch was chosen to position the lead and an anterior lead position was accepted, despite a high pacing threshold (Figure 9.8d). The total procedural time was 277 minutes.

Case example 2

A 62-year-old male with a history of permanent atrial fibrillation and heart failure (New York Heart Association (NYHA) class II–III) based on ischemic cardiomyopathy, non-sustained ventricular tachycardia, and renal failure was referred for His bundle ablation and an upgrade of his ICD to a biventricular ICD. His bundle ablation was performed without complications. The ECG prior to the procedure showed atrial fibrillation with right ventricular pacemaker rhythm (Figure 9.9a). Echocardiography demonstrated a dilated left ventricle with significant septal-to-lateral delay during right ventricular pacing (Figure 9.9b).

During the implantation procedure, only a significant posterior vein of the left ventricle was found (Figure 9.9c). No other significant posterolateral branches were observed, nor were any seen after balloon catheter obstruction (Figure 9.9d, e). An extensive attempt was made to position the left ventricular lead in the posterior vein of the left ventricle. However the lead could not be advanced because of an apparent obstruction at the ostium of the posterior vein (Figure 9.9c: arrow). After multiple laborious attempts using several guides and wires, the procedure was discontinued. The patient was referred to the cardiac surgeon for epicardial left ventricular lead placement by limited thoracotomy, which was performed a month later. Figure 9.9(f, g) demonstrates the ECG and improved left ventricular dyssynchrony after biventricular pacing.

Case example 3

This case involved a 63-year-old female with a cardiac history of heart failure (NYHA class III–IV) based on non-ischemic dilated cardiomyopathy and a mitral regurgitation, for which the patient had undergone mitral annuloplasty procedure. Echocardiography showed a left ventricular ejection fraction of 21%, a significant septal-to-lateral delay indicating left ventricular dyssynchrony, and good function of the mitral valve. The patient was referred for implantation of a biventricular ICD. Prior to implantation, a multislice CT scan was obtained from the patient for non-invasive exclusion of the presence of coronary artery disease. When the coronary venous system was examined on this scan, a marked difference in signal intensity of contrast in the right atrium as compared with the contrast in the coronary sinus was noted. Also, there was a small area that lacked contrast filling at the ostium of the coronary sinus, suggesting obstruction by a pronounced thebesian valve (Figure 9.10a, b). During the implantation procedure, it was initially not possible to advance the catheter, because the valve occluded a large part of the coronary sinus ostium (Figure 9.10c: arrow), producing the same effect of contrast attenuation as on multislice CT. After multiple attempts, a steerable catheter was eventually used to position the catheter in the coronary sinus, after which appropriate filling of the coronary venous system was obtained (Figure 9.10d). Thereafter, the left ventricular lead could be positioned without complications in a large left marginal vein. The total procedural time was 180 minutes.

These three cases demonstrate one of the limitations of cardiac resynchronization therapy – namely, that, despite the high success rates of left ventricular lead placement, there still is a small but significant group of patients in whom placement of the lead is not successful. Although the success rate for placement of a transvenous cardiac resynchronization system is relatively high (88–95% in large clinical trials), in 5–12% of patients, the procedure does not succeed due to failure to place the left ventricular lead via a transvenous approach.[14] Reasons for the failure of left ventricular lead placement include a lack of

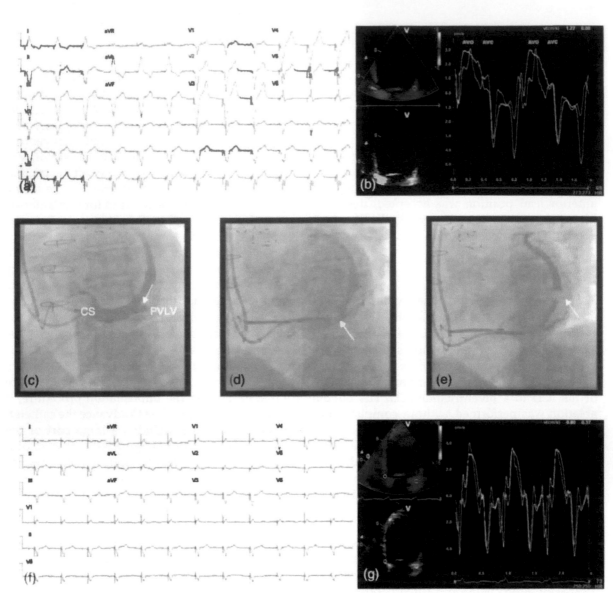

Figure 9.9 (a) ECG prior to upgrade of the ICD to a biventricular device of the patient in Case example 2, demonstrating atrial fibrillation and permanent right ventricular pacing after His-bundle ablation. (b) During right ventricular pacing, there was a significant septal-to-lateral delay (80 ms), as measured by transthoracic echocardiography. (c) Venogram obtained prior to an attempt to position the left ventricular lead. Although a significant posterior vein of the left ventricle (PVLV) was present, filling of contrast was quite slow and a valve-like structure appeared to be present at the ostium of the vein, indicated by a small slit-like area with lack of contrast filling (arrow). Cannulation of the vein was not possible. CS, coronary sinus. (d, e) Balloon occlusion (arrow) was used to reveal suitable posterolateral branches. However, no other significant branch was observed, and after extensive attempts the procedure was discontinued. (f, g) ECG and septal-to-lateral delay after epicardial placement of the left ventricular lead by limited thoracotomy. During biventricular pacing, there is no longer any significant septal-to-lateral delay (delay in peak velocity between the septum and the left ventricular lateral wall), as shown by the synchronous peak systolic velocity curves.

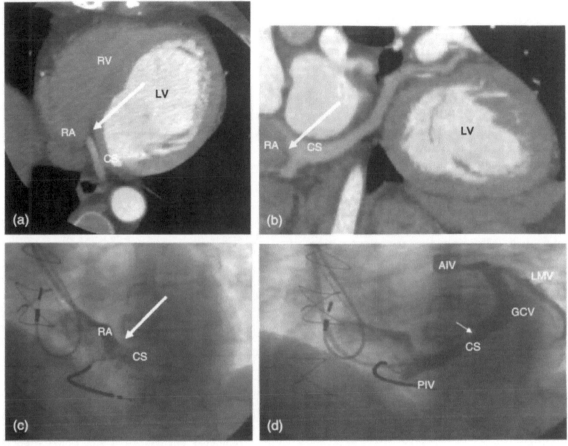

Figure 9.10 (a, b) Images obtained by cardiac multislice CT: (a) transverse view; (b) curved multiplanar reformat. Note the attenuation of contrast in the right atrium (RA) as compared with the coronary sinus (CS). A contrast blank is also observed at the ostium of the coronary sinus, in accordance with the presence of a pronounced thebesian valve at this site. (c) Venogram after contrast injection at the coronary sinus ostium. As on cardiac CT, a small area lacking contrast filling is observed (arrow), and distal from this structure the contrast density is diminished, suggesting flow impedance into the coronary sinus. (d) Situation after passing the valve with a steerable catheter: the distal coronary sinus can now be properly filled with contrast. The arrow demonstrates the 'knotted' terminal part of the cardiac vein as it continues into the coronary sinus. AIV, anterior interventricular vein; GCV, great cardiac vein; LMV, left marginal vein; LV, left ventricle; PIV, posterior interventricular vein; RV, right ventricle.

suitable side-branches,[14,15] narrowing of the coronary sinus ostium or ostium atresia,[6,16] and an inability to advance catheters through the coronary venous system.[15,17] In particular, a pronounced valve of Vieussens can be an important cause of problems when advancing the catheter into cardiac veins.[17]

These problems may result in long procedural and fluoroscopy times and an increased risk of dissection or perforation of the coronary sinus. Anatomical knowledge prior to these procedures may be helpful to distinguish patients eligible

for CRT using a transvenous approach from those who are more likely to benefit from a surgical epicardial approach.

INTEGRATION OF ANATOMY WITH ELECTROPHYSIOLOGY

In this chapter, the anatomy of the coronary venous system has been described. As is the case for many electrophysiological procedures, it has become clear that anatomy and electrophysiology cannot be seen as separate entities, but are closely related. In the case of CRT, several reports have mentioned the advantage of optimization of site selection for left ventricular pacing, for example by choosing the posterolateral vein closest to the area of latest activation for optimal results.[18] The importance of adequate vein selection in relation to the putative left ventricular pacing site is therefore important, and several authors have suggested that the pacing site should be individualized to achieve the best results.[19,20] Also, identification of areas with transmural scar tissue may guide vein selection, as these areas are less likely to respond to pacing.[21] The integration of anatomy with electrophysiology may be facilitated by using new image integration techniques, allowing the superimposition of high-resolution CT or magnetic resonance imaging (although the latter is less suitable for patients who already have a pacemaker) on electrical activation maps of the heart.[22] Some patients may benefit more from epicardial left ventricular lead implantation. High-resolution imaging techniques for accurate depiction of coronary venous anatomy may become increasingly important to identify those patients at risk of failure of left ventricular lead placement who may benefit from primary epicardial lead placement by limited thoracotomy.

ACKNOWLEDGEMENTS

The authors acknowledge Ron Slagter for producing the drawings of the embryonic and adult coronary venous system. We thank Dr Claudia Ypenburg and Dr Rutger Van Bommel for providing the images demonstrating left ventricular dyssynchrony in Case example 2 and Dr Lieselot van Erven and Dr Katja Zeppenfeld for their help in patient selection for the case examples.

REFERENCES

1. Gittenberger-de Groot AC, DeRuiter MC, Bartelings MM, Poelmann RE. Embryology of congenital heart disease. In: Crawford MH, DiMarco JP, Paulus WJ, eds. Cardiology, 2nd edn. St Louis, MO: Mosby, 2004: 1217–27.

2. Los JA. The development of the pulmonary veins and the coronary sinus in the human embryo. Thesis/Dissertation, Leiden University Medical Center, 1958.

3. Sadler TW. Langman's Medical Embryology, 10th edn. Utrecht/Antwerpen: Bohn, Scheltema & Holkema, 1988.

4. von Ludinghausen M. The venous drainage of the human myocardium. Adv Anat Embryol Cell Biol 2003;168:1–104.

5. Schneider B, Hofmann T, Justen MH, Meinertz T. Chiari's network: normal anatomic variant or risk factor for arterial embolic events? J Am Coll Cardiol 1995;26:203–10.

6. Adatia I, Gittenberger-De Groot AC. Unroofed coronary sinus and coronary sinus orifice atresia. Implications for management of complex congenital heart disease. J Am Coll Cardiol 1995;25:948–53.

7. Vrancken Peeters MP, Gittenberger-de Groot AC, Mentink MM, et al. Differences in development of coronary arteries and veins. Cardiovasc Res 1997;36:101–10.

8. Bogers AJ, Gittenberger-de Groot AC, Poelmann RE, Peault BM, Huysmans HA. Development of the origin of the coronary arteries, a matter of ingrowth or outgrowth? Anat Embryol (Berl) 1989;180:437–41.

9. Vrancken Peeters MP, Gittenberger-de Groot AC, Mentink MM, et al. The development of the coronary vessels and their differentiation into arteries and veins in the embryonic quail heart. Dev Dyn 1997;208:338–48.

10. Chauvin M, Shah DC, Haissaguerre M, Marcellin L, Brechenmacher C. The anatomic basis of connections between the coronary sinus musculature and the left atrium in humans. Circulation 2000;101:647–52.

11. Jongbloed MR, Lamb HJ, Bax JJ, et al. Noninvasive visualization of the cardiac venous system using multislice computed tomography. J Am Coll Cardiol 2005; 45:749–53.

12. Makino M, Inoue S, Matsuyama TA, et al. Diverse myocardial extension and autonomic innervation on ligament of Marshall in humans. J Cardiovasc Electrophysiol 2006;17:594–9.

13. Maric I, Bobinac D, Ostojic L, Petkovic M, Dujmovic M. Tributaries of the human and canine coronary sinus. Acta Anat (Basel) 1996;156:61–9.

14. Abraham WT, Hayes DL. Cardiac resynchronization therapy for heart failure. Circulation 2003;108:2596–603.

15. Puglisi A, Lunati M, Marullo AG, et al. Limited thoracotomy as a second choice alternative to transvenous implant for cardiac resynchronisation therapy delivery. Eur Heart J 2004;25:1063–9.

16. Khairy P, Triedman JK, Juraszek A, Cecchin F. Inability to cannulate the coronary sinus in patients with supraventricular arrhythmias: congenital and acquired coronary sinus atresia. J Interv Card Electrophysiol 2005;12:123–7.

17. Corcoran SJ, Lawrence C, McGuire MA. The valve of Vieussens: an important cause of difficulty in advancing catheters into the cardiac veins. J Cardiovasc Electrophysiol 1999;10:804–8.

18. Ansalone G, Giannantoni P, Ricci R, et al. Doppler myocardial imaging to evaluate the effectiveness of pacing sites in patients receiving biventricular pacing. J Am Coll Cardiol 2002;39:489–99.

19. Butter C, Auricchio A, Stellbrink C, et al. Effect of resynchronization therapy stimulation site on the systolic function of heart failure patients. Circulation 2001; 104:3026–9.

20. Alonso C, Leclercq C, Victor F, et al. Electrocardiographic predictive factors of long-term clinical improvement with multisite biventricular pacing in advanced heart failure. Am J Cardiol 1999;84: 1417–21.

21. Bleeker GB, Kaandorp TA, Lamb HJ, et al. Effect of posterolateral scar tissue on clinical and echocardiographic improvement after cardiac resynchronization therapy. Circulation 2006;113:969–76.

22. Tops LF, Bax JJ, Zeppenfeld K, et al. Fusion of multislice computed tomography imaging with three-dimensional electroanatomic mapping to guide radiofrequency catheter ablation procedures. Heart Rhythm 2005;2:1076–81.

10

Implantation of cardiac resynchronization devices

Samuel J Asirvatham

Introduction • General considerations • LV lead implantation • Complications associated with LV lead implantation • Specific considerations in less commonly occurring circumstances • Summary

INTRODUCTION

With the increasing use of cardiac resynchronization therapy (CRT) devices, cardiologists from varying backgrounds, including electrophysiology, interventional cardiology, and congestive heart failure specialties, require a working knowledge of the issues involved in implanting left ventricular (LV) pacing leads as part of cardiac resynchronization therapy (CRT).[1-3] Over the last few years, it has become increasingly clear not only that one needs to access the coronary venous system, but also that familiarity with navigating within this system to reach optimal pacing sites is required.[4,5] In this chapter, we will review the technical aspects of placing left ventricular (LV) pacing leads. A brief discussion of relevant gross and fluoroscopic anatomy is followed by a description of commonly encountered problems, with suggested solutions for each step of the LV lead implantation process. Since this is a significantly invasive cardiac procedure, we will also discuss potential complications and suggest techniques to minimize the recurrence of such untoward events.

The information provided in this chapter should benefit the novice implanter in improving their skills; we also hope that the more experienced implanter will benefit from the anatomical and procedural details and the description of less commonly employed maneuvers described below. In addition, we hope that the non-implanter – specifically the heart failure specialist and echocardiographer[6] – will gain from a more detailed knowledge of the implantation technique and the difficulties inherent in placing LV leads in some patients. The information contained in this section will follow a sequence similar to the implant procedure itself.

First, the implanter must have a working knowledge of techniques common to all pacemaker and implantable cardioverter–defibrillator (ICD) procedures, including vascular access and placing right-sided leads. The LV lead implantation procedure itself requires cannulating the coronary sinus, advancing the pacing wire and/or sheath into the main body of the coronary sinus or its branches, and then placing the pacing lead in a stable working position, usually in the lateral wall of the epicardial surface of the LV. For executing the procedure, the technical details that form the basis for a troubleshooting algorithm are outlined here. We hope that this will allow the implanter to decrease procedural times, while simultaneously being aware of methods to reduce complications.

GENERAL CONSIDERATIONS

Prior to attempting left ventricular lead placement, physicians should be familiar with the technique of standard placement of right-sided pacing and ICD leads. In this section, we will primarily highlight issues with standard device procedures particularly relevant to the placement of LV pacing leads. Facility with various types of vascular access and knowledge of implanting devices from both the right and left subclavian systems is necessary prior to implanting biventricular systems. Additional knowledge of alternative site placement (internal jugular, tunneling leads, etc.), lead extraction, and negotiating stenoses in the subclavian/ superior vena cava (SVC) system are increasingly required for biventricular system implanters, since these patients are frequently being 'upgraded' from existing longstanding systems, sometime with additional redundant leads.

Preimplant evaluation (Table 10.1)

A thorough analysis of patient history and available imaging is mandatory prior to placing a LV lead. If a prior coronary angiogram is available, watching for the levo phase will allow visualization of the coronary sinus and alert the implanter to specific problems such as enhanced tortuosity or an unusual angle in the LAO projection (see below) as a result of marked dilation of the LV. The echocardiogram or other imaging data should also be viewed to understand the potential effect of diastolic ventricular dimension on coronary sinus angulation and the location of ventricular scars and aneurysms. Many hours can be saved in struggling to place a lead in the midventricular lateral position if it was known previously that this segment was scarred.[7] Furthermore, detailed analysis of the echocardiogram (dyssynchrony study), as detailed elsewhere in this textbook, may yield targets for the implanter in striving for a particular possibly more beneficial location to place the pacing lead.

Vascular access

While LV pacing leads can be placed via the usual vascular routes used for standard pacemakers and defibrillators, a few specific concerns should be kept in mind. Because the LV pacing lead is often the third lead being placed, and at times

Table 10.1 Evaluation prior to LV lead implantation

Data	Use
LV end diastolic dimension	Can effect the fluoroscopic angulation of the coronary sinus in a predictable manner
Site of akinetic, dyskinetic, or aneurysmal ventricular myocardial sites.	Would avoid cannulating vein draining sites, as pacing thresholds will likely be inadequate
Severely hypokinetic myocardial location.	Anticipate prolonged capture latency even if thresholds are adequate. If leads are placed at such sites, the option of pacing the LV lead prior to the RV lead should be considered
CT, MRI, coronary angiographic data.	Coronary sinus, anomalies, tortuosity, and approximate sites of branches are useful to know prior to implantation when available

CT, computed tomography; LV, left ventricular; MRI, magnetic resonance imaging; RV, right ventricular.

extensive torque and other manipulation is required to place these leads appropriately, freedom for such maneuvers is required from the vascular route taken. It is therefore generally preferable to use either an axillary veins or an extra thoracic portion of the subclavian vein to minimize difficulty with catheter manipulation, particularly when there are multiple pre-existing leads.

Another consideration when obtaining vascular access to implant the leads is to avoid an over-the-wire reintroduction technique to obtain multiple access. The reasons for this include more significant backbleeding when three leads are introduced through the same puncture and the limited maneuverability for the guiding sheath and leads used to implant the LV pacing leads when a single puncture is made.

In patients with a previously implanted right atrial (RA) and right ventricular (RV) pacing/ICD system, the vein used for that implant may be occluded.[8] It is generally best to implant an entirely new lead system through the contralateral vein. An option, however, is to implant only an LV lead through the contralateral vein and tunnel the lead subcutaneously across the sternum to the contralateral pocket from the previous device. Since the LV pacing leads that are presently available tend to be small, tunneling may cause earlier wear and tear on these relatively fragile leads.[9]

Placing standard right heart pacing/ICD leads

The reader is assumed to be familiar with the techniques required for RA and RV lead implantation. Specific issues for the LV lead implanter include making a decision on which lead should be implanted first and the sequence for pacemaker threshold and defibrillation threshold testing following LV lead implantation.

Many patients who require LV lead implantation have left bundle branch block (LBBB). Because of the extensive catheter and lead manipulation that is sometimes required in these procedures, there is a risk of mechanical trauma to the right bundle branch, which may result in complete heart block. It is recommended that a temporary pacing wire be placed via a femoral vein. Some implanters prefer to place the RV pacing/ICD lead and the RA lead first and then attempt implantation of the LV pacing lead. The rationale for this approach is that most patients with an indication for a CRT device will have an existing indication for a standard defibrillator system. Furthermore, placement of these leads gives anatomical landmarks and orients the implanter to the fluoroscopic location of the annulus and interventricular septum. The disadvantage of this sequence for implantation, however, is that if the ventricular lead and excess redundancy is placed on the right atrial lead, the coronary sinus ostium may be obscured. Further, since the most extensive technical manipulation of the leads and sheath is required for LV lead implantation, some implanters prefer to place the LV lead first when there are fewer impediments to manipulation from occupation of the pericoronary venous ostium by the right-sided leads.

Right infraclavicular versus left infraclavicular implantation

The maneuvers described in this chapter for gaining access to the coronary sinus and then further manipulation in the coronary venous system are similarly applicable regardless of the side (right versus left subclavian) of the implant. This is because the additional curve caused by the acute angulation between the right subclavian venous system and the superior vena cava negates the effects of changing the side of implant and results in similar movement of a catheter or lead tip for a particular direction of torque application. Thus, whether a sheath or catheter is placed into the RV via the left subclavian vein or the right subclavian vein, counterclockwise torque will move the catheter tip towards the interventricular septum and (on withdrawing the catheter) atrial to the annulus onto the interatrial septum.

LV LEAD IMPLANTATION (Table 10.2)

The distinguishing feature when implanting cardiac resynchronization devices is the placement of a secure, stable, and functional LV pacing lead.[10] The steps necessary to achieve this appear straightforward: once vascular access has been obtained, the coronary sinus will need to be accessed. Typically, a guiding sheath will be placed in the proximal coronary sinus, and through this, an over-the-wire pacing lead is advanced to a second- or third-order branch of the coronary sinus to pace the lateral wall of the LV. Although the procedure is, in principle, easily executed, multiple causes of difficulty may occur, with procedural times being highly variable (40 minutes–6 hours). In this section, the fundamental anatomical knowledge required for successful execution of each step of this process is explained, followed by a discussion of solutions of potential difficulties.

Accessing the coronary sinus

Electrophysiologists who may have accessed the coronary sinus many times for mapping the mitral annulus as part of ablation procedures may find placing an LV pacing lead surprisingly onerous, at least when starting to perform

Table 10.2 Techniques for LV lead implantation

	Deflectable electrode-tipped catheters	Guiding sheath system
Deflection mechanism	Most electrode-tipped catheters have uni- or bideflection capability	Deflectable sheath with minimal deflection capacity capability
Electrograms	Readily obtainable, can be used as a surrogate for the right arterior oblique projections with large ventricular electrograms suggesting ventricular position, etc.	Not available
Use in most common cardiac sizes and anatomy	Attention must be paid to the curve placed, and torque needs to be applied	Standard curvature makes cannulation of the coronary sinus relatively straightforward
Use in unusual cardiac anatomy and asymmetric cardiac chamber enlargement	Operators can customize the curvature to suit even extreme anatomical variations	Sheath may have to be changed, and fixed curvature may work against manipulation into unusual anatomical locations for the ostium of the coronary sinus ostium and the bundle of His
Use of telescoping or inner curve sheath within the guiding sheath to choose end guidewire to select ventricular branches	–	Readily utilizable and excellent method of placing wires in a lateral vein, allowing over-the-wire leads to be placed into that venous system
Cannulating the middle cardiac vein or very posterior vein	Techniques involve the appropriate use of deflectable catheters and straight sheaths (see text)	Highly curved sheath is difficult to use in cannulating very posterior veins, with an increased likelihood of deflection
Subselection of ventricular veins	If the vein is large, the deflectable catheter can be placed in the vein, and with appropriate aligned torque the sheath can be placed into the vein of interest	Most commercially available curves on the guiding sheath are designed to seat in the coronary sinus and are difficult to manipulate into venous branches

Regardless of the technique used, sheaths and catheter/stiff wires/introducers should never be advanced without the tip of the leading system being free and fixed (benched).

this procedure. The primary reason for this difficulty is having to take into account a change in the anatomy of the coronary sinus relative to the cardiac chambers when there is significant cardiac chamber enlargement. A mental adjustment has to be made in the typical fluoroscopic views used to account for this (at times asymmetric) cardiac enlargement.

A thorough understanding of the normal anatomy and typical fluoroscopic anatomy will aid the implanter in making these adjustments, even in the most difficult cases.[11,12]

Regional and fluoroscopic anatomy

The coronary sinus is the main vein of the heart.[13] Tributaries that drain the lateral anterior and posterior walls primarily of the LV, with minor tributaries draining the RV, flow towards the mitral annulus to form the great cardiac vein (Figure 10.1). This vein gains further tributaries posteriorly and becomes the coronary sinus. The ostium of the coronary sinus is located in a fairly constant position in the inferior septal region of the interatrial septum. The ostium of the coronary sinus is bounded posteriorly as well as superiorly by the septal portion of the eustachian ridge and the tendon of Todaro. Anteriorly, atrial myocardium separates the vein from the tricuspid annulus.[14] The atrial slow-pathway input to the compact atrioventricular (AV) node, which lies directly superior to the coronary sinus roof, includes the musculature in and around the coronary sinus.

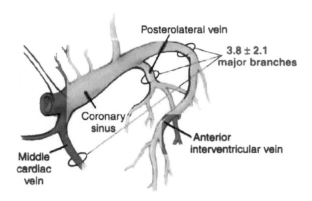

Figure 10.1 The coronary sinus has three relatively constant venous tributaries: the middle cardiac vein, the posterolateral vein, and the anterior interventricular vein. Posterior veins are also common, and arise parallel to the middle cardiac vein or branch immediately from the ostium of this vein. This figure shows the average number of ventricular venous branches that would accept a 6-French pacing lead found in an autopsy series of approximately 400 hearts (see text for details).

It is important to consider 'pure', orthogonal fluoroscopic views to best appreciate the origin and course of the coronary sinus. Since the heart is not a midline structure, but rather has its apex pointed to the left, the information usually

obtained from a standard anteroposterior projection fluoroscopically is now obtained from a left anterior oblique (LAO) projection (Figure 10.2). This LAO projection allows the implanter to immediately recognize rightward versus leftward movement of the catheter, sheath, or pacing lead. The orthogonal view to the LAO projection is the right anterior oblique (RAO) projection. As with a lateral view used fluoroscopically to examine midline structures (sinuses, face, etc.), the RAO view allows the implanter to know immediately whether a catheter, sheath, or pacing lead is advancing towards the ventricle (anteriorly closer to the sternum) or to the atrium (posteriorly closer to the vertebral column). In the figures shown, one should be familiar with standard landmarks in each of the two main fluoroscopic projections (RAO and LAO). Since the coronary sinus is an annular structure, in the RAO projection the ostium and most of the course of the coronary sinus is neither ventricular (anterior) nor atrial (posterior).[15] However, the proximal portion (since the ostium drains to the atrium) is relatively more atrial in the RAO projection, and the more distal portions of the coronary sinus are located relatively more ventricular. In the LAO projection, the vein courses (in the direction of blood flow) from the

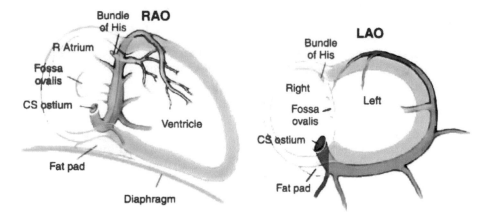

Figure 10.2 The important anatomical landmarks related to the coronary sinus in the standard right anterior oblique (RAO) and left anterior oblique (LAO) orientations. Note the epicardial fat pad at the junction of the diaphragm and the annulus close to the ostium of the coronary sinus (CS). The coronary sinus runs along the annulus, with the atrial branches being posterior and ventricular branches being anterior in the RAO projection. The relationship between the fossa ovalis and the bundle of His can also be useful during cannulation (see the text for details). In the LAO projection, the characteristic angulation from right to left and along the inferior border is seen in most hearts. With grossly dilated left ventricles, this angle is sharper (30°–60° rather than 90°) to the vertical (see the text for details).

left towards the ostium draining into the RA. A catheter that advances in the RAO projection along the annulus and advances from right to left in the LAO projection is in the coronary sinus.

One important fluoroscopic landmark is the posterior epicardial fat pad, which produces a translucency just above the diaphragm, where it meets the cardiac silhouette. This is a common landmark in the RAO projection to identify the plane of the annulus and therefore the approximate location of the ostium of the coronary sinus. Other relevant anatomical and fluoroscopic landmarks useful for the implanter depend on the cardiac subspeciality background of the implanter.[16,17] Interventionalists who are used to the fluoroscopic location of the fossa ovalis should keep in mind that the plane of the fossa ovalis in the RAO projection, which is the same plane, has a line connecting the SVC and IVC and is posterior (closer to the vertebrae) to the plane of the coronary sinus.[18] The ostium of the coronary sinus is diagonally inferior and closer to the ventricle relative to the fossa ovalis. Electrophysiologists who are used to visualizing the bundle of His catheter placed on the annulus anteriorly and on the septum should remember that the coronary sinus is directly inferior to the bundle of His location (3–5 cm) and is located relatively more atrially (posterior in the RAO projection relative to the bundle of His).[19] Once the usual location of the ostium of the coronary sinus and the course of the coronary sinus have been fixed firmly in the implanter's mind in the standard fluoroscopic views, what remains is to manipulate the guiding catheter or sheath into the vein.[20]

Several essentially equivalent techniques to cannulate the coronary sinus exist.

Technique to access the coronary sinus

Once the specific regional anatomy of the coronary sinus ostium and its subsequent course is understood,[21] the most expedient maneuvers required to cannulate the coronary sinus become evident. Regardless of the technique used, the RV should be the first target site for placing the sheath or deflectable catheter; and from there, maneuvers to keep the tip of the catheter or sheath on the septum while pulling back to a posterior and atrial location constitute the main principle for cannulation.[22] Whether a deflectable catheter or a guiding sheath with guidewires is used will depend upon the background of the implanter.

Electrophysiologists who have extensive experience with deflectable mapping and ablation catheters may prefer to use these catheters to cannulate the coronary sinus, while interventional cardiologists often prefer approaches that involve guiding sheaths and various guidewires. At the outset, it should be understood that there is no perfect system to access the coronary sinus, and neither is there a system that will work in all cases. Thus, implanters should become comfortable with one approach but periodically experiment with other approaches that may be particularly useful in a given situation. A generalization that can be useful is that appropriately but sharply curved sheaths tend to be very useful and simple to use in accessing the coronary sinus in the average case; but when the anatomy is unusual (such as in the case of a separate take off for the coronary sinus and the middle cardiac veins), a more neutral or straight sheath with a deflection mechanism on the sheath or a catheter placed through such a neutral sheath may be advisable.

Use of a deflectable catheter to cannulate the coronary sinus

Both bidirectionally and unidirectionally deflectable catheters are available for this purpose. If this approach is taken, then either a straight guiding sheath or a minimally curved guiding sheath is advanced over a wire to the RA. Before taking the wire out, it is useful to just prolapse the wire into the atrium to get an idea of the size of the atrium; this will help the implanter know how much to curve the deflectable catheter (Figure 10.3).

The deflectable catheter is then advanced through the sheath, and the sheath and catheter are placed in the basal region of the RV. The catheter may be hooked up to record electrograms at this point, and only a ventricular signal will be seen from the distal electrode. With the catheter tip placed about 2 cm distal to the tip of the sheath, a slight curve of about 10°–15° is

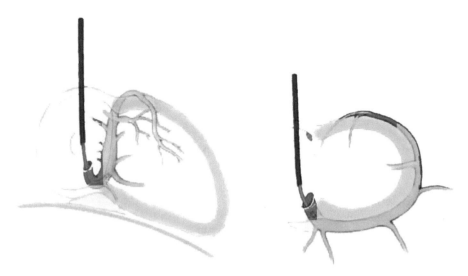

Figure 10.3 Technique for cannulating the coronary sinus with a deflectable catheter. The catheter is first placed in the right ventricle and withdrawn with a sharp counterclockwise torque. The RAO projection typical curve and movement are noted fluoroscopically on entering the ostium of the coronary sinus (see the text for details). This movement, however, can also occur if the catheter is on the tricuspid annulus – hence the importance of the LAO projection (right diagram) showing the catheter tip pointing leftward.

placed to deflect the catheter tip slightly anteriorly. Sharp counterclockwise torque is now applied to the sheath and the catheter to place it on the basal ventricular septum posteriorly. In the RAO projection, when catheter contact with the interventricular septum is obtained, an up-and-down movement will be seen (the axis of movement going from posterior near the vertebra to anterior near the sternum). As the catheter is drawn back, maintaining the sharp counterclockwise torque, the following changes should be looked for: (1) On the electrogram, an atrial signal becomes more apparent with withdrawal until nearly equal atrial and ventricular electrograms are seen. (2) In the RAO projection, a sudden change in the movement characteristics of the tip, with the tip now moving in a to-and-fro direction (atrial to ventricular), typical of an annular location, is now seen. (3) In the LAO projection, a sudden leftward movement of the catheter tip will now be visualized. The site at which these changes occur will be noted to be close to the translucent fat pad referred to above, seen in the RAO projection. These changes suggest that ostium of the the coronary sinus has been cannulated. Now, using the LAO projection,

the catheter tip is gently advanced to a more leftward site, again watching the maneuver in the LAO orientation. If the catheter advances freely, while holding the catheter tip steady ('benching' the catheter), the sheath is advanced over the catheter to engage the proximal portion of the coronary sinus.

If it is not possible to advance the catheter tip further leftward in the LAO projection, it is necessary to consider whether a proximal, atrial, or ventricular vein has been inadvertently subselected. This will be apparent on the RAO projection with a posterior orientation (towards the vertebrae) of the tip if an atrial vein is cannulated and an anterior orientation (towards the ventricle) if a ventricular vein has been cannulated. An appropriate maneuver with the catheter while withdrawing it can cannulate the main body of the coronary sinus (clockwise if an atrial vein is cannulated and further counterclockwise if a ventricular vein is cannulated). If, despite these maneuvers, the catheter tips will still not advance into the coronary sinus to allow the sheath to be placed, or repeated attempts to place the sheath cause the entire sheath and catheter system to pull out of the coronary sinus, then the following maneuvers are useful. It is likely that these problems result from is an unusually tortuous takeoff of the proximal coronary sinus. Gently manipulating the distal tip curvature of the deflectable catheter by pulling the sheath to about 3–4 cm away from the distal electrode will often allow a negotiation of this tortuosity (as discussed further below).

Use of a guiding sheath and guidewire

Similar maneuvers as described above can be used if, instead of a deflectable electrode-tipped catheter, a curved guiding sheath and guidewires and intermittent use of intravenous contrast are employed.[23] Several guiding sheaths are available in the USA and Europe for clinical use. The fundamental prerequisite of a sheath is that a sufficient primary and secondary curve allows the sheath to be balanced against the RA free wall without the curve forcing the lumen of the sheath (and thus extended wires) to point superiorly, making cannulation of the coronary sinus difficult. Most of the available sheaths can be used with equal facility in all except highly unusual cases. Here again, the principle is to place the sheath with the guidewire extended beyond the sheath into the RV. Now, with counterclockwise torque, a change in the movement of the catheter tip in the RAO projection as mentioned above will be noted. The LAO projection should be checked quickly to make sure that the tip of the sheath is pointing leftward (Figure 10.4).

Once this has been ascertained, a soft-tipped guidewire can be gently advanced to see in the LAO projection whether the wire advances leftward on in the RAO projection whether it continues to advance in the plane of the anulus that is not going anterior (ventricular) or posterior (atrial). Intermittent puffs of contrast can be used to achieve the same result – namely, to see if the contrast is injected and goes leftward in the LAO projection or along the anulus in the RAO projection. Further manipulation over a wire (or an inner second sheath) is done to seat the sheath in the proximal coronary sinus.

Causes of difficulty and potential solutions

There are several reasons why difficulty may be encountered in executing this otherwise straightforward set of maneuvers to cannulate the coronary sinus. The most frequent problems are described below, with suggested approaches to overcome them.

Large right atrium

When the RA is disproportionately large, seating a guiding catheter or finding the appropriate curve to place on a deflectable catheter can be challenging. The main problem is that the curve of a sheath or the curve resulting from deflection of a catheter rests on the lateral RA, often fairly high near the SVC–RA junction. Thus, if the lateral dimension of the RA is very large, one will

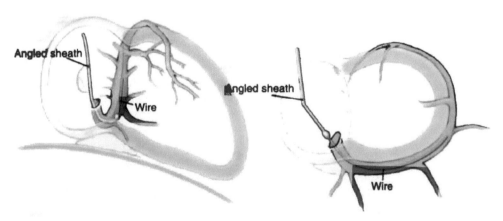

Figure 10.4 Technique of cannulating the coronary sinus with an angled sheath and guidewire. The movements described for using a deflectable catheter are demonstrated here. A curve on the sheath allows the guidewire to be directed in the plane of the coronary sinus.

not have sufficient reach to engage the coronary sinus. One method to overcome this difficulty is to use a large curved deflection catheter (extended distal curvature) and create a U-shaped curve with the distal tip lying on the interatrial septum, with the curve of the U prolapsing slightly through the tricuspid valve and the proximal portion of the catheter lying against the free wall of the atrium *anterolaterally*. A secondary deflection is now placed by deflecting the catheter tip using a bideflection mechanism to point it into the interatrial septum by gradually withdrawing the catheter, with continued 'backbend' (deflecting away from the primary curve) contact the against the interatrial septum being maintained; because the proximal portion of the catheter was placed anterolaterally, pulling back will cause its tip to travel across the fossa ovalis over the eustachian ridge and to a more anterior and inferior location (namely the region of the ostium of the coronary sinus). Once the characteristic fluoroscopic orientation and movement have been recognized, the curve is gently removed and the sheath advanced as described above. It is important to note that to successfully employ this maneuver, the guiding

sheath must be pulled well back into the SVC. Another useful maneuver is to pull the guiding sheath and catheter back into the SVC and put an exaggerated curvature on the catheter tip in order to make contact with the medial portion of the SVC and then advance the tip consistently in this medial orientation as it moves inferiorly, and then to employ a slight anterior curvature to avoid the fossa ovalis and continue to advance the catheter, constantly making contact against the septum to the anterior portion of the eustachian ridge and then into the coronary sinus. Once the coronary sinus has been engaged, however, the catheter, will have a tendency to fall out of the CS with simple further advancement. Here, the curve must be relaxed slightly and the catheter should be gently advanced without the sheath in order to seat the catheter tip in the coronary sinus, followed by advancing the sheath.

Large thebesian valve

Sometimes a large, nearly occlusive, thebesian valve is found at the ostium of the coronary sinus (Figure 10.5). This is a rare finding. However, an anatomical fact regarding the thebesian valve

(a) (b)

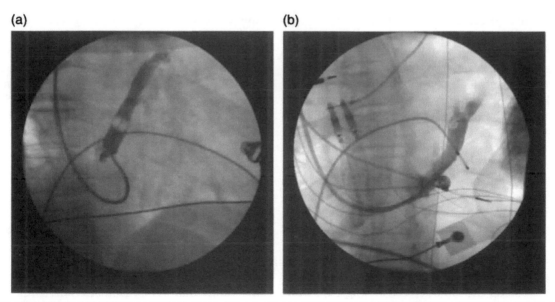

Figure 10.5 RAO (a) and LAO (b) projections of coronary venography. Note that in the RAO projection, close to the ostium of the coronary sinus, a beak-like prominent thebesian valve prevents reflux of dye into the right atrium. In the LAO projection, clear visualization of a prominent valve of the posterolateral vein (Vieussens' valve) is visualized (see the text for maneuvers to overcome difficulties in crossing such valves).

can aid in manipulation around this structure. Thebesian valves tend to be most prominent when associated with a sub-eustachian pouch, but, importantly for the implanter, thebesian valves are least prominent in the ventricular and inferior quadrant of the ostium of the coronary sinus. This is one of the main reasons why in most maneuvers to cannulate the coronary sinus, the ventricle must first be entered and from there the catheter should be drawn back into the coronary sinus. Very rarely, a fenestrated (nearly completely occluded) coronary sinus is found. In this situation, with an Amplatz-type curved sheath placed near the ostium, a floppy guidewire can be used gently to probe for the remaining ostium. Once cannulated, a low-pressure balloon can be advanced to dilate (and likely safely tear) the thebesian valve. Radiofrequency energy can also be used at the ostium, particularly near the floor, with intracardiac ultrasound guidance to help perforate a nearly occlusive thebesian valve. If radiofrequency energy is used, the roof of the coronary sinus should be avoided, because of the close proximity to the compact AV node.[24] It should be noted that sometimes a large thebesian valve may continue on as a valve of the middle cardiac vein, since similar maneuvers may be required if this vein is required for cannulation.

Large left ventricle

The primary cause of difficulty for implanters is when the LV is inordinately large, (LV end-diastolic dimension > 70 mm) resulting in change in the usual fluoroscopic orientation. In a standard LAO projection with a relatively normal sized LV or even with moderate enlargement, the course of the coronary sinus occurs *inferior* to the cardiac silhouette as the catheter advances from right to left in the LAO view. When the LV is markedly enlarged, the enlarged portion takes up a significant amount of the inferior cardiac silhouette fluoroscopically. Thus, the angulation of the coronary sinus becomes more acute, with the catheter advancing in the vein crossing the silhouette at an angle (75°–30° rather than the usual 90°, with the more acute angles occurring in the largest ventricles). Once an implanter becomes familiar with this course of the vein in the LAO view, it becomes easier

to recognize when the coronary sinus has been entered.

Presence of a sub-eustachian pouch

Sometimes, a paucity of musculature between the eustachian ridge and the tricuspid valve is found towards the septum. This gives rise to an outpouching referred to as a sub-eustachian pouch. The primary reason for difficulty when this anatomical variant is present is that when the deflectable catheter or guiding sheath is torqued in a counterclockwise fashion, on withdrawing from the ventricle, rather than engaging the coronary sinus, the cannulating device falls into the pouch (Figure 10.6). If contrast is injected at this site, there will be swirling and stasis of the contrast, giving a mistaken impression of possible perforation. If a deep pouch is found and recognized by the fluoroscopic pattern (particularly in the RAO view), then the sheath should be kept in the pouch, and a second sheath with a nearly right-angled curve or a deflectable catheter forming a right-angled deflection to the sheath tip can be advanced to engage the coronary sinus. Once engaged, the catheter tip can be advanced slightly while *simultaneously* pulling up the guiding sheath. The guiding sheath can then be advanced into the coronary sinus, following the deflectable catheter tip. Note that this maneuver is an exception to the rule whereby, when advancing the guiding sheath, the catheter tip should be benched or held in the same location. In this particular situation, the catheter tip and sheath are advanced together – as, otherwise, the tip will constantly fall out of the coronary sinus into the RV.

Advancing within the coronary sinus

Once the coronary sinus ostium has been cannulated and a sheath placed securely in the proximal portion of this vein, the next step is to advance the LV leads further into the coronary sinus and then attempting to sub-select one of the ventricular veins. This often involves retaining the ability to place a sheath further into the coronary sinus as well, and at times subselecting with a sheath into one of the ventricular veins, which is sometimes necessary in order to

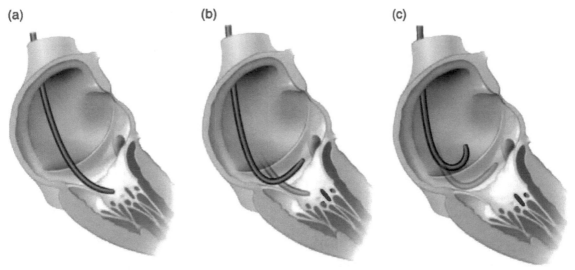

Figure 10.6 (a–c) One of the difficulties with cannulating the coronary sinus occurs when there is a large sub-eustachian pouch anterior to the eustachian ridge. When pulling back the catheter with counterclockwise torque from the ventricle, the catheter will tend to fall in to this pouch. Since the operator realizes the coronary sinus is not cannulated, he or she may mistakenly continue with clockwise torque and fall behind the eustachian ridge, and all attempts to cannulate the coronary sinus will be unsuccessful. Once the situation has been appreciated and a position in the pouch has been found, a gentle to-and-fro torque and lifting up the catheter (preferably using a deflectable catheter with back-bend), the ostium of the coronary sinus can be negotiated successfully.

get a pacing lead into one of the ventricular veins. If the implanter has used a deflectable catheter to engage the coronary sinus, it is best to use the same deflectable catheter to advance further into the coronary sinus and possibly the subselective ventricular vein. On the other hand, if a guiding sheath and guidewires have been used initially, then the wires can be advanced further into the vein, followed by advancing the sheath over the wire or, if the sheath is securely located more proximally, advancing an over-the-wire pacing lead to the distal coronary venous vasculature.

Regional and fluoroscopic anatomy

The ostium of the coronary sinus is a relatively more atrial structure as compared to the great cardiac vein and more distal tributary.[25] This is because the vein proximally empties into the atrium, but the bulk of the distal tributaries are ventricular. There is considerable variation in the luminal diameter and tortuosity of the great cardiac vein and coronary sinus. I have explained above that the proximal portion can have significant posterior tortuosity and posterior curvature and tortuosity, and both dilated and relatively stenotic segments may alternate with each other along the course of this vein.

The main consistent tributaries draining into the coronary sinus are the middle cardiac vein, running from apex to base in the posterior intraventricular groove, along with the posterior descending artery. The next branch is the posterior cardiac vein located 1–2 cm from the middle cardiac vein and draining the posterior wall of the LV. A posterolateral vein may then arise along with true lateral veins and a varying number of anterior lateral veins. The most distal branch comprises the anterior intraventricular veins, draining from apex to base on the anterior intraventricular groove.

Techniques

The primary techniques useful in helping to advance sheaths, catheters, or pacing leads along the coronary sinus are coronary sinus venography, the use of deflectable catheters, and the use of a guiding sheath with guidewires.[26]

Coronary sinus venography

Reasonable visualization of the coronary vein anatomy can be obtained by observing the levo phase (with continued cine angiography) during coronary arteriography. In fact, when arteriography has been performed for clinical reasons prior to CRT implantation, the images must be reviewed prior to implant. Specific coronary venography involves placement of a balloon occlusion catheter in the proximal coronary sinus.[27–29] After the coronary sinus has been cannulated, the end-hole balloon catheter is advanced to the proximal portion of the coronary sinus just distal to the tip of the guiding sheath. The balloon is inflated and then dye is injected through the end-hole, allowing retrograde profusion of the contrast dye into the coronary venous tree. The following technical points must be kept in mind with regard to coronary retrograde venography (Figure 10.7):

- The balloon must be fully expanded to allow good visualization of the venous branches.
- After occlusion, venography images are obtained, with continued cine angiography; the balloon must be deflated and the 'backwash' observed, as more proximal veins will only be visualized at this stage[30] (e.g., the middle cardiac vein).
- If the balloon is occluded too distally, proximal veins as well as lateral veins at the site where the balloon has been expanded will not be visualized (Figure 10.8).
- Prolonged cine angiography (5–10 s) with the balloon inflated is useful, as anastamotic flow from the distal venous branches will be seen to fill with contrast returning to the proximal coronary sinus or RA via the more posteriorly and proximally located veins (posterior cardiac vein and middle cardiac vein).
- Subselective venography can be very useful, especially in the posterior or middle cardiac vein to visualize the lateral branches of these veins that can be subselected for lead placement. Here, the guiding sheath displaced in the ventricular branch of interest and the balloon is gently expanded within this venous branch prior to contrast injection.

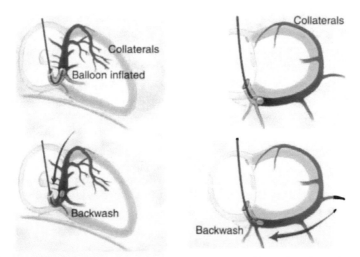

Figure 10.7 Coronary sinus angiography with an end-hole balloon catheter can be useful in identifying the ventricular veins and selecting an appropriate target vein to place the pacing lead. Careful attention to detail is important when performing coronary sinus angiography. The occlusion balloon must be placed fairly proximally to visualize the distal vessels; continued angiography is important to look for an anastomosis in collaterals, and cine imaging should be continued after the balloon is deflated to analyze the backwash that often fills retrograde into very proximal veins, including the middle cardiac vein.

(a) (b) (c)

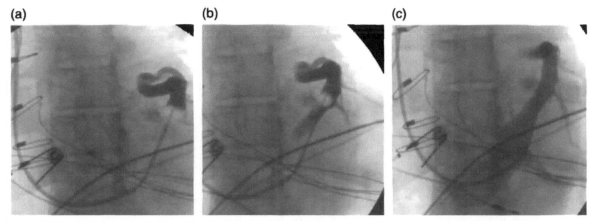

Figure 10.8 Balloon occlusion venography. (a) Too distal a balloon placement where no proximal branches are seen. (b) Full back of the balloon, with the more lateral veins now visualized. (c) Deflation of the balloon, with backwash filling an excellent large posterior vein.

Use of a deflectable catheter

When a deflectable catheter has been used to cannulate the coronary sinus in the RAO projection, the catheter should advance parallel or alongside the plane of the mitral annulus; thus, the tip of the catheter takes a gentle course from a slightly atrial location to a slightly ventricular location, with the entire catheter moving in a to-and-fro annular pattern (Figure 10.9). If resistance is met, it is possible that the tip of the catheter is now engaging either an atrial or ventricular branch or is unable to negotiate a tortuous segment. If a posterior orientation of the tip is seen using the RAO projection, sharp clockwise rotation while withdrawing the catheter and then advancing it will re-engage the main body of the coronary sinus, whereas if an anterior orientation is seen, one can simply elect to continue to advance the catheter in this orientation, likely deeper into a ventricular vein, and then place the sheath over the catheter into this vein.

Use of a guiding catheter and guidewires

If a guidewire-with-sheath approach has been used to cannulate the coronary sinus, the RAO projection can be used to see if the wire advances freely along the annulus or whether a tributary has been entered. Appropriate maneuvers as described above with the use of a deflectable catheter can be applied to re-engage the main coronary sinus or one of the ventricular veins and gently advance the guiding catheter.[31] Once the wire has been advanced into a ventricular vein, the pacing lead (in an over-the-wire system) can now be advanced over the wire by holding the wire steady (not advancing both wire and pacing leads the same time) and at times gently pulling back on the wire as the lead advances.

Causes of difficulty and potential solutions

Sometimes, the coronary sinus itself is fairly easily cannulated but there is great difficulty in advancing a guiding sheath to a stable position in the proximal coronary sinus. A frequent cause for this is a posterior angulation of the proximal coronary sinus caused by marked LV enlargement. In the RAO projection, the proximal portion of the coronary sinus close to the ostium will be directed posteriorly away from the plane of the mitral annulus. If the ostium itself has been cannulated, careful dye injection will allow the implanter to recognize this variation in coronary vein anatomy. In attempting to overcome this problem, one should not use excessive force in advancing a large guiding sheath or a

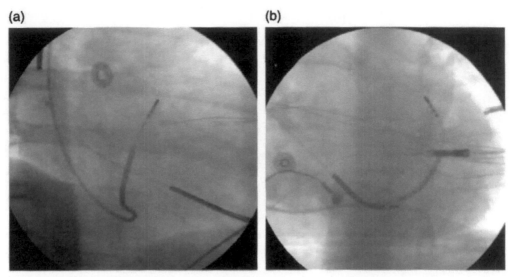

(a) **(b)**

Figure 10.9 If a deflectable catheter is used to cannulate the coronary sinus, the sheath can be advanced through fairly tortuous curves, as seen proximally in this patient. In the RAO projection (a), the catheter should advance at a very slight angle towards the ventricle. In the LAO projection (b), the catheter moves leftward and then curves around the lateral annulus and returns towards the septum. It is important that the sheath be very carefully advanced over a 'benched' deflectable catheter tip, with slow withdrawal of the catheter being required when advancing the sheath over tortuous segments or relative stenosis (see the text for details).

deflectable catheter; this will result in coronary sinus dissection and will make any further attempts to access the coronary venous system futile.

Two methods to overcome this difficulty are suggested. The first is to keep the guiding sheath close to or just at the ostium of the coronary sinus and attempt to advance a very floppy wire such as a Glide™ or Whisper™ or other highly flexible wire while monitoring fluoroscopically in the RAO projection. Initially, a posterior angulation followed by an anterior angulation of the wire's course is seen when one of the ventricular veins is entered. If there is reasonable stability of the sheath in this location, a suitable pacing lead can then be threaded over the wire, which is now in the ventricular vein, to the desired pacing position.

A second technique involves the use of a deflectable catheter. Once it has been recognized that there is a posterior or other unusual tortuosity of the vein close to its ostium, the sheath itself is maintained close to the ostium with slight

clockwise torque. The deflectable catheter with a slight curve is torqued in a counterclockwise fashion along the angulation of the proximal coronary sinus. If the sheath is also torqued parallel to the angulation (counterclockwise), the tip of the catheter will fall back to the posterior atrium. After gradually advancing the catheter, the sheath is tracked along the catheter, keeping a distance to the sheath tip of about 1 cm. Once the posterior extent of the initial angulation has been reached by the catheter, the opposite maneuver is undertaken, where now gentle counterclockwise torque is maintained on the sheath so as to avoid displacement, but with clockwise torque applied to the catheter tip to re-engage the usual plane of the coronary sinus and great cardiac vein. Once the great cardiac vein itself has been reached, similar maneuvers to those described above as performed in normal circumstances will allow the sheath to track along a 'benched' deflectable catheter.

Other important reasons for failure to advance in the coronary sinus are outlined below.

Anomalous coronary sinus origin

A rare, coronary venous anomaly involves reconstitution of an occluded proximal coronary sinus via an atrial vein that now drains into the RA relatively higher on the interatrial septum.[32] This situation is usually identified when the implanter has already experienced great difficulty in cannulating the coronary sinus and the levo phase of the coronary arteriogram is visualized to better understand this anatomical variant. To overcome this difficulty, a relatively straight sheath is used, along with a deflectable catheter, to locate the site of the bundle of His electrogram. Once this has been identified with about a 60° curve along the deflectable catheter, the catheter and sheath are torqued counterclockwise to the high intraatrial septum. The curve on the catheter is now gently released while pushing down on the sheath. This maneuver probes the higher interatrial septum for the ostium of such a vein. Once the catheter tip movement changes, entering the vein should be suspected and the sheath advanced gently over the catheter. Contrast can be injected around the catheter to confirm that one has intervenous structure. Following this, it is usually relatively straightforward to further advance the catheter tip into the main body of the coronary sinus. The sheath is then advanced over this wire and placed within the body of the coronary sinus.

Valves in the coronary sinus

Similar to the Thebesian valve at the ostium of the coronary sinus, valves can also be located at the ostia of the ventricular veins or rarely within the body of the coronary sinus itself. Common locations for valves are at the ostium of a posterolateral vein (Vieussens' valve), the ostium of the middle cardiac vein, and sometimes a valve located within the coronary sinus at the junction with the great cardiac vein, the vein of Marshall, and the posterolateral vein.[21, 33] Usually, these valves are fairly small and poorly developed and do not impede lead manipulation either into a tributary or in the main coronary sinus. When these valves are prominent and nearly occlusive, the techniques described to cross a prominent thebesian valve described above can be utilized here as well. Specifically, a deflectable catheter

with a soft tip can be advanced until resistance of the valve is met. Then, by gentle use of the deflection mechanism, all quadrants of the circumference of the vein at the site of the valve are probed with serial deflection, advancement, and withdrawal in relatively rapid succession. When the region where the valve is least developed is found, the deflectable catheter should be advanced across the valve at this opening and then the sheath advanced over the lead as well. With the sheath now kept distal to the nearly occlusive valve, a guidewire and over-the-wire pacing lead can be advanced to one of the tributaries.

Stenosis/spasm

For unknown reasons, coronary venous stenosis may occur at various sites in the coronary venous vasculature (Figure 10.10). Sometimes, a previous history of coronary sinus manipulation as part of cardiopulmonary bypass-related surgery or a history of radiofrequency ablation within the coronary venous system is obtained.[34] In most instances, however, these stenoses have no definable cause. If an abrupt narrowing in the coronary veins is noted, simple reinjection of contrast after approximately 20 minutes should first be done to see if this may have been a transient spasm involving the musculature of the proximal coronary sinus. If it appears that this is a fixed lesion, a guidewire should be passed, and over the guidewire a low-pressure inflation balloon expanded at the site of maximal stenosis to dilate the vein and allow the creation of an adequate lumen for passing a standard LV pacing lead.[35] Sometimes, multiple stenoses within the vein are noted, and serial angioplasty may be required.

Tortuosity

Excessively tortuous coronary veins can make passage of the pacing lead or sheath into the coronary sinus exceedingly difficult.[36] Once this situation has been recognized, it is generally preferable to use a deflectable catheter technique rather than a guidewire and sheath.[37] This is because if one attempts to advance a sheath over a relatively floppy guidewire and the vein is very tortuous, this may give rise to a dissection. If a wire has been advanced, however, it is very

(a) (b)

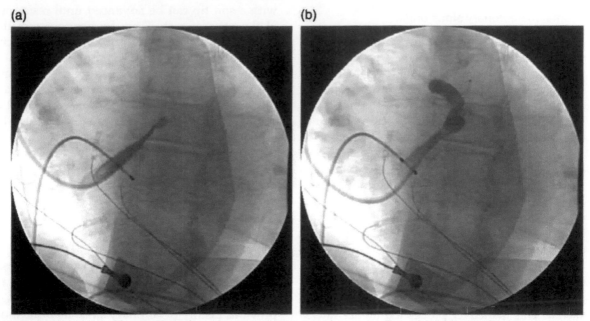

Figure 10.10 (a) Idiopathic stenosis in the midcoronary sinus is seen in some patients. (b) If this situation is recognized, low-pressure angioplasty can be performed to obtain access in the distal and mid lateral veins. Another option would be to use the middle cardiac vein, or a very posterior vein, by subselecting its lateral branches to reach the lateral wall.

reasonable to try to use this access to pass a lead over the wire to one of the ventricular branches. If this maneuver fails, it would be best to use a deflectable catheter, gently advance this catheter through a 1–2 cm tortuous segment, and then track the sheath over this relatively larger and more stable catheter (and a guidewire) up to the tip of the catheter. The maneuver is then repeated until the sheath is well placed close to the ostium of the vein of the tributary of interest for placing the LV pacing lead.

Unwanted subselection

The most common reason why a lead or sheath does not advance into the coronary vein is unrecognized subselection of one of the tributaries.[38] The novice implanter may not realize that this has happened, and if force is used in trying to advance the sheath or the pacing lead, dissection of the venous vasculature will occur. The RAO projection will readily reveal whether the pacing catheter or guidewire, or deflectable sheath has entered an atrial vein (posterior in RAO) or ventricular vein (anterior in RAO). If an atrial

vein has been selected, then *clockwise* torque while withdrawing the catheter will allow one to re-enter the main coronary sinus.[39] If the ventricular branch has been subselected, the catheter in this vein should be stabilized and attempts made to advance the sheath into this vein itself. If this occurs, then this type of access can be excellent for placing a lead through the sheath indirectly into the subselected ventricular vein. As a general rule, even if the LAO projection for fluoroscopy was used to confirm that one is going leftward into the coronary sinus, while trying to advance the catheter or sheath, the RAO projection is more informative, as described above.

Optimal placement of the pacing lead on the lateral left ventricular free wall

Early studies that required hemodynamic assessment and epicardial lead placement suggested that the ideal placement for the LV pacing lead was in the lateral midportion of the LV free wall.[40] Subsequent retrospective studies with endovascular implantation have given mixed results,[41] but, in general, attempting to place the LV lead on the free wall as far away as possible from the RV pacing lead is a common practice. Clearly, exceptions to this goal for implant exist, including situations where the lateral LV is scarred or aneurysmal or data from echocardiographic studies (as discussed elsewhere in this textbook) suggest a non-lateral wall site as an optimal pacing site. Because of this generally desirable location for placing a stable LV pacing lead, thorough knowledge of the venous anatomy for the lateral wall and the techniques available to subselect the veins of interest is required.

Regional and fluoroscopic anatomy

The venous drainage of the lateral LV free wall is complex and parallels the arterial supply to this region of the heart.[42] Several branches of the main coronary arteries, including the diagonals, the obtuse marginals, the posterolateral branches of the right coronary system, and (in some patients) a separate intermitted ramus artery, contribute to the arterial supply of this region. Similarly, the venous drainage from this site may include a distinct lateral vein, branches of a posterolateral or posterior vein,[25] branches of the anterior intraventricular and anterolateral veins, and (in some patients) lateral tributaries of the middle cardiac vein (Figure 10.11).

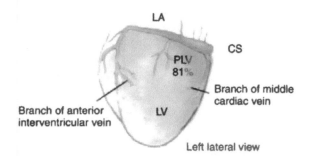

Figure 10.11 The varied venous drainage of the lateral left ventricle (LV). A posterolateral vein (PLV) is found in about 80% of hearts, but the lateral wall is drained by multiple venous tributaries, including branches of the anterior interventricular vein, the posterior veins, and the middle cardiac veins. Separate lateral veins may also be found (see the text for details). CS, coronary sinus.

Because of this varied and diverse venous drainage pattern to the lateral wall, an important dictum for the implanter to bear in mind is that the target should not be cannulation of a lateral vein, but to get a pacing lead on the lateral wall.[43] In other words, whether one reaches the midportion of the lateral wall via a separate lateral vein or via an anastomotic tributary via an anterior vein or posterior vein, the eventual pacing site and pacing sequence for the heart are identical.

The true lateral wall of the left ventricle is difficult to identify fluoroscopically. One of the problems that has plagued the interpretation of retrospective data when trying to assess responder status to cardiac resynchronization and lead position has been a difficulty with interpreting lead position fluoroscopically. In a standard anteroposterior (AP) projection, it is extremely difficult to distinguish anterolateral, lateral, and even posterolateral locations, even with the orthogonal lateral view or with orthogonal RAO and LAO views. The same lead position may be anterolateral in patients with some types of cardiac enlargement, while it may be on the lateral midportion in patients with less or different cardiac enlargement. Nevertheless, it is generally best to use the RAO and LAO projections as detailed above to estimate the lateral location for the pacing lead. An estimate of the correction that needs to be made in interpreting the X-ray in the LAO projection with markedly enlarged hearts can be obtained by analyzing the fluoroscopic appearance of the right-sided apical pacing or ICD lead. In a standard LAO projection, the RV lead does not 'break the plane' of the midline (interventricular septum). If the lead is seen to go significantly leftward, this suggests that the RV apex is located more posteriorly and to the left than usual, and thus the lateral wall of the ventricle will appear to be in a more anterior location in the LAO and left lateral projections (counterclockwise cardiac rotation). A few electrocardiographic clues are also worth noting at this point to use in conjunction with fluoroscopic interpretation. First, counterclockwise rotation of the heart should be suspected if there is progressive S-wave deepening from lead V1 to V3. Secondly, with a lateral pacing site, one should nearly always expect to see a QS deflection in the paced morphology in lead 1. If lead 1 is not negative, this suggests that the lead is either very posterior or on the septum, and more careful analysis of the X-ray and perhaps echocardiographic patterns of activation should be performed.[44]

Techniques

Primary techniques with which the implanter should be familiar in order to get a lead to the lateral wall or to a particular desirable site are techniques to subselect a vein or an anastomotic branch using a deflectable catheter and secondly the use of telescoping sheaths (sheaths within sheaths) and guidewires.

Subselection with a deflectable catheter and sheath

If a deflectable catheter has been used to cannulate the coronary sinus and then aid the advancement of the guiding sheath into a stable location in the proximal coronary sinus, the same system can be used to subselect a ventricular vein of interest (Figure 10.12). Counterclockwise torque will have been used to gain access to the coronary sinus. The implanter should advance the deflectable catheter to the most anterior location possible, taking the precautions described in the previous section. Once a good anterior location has been obtained with the catheter tip, a slight curve is placed using the deflection mechanism, simultaneously torquing the deflectable catheter in a *clockwise* fashion. In the RAO projection, this maneuver will cause the tip of the deflectable catheter to point anterior towards the LV.[45] Maintaining this torque, the catheter is then gently moved back towards the coronary sinus ostium. With the curved tip pointing anterior, moving back towards the ostium, if a large enough ostium of a ventricular vein is met during the maneuver, the tip of the catheter will fall into the vein. In the RAO projection, this movement of the catheter tip 'plunging' into a more ventricular location produces a characteristic movement and allows the implanter to

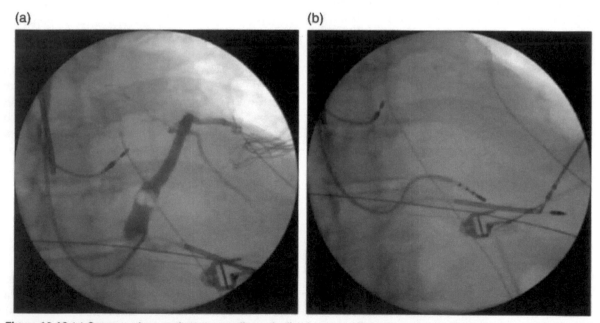

(a)   (b)

Figure 10.12 (a) Coronary sinus angiogram revealing only distal venous tributaries and a small shadow of a proximal middle cardiac vein. (b) With gentle clockwise rotation of the catheter tip and withdrawal towards the ostium of the coronary sinus, a large posterolateral vein draining the lateral left ventricular free wall is entered and the sheath is advanced carefully into this vein, holding the catheter tip steady while pulling back slightly while advancing over this curvature. Note that, because of the balloon location, this branch was not seen on initial venography.

know that the vein has been subselected. The guiding sheath must now be advanced, with care being taken to keep *the same torque* on the guiding sheath as has been placed on the catheter. If this simple precaution is not implemented, then advancing the sheath will cause the tip of the catheter in the subselected vessel to prolapse back into the main body of the coronary sinus. With the torque on the catheter and sheath identical, the sheath is advanced into the ventricular vein draining the lateral wall. This will usually allow the deflectable catheter to advance further into a large ventricular vein, and the sheath can be further advanced to a stable location in this vein. The deflectable catheter is now removed and a pacing lead can be placed directly into this vein, advancing the lead into a second- or third-order branch, producing a stable position. This maneuver is ideal for non-over-the-wire pacing leads, particularly larger-diameter leads, which are useful in patients with a very large venous system. The sheath is then peeled or slipped away, leaving the lead in position.

Telescoping sheaths and the use of over-the-wire leads

Once the sheath has been placed in the coronary sinus, an over-the-wire lead can be directly advanced into a lateral ventricular vein.[46,47] Sometimes, simply advancing the lead while maintaining slight clockwise torque on the sheath so that the lead will be forced to proceed anteriorly, usually into a ventricular vein, is successful. At other times, the lead is advanced to the midportion of the coronary sinus and a flexible wire is advanced, first probing with different sheath orientations to find a ventricular vein; once the wire is seen to go into the ventricular vein, the lead advances over it into a wedge position usually in a second or third order branch of this vein.

Often, however, simple advancement of a wire or lead will cause the lead to track to a very anterior, likely undesirable, position.[46,48] In this situation, the use of a telescoping sheath system is highly effective for placing the lead in a less anterior lateral ventricular vein. Through the guiding sheath placed in the proximal coronary sinus, a sharply curved secondary sheath is advanced into more distal locations of the coronary sinus. Several such curved sheaths are available, usually with a near 90° angle at the tip of the sheath. The inner sheath with the right-angle is now rotated (clockwise) to about a straight anterior position on the RAO projection. A floppy guidewire is repeatedly advanced and withdrawn through the tip of this sheath, directed toward the LV. This to-and-fro movement of the wire continues while the implanter slowly withdraws the inner sheath as a ventricular vein is encountered; the wire will move in through the ventricular vein, allowing several options to place the lead.[31] In one iteration, once the guidewire has cannulated the ventricular vein of interest, the inner sheath is removed and the pacing lead is threaded over this wire in an attempt to get it into the vein of interest at a stable pacing site. In another method, once the wire has actually been placed inside the lateral vein, the inner sheath is tracked along this wire into this vein subselecting it. Using this for support, the main guiding sheath is tracked over the inner guiding sheath into the vein of interest, and (as noted in the description above), using a deflectable catheter, once the sheath is in this location and stable, pacing leads can easily be advanced into this vein into a stable wedged position.

Removing the guiding sheath

Several methods exist for removing the guiding sheath.[31] These include slitting of the guiding sheath, peeling it, and removing it over the pacemaker lead. In trying to remove a guiding sheath over a pacemaker lead pacing the LV, there is a high risk of dislodgment, so that most systems today involve either slitting or peeling of the sheath over the lead.

Slitting a sheath

Although several types of slitters are available, the general principles are the same. First, the lead position in the ventricular venous system should be assessed. If multiple curves have had to be negotiated, either in the proximal coronary sinus or because of tortuosity at the takeoff of the lateral ventricular vein, it is best to slit the lead with a relative floppy wire in place. On the other hand, if a wedged position has been obtained without excessive curvature, a stylet or stiffer wire can be placed all the way to the tip of the lead. If the coronary sinus itself is fairly straight, but an anastomotic branch was used to get to the lateral wall, then a stiffer wire or stylet should be placed in the main body of the coronary sinus. The slitting blade should be attached securely to the lead close to the hub of the sheath. Meticulous attention must be paid to the implanter's hand position. The hand that holds the slitting blade (now secured to the lead) should be balanced against the patient's body and should not move either towards or away from the patient during the slitting maneuver. It is equally important that the other hand (usually the left), which is going to now pull back the sheath against the blade slitting it, should also be stable and the entire slitting maneuver performed in one smooth motion.

Common errors include rotating the sheath to get a comfortable hand position; this should be avoided, as doing so may pull the lead out of the ventricular vein or tributary. Another error is to stutter or repeatedly stop while slitting the sheath. If the sheath is split partway, the implanter should stop to look fluoroscopically. When stopping midway, the sheath may straighten – particularly when just coming out of the ostium of the coronary sinus – and push the lead down toward the inferior vena cava, causing dislodgement. If a smooth maneuver has occurred and the lead is slitting well, an angle of about 30° between the sheath now being pulled towards the operator and the lead should be maintained to avoid entanglement of the proximal portions of the lead as the sheath is being slit back. The slitting blade is then detached from the lead; the lead can now be secured to its sleeve and the sleeve to the underlying pectoral muscle. If a stylet has been placed into the lead, removal of this stylet should also be in smooth single motion. Watching fluoroscopy is not necessary during the slitting maneuver; however, if it is done, the tip of the lead should be watched to see that the motion of this lead does not change as the slitting occurs. The portion of the lead near the tricuspid valve should also be watched carefully. If a loop of the lead in this location is seen to prolapse either into the inferior vena cava or into the tricuspid valve, then excess slack is present; the slitting

maneuver should be halted and the lead pulled back slightly until this excess slack is removed.

Peeling sheaths Similar principles are used when a peelaway sheath needs to be removed. Here it is best to have an assistant stabilize the lead and instruct the assistant not to push the lead in or pull it out, but maintain gentle pressure against the sheath as it is being peeled back. Once again, smooth movement is important to prevent a stutter stop-type movement that could cause the lead to pull out.

Causes of difficulty and potential solutions

Several potential problems may arise in trying to optimally place an LV lead. It may be difficult to thread a pacing lead through a target vein, as judged by the operator. Potential reasons include an acute take off of the tributary or excessive tortuosity proximally. Sometimes, the vein is too small. At other times, it is so large that pacemaker lead contact with the myocardium is poor. The phrenic nerve often crosses the LV near its lateral wall and must be avoided. In this section, we will analyze the most common causes of inadequate lead position or the inability to place an optimal LV pacing lead.

Lead stability and choice of pacing lead

Ideally, once a vein draining the lateral wall of the LV has been cannulated, the lead must be wedged into a stable position. This can be done in one of two ways. First, the lead is advanced into the vein until the lead diameter is greater than the distal portion of the vein. The operator should observe for fluoroscopic lead movement with a cardiac silhouette in each cardiac cycle. If a differential mobility (i.e., the lead tip is moving in one axis while the cardiac silhouette at that site is moving in another) is noted, the lead is not in a wedged position. In the second method, if the lead is much smaller than the distal branches of the vein, it should be maneuvered into a tributary of the main vein of interest, and, if possible, maneuvered further into a subtributary or third-order branch. The eventual orientation of the lead tip in this ideal situation will be parallel to the main portion of the lead in the ventricular

(a) (b)

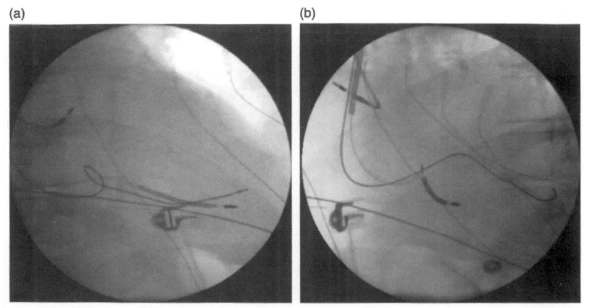

Figure 10.13 Methods to improve the stability of left ventricular pacing leads. (a) Optimal torque placement to allow good catheter tip movement, including deep respiration, required the creation of a loop in a wide coronary sinus. If a loop is recognized, then every effort should be made to perform respiratory maneuvers, and if possible shoulder shrugs, in order to see that the loop is in fact aiding stability. (b) 'U'-shaped positioning with subselection of a branch perpendicular to the main ventricular vein and then subselection of a third-order branch moving back towards the annulus is an excellent radiographic correlate of lead stability.

vein, but with the lead tip pointing to the base (U-shaped placement). It is usually adequate, however, to have the lead cannulate a second-order branch, with the lead tip now being perpendicular to the main portion of the lead in the ventricular vein (L-shaped positioning). Regardless of the final lead tip position, once it is felt that it is stable, the appropriate amount of slack should be given to the lead. If there is inadequate slack on the lead, then it will be round that every time the patient takes a deep inward breath, the lead tip will move slightly to a more proximal position (Figure 10.13). If there is too much lead slack, it will be seen that, on expiration, there is a prolapsing segment of the lead across the tricuspid valve or into the inferior vena cava.

Choice of pacing lead

Many types of LV pacing leads are now available.[46] Essentially, these are either stylet-driven leads, which tend to be of larger French size and diameter, or over-the-wire leads. The latter, in turn, may be relatively straight leads (with or

without small tines) or leads with prominent corkscrew-type curvature, proximal to the lead tip. Although manufacturers often suggest specific leads for specific circumstances or have tried to design leads intended for certain angiographic venous appearances, no clear prospective method is consistent in predicting which lead will produce the most stable lead position in the vein. This is because thresholds may be quite different in proximal and distal portions of the vein, and proximity of the phrenic nerve may cause the operator to select a more basal or more apical location – factors that cannot be determined from simple angiography. The implanter must be willing to try to maneuver any lead to a good stable wedged position as described above. If this does not work – for example in large veins – then, switching to a stylet-driven lead or leads with proximal tertiary curvatures may be necessary.

Valves

Just as valves may guard the ostium of the coronary sinus or a specific ventricular vein,[33] as described above, they may also be found

(a)　　　　　　　　　　　　　　　　(b)

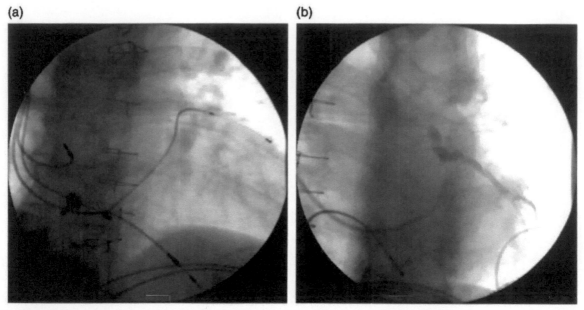

Figure 10.14 (b) The usual circumstance of multiple valves in a large lateral vein. In such circumstances, (a) a stylet-driven lead can be used to negotiate these relatively large valves and obtain an adequate pacing lead position (see text for alternate methods to deal with valves).

within the straight portion of a ventricular vein (Figure 10.14). If an alternative vein or anastomotic system is available. The desired ventricular site (usually the lateral wall), should be chosen. If a vein with multiple valves is the only available method and simple attempts at prolapsing a wire or lead are ineffective, then the following maneuver should be employed. The deflectable catheter should be advanced to the coronary sinus, and a curve should be applied and turned clockwise as described above to engage the ostium of a lateral vein. Once engaged, the catheter should be advanced with gentle pressure and constant forward movement of the sheath to provide stability across the valvular structure. The sheath is then advanced as distally as possible into this vein over the deflectable catheter. The catheter is then removed and a stylet-driven or larger-diameter over-the-wire lead is placed at the tip of the sheath and moved to a wedged position. The sheath is then withdrawn while gentle pressure on the lead is maintained. While the sheath is being withdrawn, it is best to place a soft stylet all the way to the tip of the lead while moving the sheath back in this situation.

Aneurysmal or variceal veins

In patients with congestive heart failure, there can be considerable enlargement of the coronary veins.[49] While this may make it easy to get a wire or pacing lead into the vein, the vein may be so large that the lead tip does not make adequate contact with the myocardium. It is then difficult to get good pacing thresholds, even though the myocardium below may be quite viable. This situation is suspected on fluoroscopy typically in the LAO projection, where the tip of the lead will be found to be moving in a haphazard fashion and not synchronous with the cardiac silhouette movement. In this circumstance, three options can be employed:

- Specific cannulation of a secondary or tertiary branch of the vein can be attempted to try and wedge the lead into these typically smaller branches.
- The lead may be advanced further towards the apex of the heart and then from the apex through another anastomotic branch that may climb back up to the lateral wall either slightly more posterior or slightly more anterior to the initial vein cannulated.

- Larger stylet-driven leads or a lead with prominent curvature can be placed in an attempt to get a better wedged position.

Increased pacing thresholds

Sometimes, an implanter may find an ideal vein and get what appears to be an excellent wedged position on the midlateral wall only to find that the pacing thresholds are unacceptably high or capture is not present even at the highest output. Here, if a thorough preimplant evaluation had been done, whether or not a myocardial scar is present in this location, this would have been known to the implanter. If there was no echocardiographic documentation of scar at the site where the implanter feels he or she has wedged the lead, then the possibility of a very localized area of non-viable myocardium should be considered. Here, pacing with a different vector configuration should be employed – for example from a proximal electrode of a bipolar LV lead (cathode) to the proximal ring or coil of the RV ICD lead, which can give excellent thresholds with a very similar pacing vector. Most importantly, however, the implanter should consider the possibility that the lead position is not stable and properly wedged. Careful fluoroscopic evaluation should be done – primarily to document that the lead tip moves with the cardiac silhouette. If there is any doubt, and the vein was not extremely difficult to subcannulate, then the smaller pacing lead should be removed and a larger stylet-driven lead placed into the subselected vein to obtain better contact.[48]

Increased capture latency

This problem is similar to that described for increased pacing thresholds, except that it can be difficult to detect. Here, the implanter has successfully negotiated a lateral vein or an anastomotic branch to reach the lateral wall. A fluoroscopically wedged position is obtained and the pacing threshold is excellent. All of these features would suggest an optimal lead position. However, when biventricular stimulation is performed, the QRS morphology and echocardiographic pattern of mechanical activation is very similar to right ventricular pacing alone. This is because of unhealthy myocardial tissue at

the site of the pacemaker lead placement, and while the threshold may be acceptable, too much delay occurs between the time of pacing to the onset of the QRS complex. The initial captured myocardium is insufficient to generate a deflection on the QRS complex, and inordinate delay occurs as the initial wavefront has to propagate through partially scarred tissue to eventually exit to relatively healthy myocardium and generate the encryption seen on the surfaced 12 lead ECG as the QRS complex. In this situation, if biventricular simultaneous pacing occurs, a large portion of the ventricle is already depolarized by the RV pacing wavefront, and there is no evidence either electrically or mechanically of pacing from the LV lead (Figure 10.15). Sometimes, the situation can be resolved by setting an offset for the LV lead – often as much as pacing from this lead 50–70 ms prior to stimulating via the RV lead. An important clue to the implanter that this situation may occur is that when placing the lead in such a location there is a long delay from the stimulus artifact to the onset of the QRS complex (capture latency). If other lead positions in or near the lateral wall

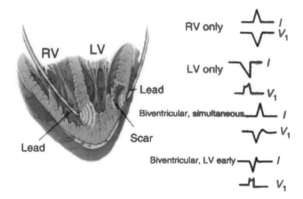

Figure 10.15 This figure illustrates the principles of detecting capture latency. Sometimes, pacing lead location in the lateral wall of the left ventricle (LV) is completely ineffective for resynchronization. Even though capture thresholds may be excellent as can be seen in this figure, the presence of neighboring scar and slow-conducting tissue in the left ventricle results in a right ventricular paced morphology with simultaneous biventricular stimulation to the situation can be corrected by either slightly moving the lead to a more arterior or posterior location or by providing an offset, whereby the left ventricle is stimulated earlier than the right ventricle.

have not yet been tried, this should be attempted. If not, a device that allows a strong LV offset (LV earlier than RV) can be resorted to.

Anodal stimulation

Sometimes, excellent pacing thresholds without undue capture latency are obtained with a stable lead position in the lateral LV wall. However, biventricular stimulation (particularly using an LV configuration with either the proximal or distal LV electrode as the cathode and the RV ring electrode or ICD-RV coil as the anode) may result in a paced morphology and echocardiographic activation pattern consistent with stimulation from the RV lead alone. This phenomenon may be the result of anodal stimulation where (despite configuring the LV electrode as the cathode) stimulation proceeds from the ring electrode (or RV coil) although this electrode is the anode.[50] In some patients, anodal stimulation may occur at higher pacing output, while in others it may occur close to the threshold. The major disadvantage of anodal stimulation is that biventricular stimulation in such situations is effectively two-site stimulation (closely spaced)

from the RV only. When testing the LV lead, the QRS morphology should be monitored to assess the true threshold. For example, if the LV threshold when configured as LV tip to RV ring is found to be 0.5 V at 0.5 ms, on closer scrutiny, one may find that at 3 V at 0.5 ms the paced morphology changes in lead 1 from negative to positive, unless two distinct thresholds are present: 3 V at 0.5 ms is loss of true LV stimulation, and 0.5 V at 0.5 ms is loss of all capture – specifically anodal stimulation. If the implanter recognizes this phenomenon, bipolar stimulation from the LV lead should be tried, and if this is not possible because of the type of pacing lead or poor capture in this configuration, then the lead should be moved to another stable location on the LV lateral wall.

Absent lateral vein

When significant lateral veins are absent, the implanter can utilize an anastamotic vein or access the middle cardiac vein or other posterior vein to access the lateral wall.[51]

The vast majority of hearts show multiple veins draining the lateral wall (Figure 10.16). Sometimes the true lateral vein is small, atretic, or with an

(a) (b)

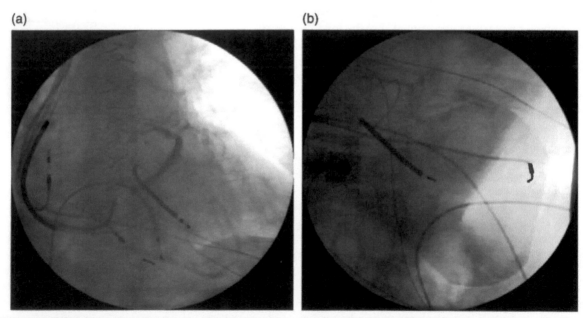

Figure 10.16 This figure illustrates the use of collateral veins to pace the lateral wall. (b) An angiogram showing complex atretic lateral veins. We note, however, multiple collateral veins (some quite large), extending from the middle cardiac vein and posterior veins to the lateral wall. (a) A pacing lead is placed through one of these anastomotic vessels to obtain an excellent location in the lateral wall.

unusual takeoff making cannulation difficult. In these circumstances, either a more posterior vein or an anterolateral vein can be cannulated, and with the use of soft wires a lateral and anastomotic branch or tributary or second-order tributary draining the lateral wall can be subcannulated and the pacing lead advanced to a wedged position at the site. Once again, the implanter should keep in mind that it is not the vein that is the target, but the location on the lateral wall (Figure 10.17). Of course, if phrenic nerve stimulation or a poor pacing threshold was the reason for the inability to get an adequate site in the lateral wall (Figure 10.18), then using the anastomotic branches will be of no use, as the eventual location of the pacing lead is in a similar territory. In these circumstances, another site, either more anteriorly, posteriorly, or perhaps more apically, should be chosen.[52]

Accessing the middle cardiac veins

An important fallback option with which operators should be familiar is the use of methods to cannulate the middle cardiac veins and then subselect the lateral branch to access the LV

free wall. The following maneuver yields a high chance of successfully accomplishing middle cardiac vein cannulation.

Once the sheath has been placed in the proximal portion of the coronary sinus, a deflectable catheter with a slight curve is placed in the main body of the coronary sinus. The catheter is torqued clockwise so that the tip of the catheter points to the ventricle. The catheter is then gradually drawn back in a maneuver similar to that described for subselection of a posterolateral vein, without falling into the posterior or posterolateral vein (if the catheter falls into one of these veins, it is pulled out and the drawback maneuver continues). On approaching the ostium of the coronary sinus, the curve is slightly relaxed and the catheter and the guiding catheter are disengaged from the coronary sinus and pulled up to the RA. Continued clockwise torque is applied as the catheter is pulled back, with to-and-fro movements near the ostium of the coronary sinus. As this maneuver progresses, the catheter will fall into what appears to be a venous structure. Fluoroscopically, it can be difficult to determine whether one

(a) (b)

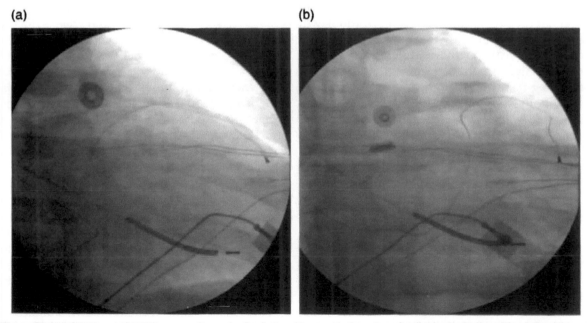

Figure 10.17 RAO (a) and LAO (b) images of a pacing lead placed in an anterior vein and subselectively placed in a lateral branch that drains the lateral wall of the LV. An identical location will be obtained if a lateral vein or a tributary of a posterolateral vein is used. The aim for the implanter is where the lead winds up in pacing the lateral ventricular wall and not the vein that is chosen to get there!

(a) (b)

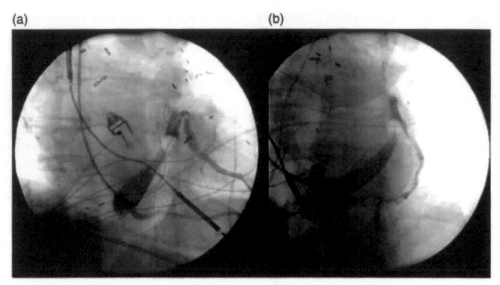

Figure 10.18 RAO (a) and LAO (b) projections during coronary venography, showing a large anastomotic branch between the lateral and middle cardiac venous systems. If the sharp tortuosity and angulation at the take-off of the lateral vein cannot easily be negotiated, then cannulating the posterior vein with the techniques described in the text and subselecting a lateral branch can yield excellent results, with a lower chance of dissection, in less time.

has entered the middle cardiac vein (desirable) or is positioned within the posterior wall of the right ventricle (undesirable, risk of perforation).[53] A gentle attempt at catheter manipulation (applying various curves or torque) will enable the operator to know whether the catheter is truly in the middle cardiac vein – specifically, further clockwise torque or torquing the catheter with a curve in place will not significantly affect either the lead position or the final location within the vein. Once the deflectable catheter is well seated in the middle cardiac vein, the guiding sheath is pulled back to the RA and a relatively straight course is maintained between the deflectable catheter and the guiding sheath. The sheath is then gently advanced into the middle cardiac vein, the deflectable catheter is removed, and the pacing lead is manipulated to a lateral branch of this vein. This maneuver can be very useful when no lateral veins or good anastomotic branches from the posterior or anterior circulation are noted.

Phrenic nerve stimulation

One of the most difficult problems to overcome with left lateral lead placement is extracardiac stimulation. This may take the form of direct diaphragmatic stimulation, left phrenic nerve stimulation, or intercostal stimulation. The left phrenic nerve crosses typically anterior and just lateral to the LA appendage and crosses the ventricle. Basally, in a lateral location, the course of this nerve is variable, and the proximity to the myocardium depends on the degree of ventricular enlargement and the amount of epicardial fat. If a particular tributary of the coronary sinus that was used to place the LV lead results in phrenic nerve stimulation, it is usually best to choose another region of the lateral wall, either more anteriorly or posteriorly, than to try to 'microposition' within that same tributary. Even if one finds a particular pacing output or specific location within a vein site that only intermittently or only at high-output causes phrenic stimulation, the risk of extracardiac stimulation after the patient is mobile and standing is high. If no other option is available, the following maneuvers can be considered to minimize the chance of phrenic stimulation at a site close to the phrenic nerve:

- An intramyocardial perforating vein can be subcannulated. Here, a telescoping sheath is advanced into the lateral or other ventricular vein and, on using a guidewire with the tip of a right-angled sheath pointing towards the ventricular myocardium (not away from, but towards the epicardium) as the wire is advanced, brief ventricular ectopy will often be seen. The pacing lead is then threaded over the wire to this intermyocardial location with less likelihood of phrenic stimulation.

- A different pacing configuration (e.g., switching to another paced vector such as with the proximal LV electrode (negative) to the right ventricular ring electrode (positive) may be associated with less phrenic stimulation.
- Cannulation of a second- or third-order branch of a ventricular vein can be used to move the lead slightly more posterior or slightly more anterior, but in a very strongly wedged position such that the implanter feels the chance of even microdislodgement is very low. Once again, we should emphasize that it is best to avoid the region or vein

near a site where phrenic nerve stimulation was obtained, while remembering the options discussed above in cases where no other pacing site is possible (Figure 10.19).

Sometimes, even with the best efforts to place a lead in a stable location on the lateral wall, pacing thresholds or phrenic nerve stimulation may be poor, or there may be a simple inability to access the veins draining this region of the LV free wall. Here, a decision needs to be made whether to refer the patient for surgical epicardial lead implantation or accept a less than ideal location for the endocardial coronary sinus lead, either in the anterior lateral portions of the LV free wall or in a posterior portion of the LV.[54] The criteria that should be used to make this decision are as follows:

- If the reason for the inability to place a lead on the lateral wall was multiple sites of phrenic stimulation or very poor thresholds despite good lead position, and a correlated

(a) (b)

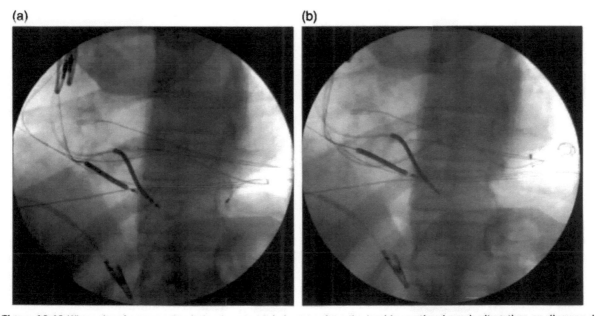

Figure 10.19 When phrenic nerve stimulation is noted it is best to place the lead in another branch altogether, as discussed in the text. Sometimes, as in this patient, direct diaphragmatic stimulation is noted when the lead tip in a given branch points further inferiorly. Wedging the lead tip in a more superior orientation by subselecting a second- and third-order vein overcomes this difficulty, while maintaining an excellent lateral venous pacing site.

echocardiographic presence of a scar at this site, it is unlikely that an epicardial implant will directly overcome this problem. If the myocardium of the lateral wall is extremely poor, placing an epicardial lead at this location will not change the threshold. Although the phrenic nerve can be manipulated surgically, often the surgeon will place the epicardial lead in a slightly more anterior position not dissimilar to what may have been performed with an endovascular approach.[55]

- If the primary reason for the inability to place the lead in the lateral wall was inability to access one of the lateral veins or tributaries or anastomotic branches, and echocardiographically the lateral wall appears to be an ideal site to place the pacing lead, the patient is likely to benefit from an epicardial approach.

- If the patient's clinical situation is precarious and there is a history of previous cardiac surgery (where multiple adhesions may be present), it is probably best to accept a slightly anterior or posterior location rather than subject the patient to an operative procedure.

Newer methods to place epicardial leads are being developed, including using subxiphoid pericardial access, limited thoracotomy, and thoracoscopy. LV epicardial pacing leads have also evolved, with more secure and reliable leads becoming available.

COMPLICATIONS ASSOCIATED WITH LV LEAD IMPLANTATION

In addition to the complications known to occur with standard pacemaker and ICD procedures (pneumothorax, SVC perforation, RV perforation, infection, pocket hematoma, etc.) some untoward events occur specifically with LV lead implantation.[56] Usually, with careful lead and sheath manipulation and an accurate knowledge of cardiac and venous anatomy, these complications can be avoided. Nevertheless, even with the utmost caution, complications may occur, and the implanter should be familiar with methods to promptly recognize and treat the patient should they occur[57] (Table 10.3).

Table 10.3 Avoiding complications with left ventricular lead implantation

1. Watching catheter/sheath/lead movement in the left anterior oblique and right anterior oblique fluoroscopic projections
2. 'Benching' (holding secure) deflectable catheters or introducers when advancing a guiding sheath
3. Gently pulling back on deflectable catheters/introducers or guidewire when advancing a guiding sheath in the venous system
4. Understanding when inadvertent subselection of an atrial or ventricular vein has occurred, and avoiding further attempts to advance the catheter/sheath or pacing lead
5. Recognizing unusual tortuosity in the venous system or acute take-off of ventricular veins, and using the appropriate maneuver to overcome this difficulty (see text)
6. Observing for characteristic movements of the tip of a lead or a guidewire when making optimal myocardial contact (moving with the cardiac silhouette), or without myocardial contact (to-and-fro movement of the lead tip distinct from that of the heart), and lead or wire perforation (excessive mobility of the lead tip or wire suggests entry to the pericardial space).
7. If perforation or entrance to the pericardium of a wire is suspected, avoiding attempts to advance the guiding sheath.
8. Avoiding forceful dye injection when the tip of the guidewire does not advance further in the venous system (dissection, subselection of an atrial vein)

Perforation

Perforation may occur through the coronary sinus, in the great cardiac veins, or in one of the ventricular branches or their subbranches. Potential steps during the implantation procedure where the risk of perforation is high include attempts to pass a deflectable catheter or sheath deeper into the coronary sinus despite a highly tortuous proximal portion. When trying to wedge a pacing lead into a second- or third-order ventricular venous branch, the lead may perforate through the thin-walled veins. Another time when perforation may occur is during attempts to cannulate the middle cardiac veins and with the downward (posterior) to-and-fro movements of the catheter or lead in trying to access the middle cardiac vein – either this vein itself or the posterior wall of the RV may be perforated. If perforation of a vein occurs, the patient must be monitored closely for cardiac tamponade. In general, distal coronary vein perforations are well tolerated, even when the sheath penetrates through the vein. However, more proximal veins – and importantly the great cardiac vein – when perforated may lead to sudden cardiac collapse from tamponade. The effusions may be contained posteriorly (including effusions tracking into the oblique sinus), particularly when the patient is lying down.

Dissection

Coronary venous dissection sometimes occurs during attempts to engage the coronary sinus or when trying to advance catheters, sheaths, or pacing leads further into the vein and into the ventricular branches. The exact histopathological nature[15] of venous dissection has not been described clearly, but this term is applied to a fairly characteristic angiographic appearance. Often, what is noted is difficulty in advancing a catheter, guidewire, or pacing lead through a portion of the coronary sinus where one does not expect such difficulty (e.g. the coronary sinus itself, or the great cardiac vein). When contrast is injected, there is staining of the vessel wall and progressive reduction in the size of the venous lumen. Sometimes the staining is minimal and the implant procedure otherwise proceeds as usual. In some instances, however, there is complete luminal occlusion, and the procedure has to be aborted. In such cases, reattempting the implant in 2–3 months' time has been successful – apparently because of resolution of the dissection.

The primary causes of dissection include attempting to advance a large guiding sheath into a tortuous vein without an adequate-sized guiding catheter within the lumen of the guiding sheath. As described above, if a deflectable catheter has been used to gain access to the coronary sinus, the catheter itself should be kept still (benched) or pulled back slightly while advancing the sheath. Dissection may occur if there is inadvertent forward pressure on the catheter as the sheath is being advanced, causing perforation or dissection distally, or if an inadequately sized catheter (or no catheter) is within the sheath as it is being advanced (the sheath may then be angled against the vessel wall, scraping its endothelial surface). Another less widely recognized (but equally important) cause of dissection occurs when there has been inadvertent subselection of an atrial vein by a guiding catheter, sheath, or guidewire. With inadvertent subselection, the guiding catheter may be lodged within a relatively small atrial vein. If a sheath is advanced further into the main body of the coronary sinus, an unwanted shearing force is created at the junction of the coronary sinus and the atrial vein, and dissection may occur.

If coronary vein dissection is recognized at implant, a floppy guidewire should be advanced from the proximal portion of the coronary sinus and into the true lumen to a distal branch of the coronary venous system. If the wire advances freely into a lateral or anterolateral vein, then, with no further attempts at angiography or to move the sheath, a lead should be threaded over this wire into the desired ventricular branch. Complete luminal occlusion has occurred, and the site of this deflection/occlusion is fairly distal, when access is to the more proximal lateral and posterolateral vein. However, if a proximal dissection has occurred, the technique described above to cannulate the middle cardiac vein can be very useful, and can be utilized with further subselection of the lateral branches of this vein, even with very proximal dissections and occlusions.

There are no reported pathological sequelae of coronary vein dissection other than the difficulty with implantation. This is presumably because of anastomotic venous drainage that occurs between the branches of the coronary veins and the Thebesian venous system (see below).

Ventricular arrhythmia

In some patients, premature ventricular contractions and non-sustained ventricular tachycardia may occur while advancing the lead. These presumably occur because of subselection of a perforating intramyocardial vein and are generally not associated with clinical arrhythmia or other complications. Although not technically an implant complication, some patients may develop increased ventricular arrhythmia, the presumed etiology of this phenomena is that ventricular pacing at certain sites on the epicardium may more easily induce re-entrant tachycardia. If the phenomenon is recognized during the implant procedure – specifically during threshold testing – the lead should be moved to a neighboring myocardial area to see if it persists. Implant electrophysiological testing using the LV and RV leads can also be performed.

Worsening of congestive heart failure

Some patients report worsened congestive heart failure after biventricular lead implantation. This is generally not a complication of the implant per se, and its causes include inappropriate timing with the pacemaker between the atrial lead and the ventricular lead or between the two ventricular leads. However, if an extreme increase in capture latency is noted during the implant procedure, or marked intraatrial conduction delay from the chosen atrial pacing site is seen, such untoward effects may be anticipated and either the atrial or the LV lead should be moved to another location. If during the implant procedure, in the immediate postimplant procedure, adverse hemodynamic parameters (lower blood pressure) or subjective dyspnea are reported, extracardiac stimulation, perforation, or effective simultaneous atrioventricular pacing should be looked for and corrected as appropriate.

SPECIFIC CONSIDERATIONS IN LESS COMMONLY OCCURRING CIRCUMSTANCES

Right-sided implantation

As mentioned briefly earlier in this chapter, because of an additional right-angled curve in the venous system between the subclavian/brachiocephalic vein and the superior vena cava (SVC) occurring with right-sided implants (with a sharper curvature than experienced from the left brachiocephalic system), the maneuvers required to cannulate the coronary sinus or subselect ventricular veins discussed above are identical for right- and left-sided implants. However, some important differences remain. The main issue is with the use of guiding sheaths to help cannulate the coronary sinus. Most guiding

sheaths that are presently available are designed for left-sided implants, and help 'balance' the sheath at the SVC–RA junction on the right or lateral portion of the SVC. If a similar sheath is used from the right side, then, because of the difference between the two sides in the heights of the brachiocephalic and subclavian veins entering the SVC, the sheath will balance at a lower site and on the septal wall (the left side of the SVC), directing the sheath to the lateral wall of the tricuspid annulus. If the operator tries to compensate for this by torquing the sheath to make the lumen point towards the coronary sinus, then the beneficial balance of the sheath on the SVC or RA wall is lost, again causing the tip of the sheath to point too superiorly. Thus, either specific sheaths designed for right-sided implantation or a neutral sheath and deflectable catheter tend to be more beneficial in cannulating the coronary sinus. The author's preference is to use a very slightly curved guiding sheath and a deflectable catheter. The catheter and sheath are both advanced to the tricuspid annulus near the septum, and a 'back-bend' is then applied on the catheter to gain contact to the posterior wall. In this position, sharp counterclockwise torque is applied to the system, withdrawing the catheter to cannulate the coronary sinus. Once cannulated, a slightly curved sheath should be advanced just into the coronary sinus, with the torque on the guiding catheter and sheath remaining identical. The catheter is then removed, and the sheath can be used to access the veins as described above.

Congenital heart disease

A detailed discussion of venous anatomy and lead postioning in various congential anomalies is beyond the scope of this textbook, and is infrequently encountered in clinical practice.[32] Guiding principles for situations that occur more commonly are detailed below.

Peristent left superior vena cava

During fetal development, a left SVC is present that drains into the coronary sinus. This structure persists in about 1% of the adult population. A proportion of patients with a persistent left SVC may not have a right SVC or may not have anastomoses between the two SVCs. In such situations, when performing a left-sided CRT implant, the sheath and leads will enter the left SVC and directly into the coronary sinus. An anatomical fact worth noting is that the left SVC (or its vestigal remnant, the vein of Marshall) occurs in the same vertical axis as the posterolateral vein draining the ventricular myocardium.[58] Thus, when the coronary sinus is entered, if a wire is advanced from the left SVC itself, the posterolateral vein may be cannulated (if no Vieussens' valve is present), and the lead can be placed in this vein. Because of the angulation between the left SVC and the coronary sinus and the fact that the coronary veins can be massively enlarged when a left SVC is present, lead stability is a major issue when implanting a left-sided lead in these patients. The author's preference in this situation has been to enter the coronary sinus with a deflectable catheter, and then to angle the catheter to the more distal portions of the coronary sinus (not towards the ostium) and place a slightly curved sheath to enter the coronary sinus, but to point the tip of the sheath away from the ostium and towards the distal vessels.[59] Often, this maneuver provides stability to attempt subselection of various anterolateral veins and anastomotic branches. Once the sheath has been deployed in the manner described above, the lead can be advanced to an anterior or anterolateral vein and subselect veins draining the lateral wall. Larger, perhaps stylet-driven, leads are preferable in these large venous systems. The lead should be advanced to at least a third-order branch, preferably producing a U-shaped pattern (a lead in the main body of the vein subselects a right-angled branch and then subselects a right-angled branch of the secondary branch going back towards the annulus), as mentioned above.

If the operator prefers to place a sheath closer to the ostium of the coronary sinus, a straight sheath should be used and preferential cannulation of the middle cardiac vein or a posterior vein attempted.

Anomalous origin of the coronary sinus

Sometimes, the ostium of the coronary sinus is occluded by either a thebesian valve or another cause of stenosis. An atrial vein draining onto the interatrial septum or a ventricular vein anastomosing with the thebesian vein network (see below) may enter the region of the tricuspid valve. RA angiography as well as the levo phase of coronary arteriography can be used to visualize the drainage pattern of these anomalous veins, and a deflectable catheter can be used to cannulate the orifice using similar techniques detailed above for overcoming difficulty because of a large RA. It can be beneficial to place the deflectable catheter and sheath in the region of the coronary sinus while coronary arteriography is being performed, and with continued fluoroscopy during the levo phase, the anomalous origin can be visualized and attempts made to cannulate the vein. One rare anomaly of the coronary sinus is when all of the ventricular veins drain into one large vein emptying into the proximal coronary sinus, while a similar parallel vein drains the atrial branches. This should be suspected if on angiography only atrial branches are seen. If this occurs, the sheath should be withdrawn closer to the proximal coronary sinus and slight clockwise torque applied to enter the ventricular portion of this vein.

Finally, in some patients, following cardiac surgery (e.g., for Ebstein's anomaly) the coronary sinus ostium may be found below the tricuspid valve.[60] In these cases, the deflectable catheter or guiding sheath should be advanced to the RV and sharp counterclockwise torque applied with continuous brief dye injections or probing with a catheter on the ventricular myocardium until the vein is entered.

Non-coronary sinus endocardial pacing lead deployment

In certain uncommon instances, the coronary sinus is either occluded or completely covered by a occlusive thebesian valve. Although epicardial lead implantation can be performed in this situation, sometimes alternative venous drainage can be used. An intramyocardial plexus of veins called thebesian veins (not to be confused with the thebesian valve) may be used.[61] In the normal heart, these veins drain the RV myocardium, but with an occluded coronary sinus they may drain a large portion of the LV myocardium as well.

Table 10.4 Overcoming difficulties with left ventricular lead implantation

	Reason for difficulty	Solution
Accessing the coronary sinus		
Prominent sub-eustachian pouch	Guiding sheath or catheter prolapses into pouch	• Use of large curved guiding sheath balanced on high RA • Deflectable catheter with back bend moved into coronary sinus from higher interatrial septum (see text for details)
Prominent thebesian valve	May be nearly occlusive, not allowing access	• Enter from inferior and ventricular portion, where thebesian valve is least prominent. • Use of radiofrequency energy • Guidewire and balloon dilation of coronary ostium
Large LV	Coronary sinus fluoroscopic appearance different in LAO projection	• Understand that angle formed between coronary sinus and inferior cardiac silhouette becomes larger with larger LV
Large RA	Failure of guiding catheter or sheath to reach interatrial septum and ostium of coronary sinus	• Use of large curved guiding sheath • Looping of large curved deflectable catheter and using back bend to probe septum for coronary sinus • Finding fossa ovalis, or bundle of His, and working inferiorly to reach coronary sinus from roof
Advancing within the coronary sinus Stenosis/spasm	Narrowing of lumen not allowing a guiding sheath to advance	• Passing guidewire and performing low-pressure balloon dilation • Accessing ventricular branches proximal to stenosis/spasm and subselecting lateral branches of proximal posterior vein
Valves in the coronary sinus	Curling up of guidewires and difficulty inadvancing a deflectable catheter	• Using stiffer guidewire • Using deflectable catheter, probing for opening of a semiocclusive valve • Using a ventricular vein proximal to valve, and subselecting lateral branches of proximal posterior vein to access lateral wall
Excessive tortuosity	Wires/sheath/deflectable catheters may cause dissection with force applied perpendicular to tortuous segment	• Use soft guidewires with constant venography to assess direction of tortuosity and advance guidewire, or deflectable catheter, and sheath at angles alternating with each other (see text for details)
Inadvertent subselection of an atrial vein by a leading catheter or guidewire	Dissection of perforation occurs if sheath is advanced with lead tip, or wire tip, lodged in an atrial branch	• Understand atrial and ventricular orientation of lead/wires/catheters in RAO projection
Placement of the pacing lead on lateral LV Lead instability	Potential for dislodgement; changing pacing vector; changing pacing threshold; ventricular ectopy	• Wedging lead into a second-order branch • Understanding fluoroscopic appearance of under- and over-slacked leads (see text)

Table 10.4 Overcoming difficulties with left ventricular lead implantation—cont'd

	Reason for difficulty	Solution
Absent lateral veins	Problem with placing lead in desired midlateral free-wall location	• Using second- and third-order branches of veins to produce 'U-shaped' or 'L-shaped' lead tip (see text) • Using posterior or anterior veins and subselecting anastomotic branches that drain the lateral wall • Using middle cardiac vein and understanding specific cannulation maneuver for this vein (see text)
Extensively diseased myocardial tissue on free wall	Increased pacing thresholds; increased capture latency	• Maximizing tissue contact • Placing leads slightly anterolateral or slightly posterolateral to lateral scar • Understanding inappropriate paced morphologies on ECG even with good capture thresholds (see text)
Small/atretic lateral ventricular veins	Risk of dissection and difficulty placing a vein in distal or midportion of the free wall	• Using anastomotic branches or second-order branches from anterolateral or posterolateral circulation
Large/variceal ventricular veins	Inadequate myocardial contact as lead is free in large ventricular vein	• Using larger stylet-driven leads • Using larger over-the-wire leads with prominent proximal 'corkscrew' curvatures • Subselection of second-, third-, or fourth-order branches until smaller veins are reached
Phrenic nerve stimulation	Optimal pacing site if in proximity of phrenic nerve may result in positional or intermittent diaphragmatic stimulation	• Change configuration option (e.g., proximal rather than distal bipolar LV lead electrode as the cathode) • Avoid repositioning lead in same main venous branch • Avoid using lower output (> capture threshold but < phrenic nerve threshold), but rather reposition lead in another ventricular vein

ECG, electrocardiogram; LAO, left arterior oblique; LV, left ventricle; RA, right atrium; RAO, right arterior oblique.

RV angiography, if performed, can identify the ostia of these veins. If one of them is large, a deflectable catheter and sheath can be used to cannulate it and thread the lead and wire to a lateral branch draining the LV. If ventricular ectopy is noted when trying to advance the lead, then it is likely that a normal thebesian vein without anastomosis to the lateral wall has been cannulated, and the lead should not be left in this location because of possible ventricular arrhythmia. Gentle selective venography can identify branches to the lateral wall allowing the pacing lead to be placed at an adequate site the lateral wall. Other veins that should be mentioned in this context are the subdiaphragmatic, pericardiophrenic, and suprasplenic veins, which drain either the pericardial structures or (in the case of the subdiaphragmatic veins) the subdiaphragmatic and suprasplenic tissues.[62] The veins run from left to right and drain into the inferior vena cava about 1 cm below the floor of the coronary sinus. In some patients, these veins can be quite large and it is possible to cannulate them. In fact, leads placed in these veins can provide reasonable ventricular sensing and ventricular capture. However, the risks of diaphragmatic stimulation, even if not seen on implantation, are very high and the vein should not be used to place a pacing lead. The main reason to be aware of these veins is to understand any unusual angiographic or fluoroscopic patterns encountered during the implantation procedure. The best differentiating feature between the subdiaphragmatic vein and the lateral branches of the middle cardiac vein (which they are often confused) is to observe the effect of respiration. Branches of the middle cardiac vein will move with the cardiac cycle, with few differences in the mobility of the lead with respiratory variation. On the other hand, a lead placed in a subdiaphragmatic vessel will move with the cardiac motion, but only in expiration, where the inferior wall of the heart and diaphragm are close together. With deep inspiration, the motion of the lead changes and becomes much less pronounced.

SUMMARY

The procedure of implanting an LV lead is straightforward in principle. Vascular access is obtained, and then the sheath or lead delivery system is placed in the RA posteriorly, the coronary sinus is cannulated, the sheath is advanced within the coronary sinus, and a pacing lead advanced to a secure position on the lateral wall through one of the lateral veins. While this uncomplicated sequence of implantion is ideal, several potential difficulties do arise. In this chapter, we have reviewed the relevant anatomy, including fluoroscopic anatomy, to allow each implanter to develop his or her system to troubleshoot these difficult situations. Recommendations for specific maneuvers to overcome common causes of difficulty have also been described (and are summarized in Table 10.4). As newer guiding sheaths, leads, and information from the heart failure and echocardiographic literature emerge telling us more about the best way and where to place the leads, some of the difficulties involved and techniques to overcome these problems described above will hopefully have become obsolete.

REFERENCES

1. Gras D, Leclercq C, Tang AS, et al. Cardiac resynchronization therapy in advanced heart failure: the multicenter InSync clinical study. Eur J Heart Fail 2002;4:311–20.
2. Casey C, Knight BP. Cardiac resynchronization pacing therapy. Cardiology 2004;101:72–8.
3. Ross HM, Kocovic DZ. Cardiac resynchronization therapy for heart failure. Curr Treat Options Cardiovasc Med 2004;6:365–70.
4. Asirvatham SJ, Hayes DL. Biventricular device implantation. In: Hayes DL, ed. Resynchronization and Defibrillation for Heart Failure: A Practical Approach. Oxford: Blackwell/Futura, 2004:139–62.
5. Auricchio A, Klein H, Tockman B. Transvenous biventricular pacing for heart failure: Can the obstacles be overcome? Am J Cardiol 1999;83:136D–42D.
6. Asirvatham SJ. Biventricular device implantation. In: Hayes DL, ed. Resynchronization and Defibrillation for Heart Failure: A Practical Approach. Oxford: Blackwell/Futura, 2004:99–137.
7. Goitein O, Lacomis JM, Gorcsan J 3rd, Schwartzman D. Left ventricular pacing lead implantation: potential utility of multimodal image integration. Heart Rhythm 2006; 3:91–4.
8. Oginosawa Y, Abe H, Nakashima Y. The incidence and risk factors for venous obstruction after implantation of transvenous pacing leads. Pacing Clin Electrophysiol 2002;25:1605–11.
9. Magney J, Flynn D, Parsons J. Anatomical mechanisms explaining damage to pacemaker leads, defibrillator leads, and failure of central venous catheter adjacent to the sternoclavicular joing. Pacing Clin Electrophysiol 1993;16:373–6.
10. Leon A, Delurgio D, Mera F. Practical approach to implanting left ventricular pacing leads for cardiac resynchronization. J Cardiovasc Electrophysiol 2005;16: 100–5.
11. Daoud EG, Kalbfleisch SJ, Hummel JD, et al. Implantation techniques and chronic lead parameters of biventricular pacing dual-chamber defibrillators. J Cardiovasc Electrophysiol 2002;13:964–70.
12. Ho S, Sanchez-Quintana D, Becker A. A review of the coronary venous system: a road less traveled. Heart Rhythm 2004;1:107–12.
13. Grzybiak M. Morphology of the coronary sinus and contemporary cardiac electrophysiology. Folia Morphol (Warsz) 1996;55:272–3.
14. Artrip JH, Sukerman D, Dickstein ML, Spotnitz HM. Transesophageal echocardiography guided placement of a coronary sinus pacing lead. Ann Thorac Surg 2002; 74:1254–6.
15. Asirvatham S, Packer D. Evidence of electrical conduction within the coronary sinus musculature by noncontact mapping. Circulation 1999;100(Suppl 1):I-850.

16. Asirvatham SJ, Bruce CJ, Friedman PA. Advances in imaging for cardiac electrophysiology. Coronary Artery Dis 2003;14:3–13.

17. Gerber T, Sheedy C, Bell M, et al. Evaluation of the coronary venous system using electronbeam computed tomography. Int J Cardiovasc Imaging 2001;17:55–75.

18. Altun A, Akdemir O, Erdogan O, Aslan O, Ozbay G. Left ventricular pacemaker lead insertion through the foramen ovale – a case report. Angiology 2002;53:609–11.

19. Shalaby AA. Utilization of intracardiac echocardiography to access the coronary sinus for left ventricular lead placement. Pacing Clin Electrophysiol 2005;28:493–7.

20. Nazarian S, Knight B, Dickfeld T. Direct visualization of coronary sinus ostium and branches with a flexible steerable fiberoptic infrared endoscope. Heart Rhythm 2005;2:844–8.

21. von Ludinghausen M. Clinical anatomy of cardiac veins. Surg Radiol Anat 1987:159–68.

22. Gulotta S. Transvenous cardiac pacing. Techniques for optimal electrode positioning and prevention of coronary sinus placement. Circulation 1970;42:701–18.

23. Al-Khadra AS. Use of preshaped sheath to plan and facilitate cannulation of the coronary sinus for the implantation of cardiac resynchronization therapy devices: preshaped sheath for implantation of biventricular devices. Pacing Clin Electrophysiol 2005;28:489–92.

24. Maros T, Racz L, Plugor S, Maros T. Contributions to the morphology of the human coronary sinus. Anat Anz 1983;154:133–44.

25. Asirvatham S. Anatomy of the coronary sinus. In: Yu C, Hayes D, Auricchio A, eds. Cardiac Resynchronization Therapy: Oxford: Blackwell Futura, 2006.

26. Ollitrault J, Ritter P, Mabo P, et al. Long-term experience with a preshaped left ventricular pacing lead. Pacing Clin Electrophysiol 2003;26:185–8.

27. Maurer G, Punzengruber C, Haendchen R, et al. Retrograde coronary venous contrast echocardiography: assessment of shunting and delination of regional myocardium in the normal and ischemic and canine heart. J Am Coll Cardiol 1984;4:577–86.

28. Sethna D, Moffitt E. An appreciation of the coronary circulation. Anesth Analg 1986;65:294–305.

29. Gilard M, Mansourati J, Etienne Y, et al. Angiographic anatomy of the coronary sinus and its tributaries. Pacing Clin Electrophysiol 1998;21:2280–4.

30. Melow D, Prudencio L, Kusnir C, et al. Angiography of the coronary venous system. Used in clinical electrophysiology. Arq Bras Cardiol 1998;70:409–13.

31. Pepper C, Davidson N, Ross D. Use of a long preshaped sheath to faciliate cannulation of the coronary sinus at electrophysiologic study. J Cardiovasc Electrophysiol 2001; 12:1335–7.

32. Zanoschi C. [Malformation of the coronary sinus]. Rev Med Chir Soc Nat Iasi 1986;90:749–52. [in Romanian]

33. Duda B, Grzybiak M. Variability of valve configuration in the lumen of the coronary sinus in the adult human heart. Folia Morphol (Warsz) 2000;59:207–9.

34. Hansky B, Lamp B, Minami K, et al. Coronary vein balloon angioplasty for left ventricular pacemaker lead implantation. J Am Coll Cardiol 2002;40:2144–9.

35. Sandler DA, Feigenblum DY, Bernstein NE, Holmes DS, Chinitz LA. Cardiac vein angioplasty for biventricular pacing. Pacing Clin Electrophysiol 2002;25:1788–9.

36. Lawo T. [Anatomy, special features and angiographic assessment of the coronary sinus]. Herzschrittmacherther Elektrophysiol 2006;17(Suppl 1):I1–6. [in German]

37. D'Cruz I, Shala M, Johns C. Echocardiography of the coronary sinus in adults. Clin Cardiol 2000;23: 149–54.

38. Duda B, Grzybiak M. Main tributaries of the coronary sinus in the adult human heart. Folia Morphol 1998;57:353–9.

39. Cendrowska-Pinkosz M, Urbanowicz Z. Analysis of the course and the ostium of the oblique vein of the left atrium. Folia Morphol (Warsz) 2000;59:163–6.

40. Gasparini M, Mantica M, Galimberti P, et al. Is the left ventricular lateral wall the best lead implantation site for cardiac resynchronization therapy? Pacing Clin Electrophysiol 2003;26:162–8.

41. Cha YM, Rea RF, Asirvatham SJ, et al. Responders of cardiac resynchronization predicts long-term survival. J Card Fail 2006;12(6 Suppl 1):S46 (Abst 152).

42. Talreia D, Gami A, Edwards W, et al. Coronary venous drainage of the lateral left ventricle: implications for biventricular pacing. Pacing Clin Electrophysiol 2003;26(2 part II):S135 (Abst 539).

43. Asirvatham SJ, Talreja DR, Gami AS, Edwards WD. Coronary venous drainage of the lateral left ventricle: Implications for biventricular pacing. Circulation 2001;104(17 Suppl):II619.

44. Hayes DL, Wang PJ, Sackner-Bernstein J, Asirvatham SJ. In: Hayes DL, ed. Resynchronization and Defibrillation for Heart Failure: A Practical Approach. Oxford: Blackwell/Futura; 2004:209–28.

45. Ortale J, Gabriel C, Marquez C. The anatomy of the coronary sinus and its tributaries. Surg Radiol Anat 2001;23:15–21.

46. Ellery S, Paul V, Prenner G, et al. A new endocardial 'over-the-wire' or stylet-driven left ventricular lead: first clinical experience. Pacing Clin Electrophysiol 2005;28(Suppl 1):S31–5.

47. Geske JB, Goldstein RN, Stambler BS. Novel steerable telescoping catheter system for implantation of left ventricular pacing leads. J Interv Card Electrophysiol 2005;12:83-9.

48. Sack S, Heinzel S, Dagres N, et al. Stimulation of the left ventricle through the coronary sinus with a newly developed 'over-the-wire' lead system – early experiences

with lead handeling and positioning. Europace 2001;3:317–23.

49. Potkin B, Roberts W. Size of coronary sinus at necropsy in subjects without cardiac disease and in patients with various cardiac conditions. Am J Cardiol 1987;50: 1418–21.

50. Abe H, Oginosawa Y, Kawakami K, Nagatomo T, Nakashima Y. Clinical advantage of neutral anode positioning feature in recent pacemaker generator. J Uoeh 2003;25:13–22.

51. Meinertz T. A study of coronary sinus, the middle cardiac vein and the aortic arch as well as ductus Botalli in a number of mammal hearts. Gagenbaurs Morthol Jahrb 1966;109:473–500.

52. Yoda M, Hansky B, Schulte-Eistrup S, Koerfer R, Minami K. Left ventricular pacing through the anterior interventricular vein in a patient with mechanical tricuspid, aortic and mitral valves. Ann Thorac Surg 2005; 80:328–30.

53. Kozlowski D, Kozluk E, Piataowska A, et al. The middle cardiac vein as a key for 'posteroseptal' space – a morphological point of view. Folia Morphol (Warsz) 2001;60:293–6.

54. Kleine P, Gronefeld G, Dogan S, et al. Robotically enhanced placement of left ventricular epicardial electrodes during implantation of a biventricular implantable cardioverter defibrillator system. Pacing Clin Electrophysiol 2002;25:989–91.

55. Mair H, Sachweh J, Meuris B, et al. Surgical epicardial left ventricular lead versus coronary sinus lead placement in biventricular pacing. Eur J Cardiothorac Surg 2005;27:235–42.

56. Gasparini M, Lunati M, Bocchiardo M, et al. Cardiac resynchronization and implantable cardioverter defibrillator therapy: preliminary results from the InSync Implantable Cardioverter Defibrillator Italian Registry. Pacing Clin Electrophysiol 2003;26:148–51.

57. Niu HX, Hua W, Wang FZ, et al. Complications of cardiac resynchronization therapy in patients with congestive heart failure. Chin Med J (Engl) 2006;119:449–53.

58. Asirvatham S, Johnson SB, Wahl MR, Roman-Gonzalez J, Packer DL. Can the ligament of Marshall be ablated with energy delivery at the ostium of the left-sided pulmonary veins? Circulation 2000;102(18 Suppl):II484.

59. Santoscoy R, Walters H, Ross R, Lyons J, Hakimi M. Coronary sinus ostial atresia with persistent left superior vena cava. Ann Thorac Surg 1996;61:879–82.

60. van Gelder BM, Elders J, Bracke FA, Meijer A. Implantation of a biventricular pacing system in a patient with a coronary sinus not communicating with the right atrium. Pacing Clin Electrophysiol 2003;26:1294–6.

61. Ansari A. Anatomy and clinical significance of ventricular Thebesian veins. Clin Anat 2001;14:102–10.

62. Vaseghi M, Cesario DA, Ji S, et al. Beyond coronary sinus angiography: the value of coronary arteriography and identification of the pericardiophrenic vein during left ventricular lead placement. Pacing Clin Electrophysiol 2005;28:185–90.

11

Optimization of atrioventricular delay during cardiac resynchronization therapy

S Serge Barold, Arzu Ilercil, Stéphane Garrigue, and Bengt Herweg

Atrioventricular delay • Prolonged AV delay • Short AV delay • Optimal AV delay • Invasive and non-invasive determination of LV dP/dt$_{max}$ • Echocardiography • What is the best echocardiographic method to optimize AV delay? • Alternative techniques to echocardiography • AV optimization during activity • Long-term evaluation of AV delay • Fusion with spontaneous ventricular activation: beneficial or harmful? • Intra- and interatrial conduction delay • Late atrial sensing (intraatrial conduction delay) • Effect of rate smoothing on AV delay • Device-based automatic optimization of AV delay • AV optimization in major trials • Potential of device-based automatic optimization of AV interval

ATRIOVENTRICULAR DELAY

The atrioventricular (AV) interval during AV sequential pacing influences left ventricular (LV) systolic performance by modulating preload. However, the value of AV optimization in patients with severe congestive heart failure (CHF) has been questioned because the high LV filling pressure may minimize the preload contribution of atrial systole. The majority of the acute and long-term benefit from cardiac resynchronization therapy (CRT) is independent of the programmed AV interval.[1] The influence of the AV delay appears to be less important than the proper choice of LV pacing site.[2] Nevertheless, programming of the left-sided AV delay is important in CRT patients. Appropriate AV interval timing can maximize the benefit of CRT, and if programmed poorly, it has the potential to curtail the beneficial effects. Optimization will not convert a non-responder to a responder, but may convert an under-responder to improved status.

The optimal AV delay in CRT patients exhibits great variability from patient to patient.[1,3] This suggests that an empirically programmed AV delay interval is suboptimal in many patients. Thus, empiric programming of the AV delay is generally not recommended.

Optimized AV synchrony is achieved by the AV delay setting that provides the best left atrial (LA) contribution to LV filling, the maximum stroke volume, shortening of the isovolemic contraction time, and the longest diastolic filling time in absence of diastolic mitral regurgitation (in patients with a long PR interval)[4,5] (Figures 11.1 and 11.2).

In clinical practice, there are many techniques for optimizing the AV delay in CRT patients, as well as great variability in their use. These include invasive techniques (LV or aortic maximum rate of LV pressure generation (dP/dt_{max})) and non-invasive techniques (largely echocardiography).[1,3,6] LV dP/dt is one of the most sensitive indices of contractility, and is often recorded with cardiac catheterization.[3,6] It is the rate of increase of intraventricular pressure during isovolumetric contraction (determined from the slope of the waveform during systole), and represents the change in LV pressure as a function of time. AV optimization in DDD(R) pacemakers has traditionally been achieved using non-invasive Doppler echocardiography, which still remains widely used in CRT patients for acute and long-term hemodynamic assessment. Recently applied Doppler echocardiographic methods for AV optimization in CRT

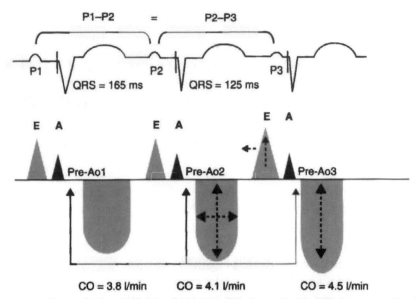

Figure 11.1 Consequences of optimization of AV delay during biventricular pacing at stable heart rate. The QRS complex resulting from P1 is wide due to apical right ventricular pacing (165 ms). The aortic pre-ejection time interval (Pre-Ao1) is long; the aortic systolic phase is also long due to the wide QRS complex. The second QRS complex resulting from P2 is narrowed due to biventricular pacing, leading to a shorter aortic pre-ejection time interval (Pre-Ao2) compared with Pre-Ao1. Consequently, the duration of the aortic systolic phase is reduced, and the E-wave corresponding to P3 occurs earlier (compared with P1 and P2) with a greater amplitude, indicating a better LV filling phase. Pre-Ao3 is even shorter than Pre-Ao2 due to the addition of an AV delay optimization during P3, resulting in a greater cardiac output (CO) during P3 compared with the one obtained during P2, in which biventricular pacing was delivered without AV delay optimization. (Reproduced from Bax JJ et al. J Am Coll Cardiol 2005;46:2168–82.[5]).

patients vary substantially in performance.[6] They include analysis of mitral, LV outflow tract (LVOT), and aortic blood flow velocity profiles using conventional pulsed and continuous-wave Doppler techniques and determination of dP/dt as derived from the continuous-wave Doppler profile of mitral regurgitation.[5-9] Non-echocardiographic techniques include radionuclide angiography,[10] impedance cardiography,[11,12] plethysmography,[13-15] and data from a peak

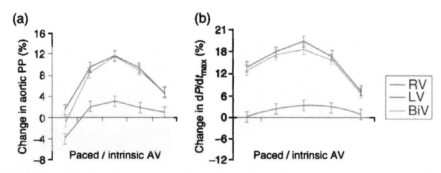

Figure 11.2 (a,b) AV delay optimization. Average percentage change in systolic parameters as a function of five normalized AV delays for each pacing chamber – right ventricle (RV), left ventricle (LV), and biventricular (BiV) – in 20 patients with a QRS complex 180 ± 22 ms: (a) changes in aortic pulse pressure (PP); (b) changes in maximum rate of increase of LV pressure (dP/dt_{max}). Tested AV delays were normalized to the patient's PR interval minus 30 ms. Data points are shown with SE bars. Parts (a) and (b) reproduced from Auricchio A, et al. Circulation 1999;99:2993–3001.[1]

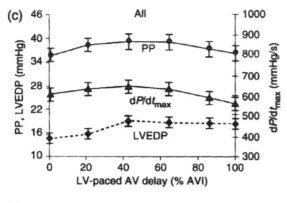

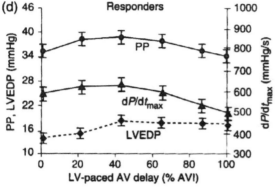

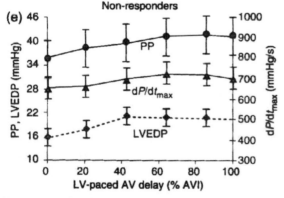

Figure 11.2—Cont'd (c–e) AV optimization. Average aortic PP, LV dP/dt$_{max}$, and LV end-diastolic pressure (LVEDP) obtained during LV stimulation at each tested AV delay and at baseline (i.e., 100%) for the entire patient population (c), the responder subgroup (d), and the non-responder subgroup (e). Actual AV delays were normalized to baseline intrinsic AV interval (AVI) to simultaneously represent both the effect of short AVIs and pre-excitation present in the individual patients. The responders and non-responders are defined in the text. Parts (c–e) reprinted from J Am Coll Cardiol, Vol 39, Auricchio A, Ding J, Spinelli JC, et al. Cardiac resynchronization therapy restores optimal atrioventricular mechanical timing in heart failure patients with ventricular conduction delay. 1163–1169;2002. With permission from The American College of Cardiology Foundation.[3]

endocardial acceleration sensor incorporated into a pacing lead.[16] The best method of measuring or assessing the effects of AV interval programming in terms of accuracy, cost, rapidity, ease, and perhaps automaticity remains to be defined.

The optimal AV interval determined for biventricular stimulation may differ from the optimal AV interval to achieve CRT with LV stimulation alone. Timing of mechanical left atrial (LA) to LV events during CRT may differ markedly, depending upon whether the right atrium (RA) is sensed or paced. Thus, AV interval programming becomes even more complex if the patient is expected to alternate between atrial sensed and paced events. Unfortunately, the findings of most studies may not be applicable during upright posture or during exercise. In patients with normal AV conduction (i.e., normal PR interval on the surface electrocardiogram (ECG)), it is generally recommended to first ensure complete biventricular capture without fusion, and then shorten the AV delay compared with the spontaneous PR interval. In some patients, fusion with spontaneous QRS complex may yield superior hemodynamic benefit (as discussed later), although this approach for AV optimization is not as yet generally accepted (this is discussed later). Finally, in some CRT patients, optimization of the AV interval may be impossible due to the inability to prolong the AV delay sufficiently without losing CRT.

PROLONGED AV DELAY

Prolonged AV conduction is not uncommon in CHF patients. In this situation, atrial systole occurs too early in diastole, compromising ventricular filling and leading to decreased cardiac output, which is poorly tolerated in CHF patients. Transmitral blood flow velocity profiles obtained by pulsed-wave Doppler echocardiography can be used to assess the temporal relationships of diastolic and systolic events, including early diastolic filling (E wave), atrial contraction (A wave), and the onset of ventricular contraction. Atrial contraction in early diastole is superimposed upon the early LV filling phase rather than preceding isovolumic LV contraction (Figure 11.3). There is therefore delay of

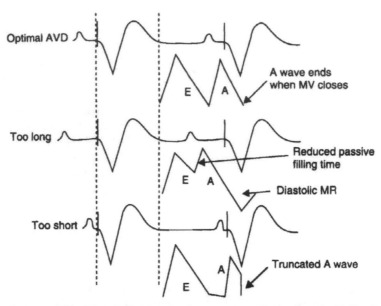

Figure 11.3 Schematic diagram of the effect of AV delay duration on echocardiographic mitral inflow tracings. Note that when the AV delay is optimal, the mitral valve closes at the end of the mitral A wave. If the AV delay is too long, the A and E waves become fused and the duration of diastolic filling is reduced. Late diastolic mitral regurgitation (MR) may occur. If the AV delay is too short, the A wave is truncated as the mitral valve (MV) closes before active filling from atrial contraction has completed. (Reprinted from Saunders; Ellenbogen KA, Kay GN, Wilkoff BL, et al. Device therapy for Congestive Heart Failure: 232–293. (2003). With permission from Elsevier.

the E wave, with resultant fusion between the E and A waves producing shortening of the LV diastolic filling time. The delay in AV conduction induces diastolic mitral regurgitation. In a normal heart, atrial systole occurs immediately before ventricular systole. In the setting of a long AV delay, the atrium begins to relax and atrial pressure drops after atrial systole. The mitral valve remains open because LV contraction is delayed. With the mitral valve open, the LV end-diastolic pressure (LVEDP) rises and exceeds the LA pressure, thereby producing diastolic mitral regurgitation, a decrease in preload (LVEDP) at the onset of LV systole, and, ultimately, a decrease in LV dP/dt_{max} and cardiac output. Programming an optimal AV/PV delay helps to eliminate diastolic mitral regurgitation.

SHORT AV DELAY

A short AV delay results in an earlier E wave, and therefore, a longer LV filling duration.

However, it compromises the LA contribution to LV filling because the terminal portion of LV filling is interrupted by LV contraction (early mitral valve closure) (Figure 11.3). The E and A waves are separated, but the A wave is truncated or absent. The low LVEDP and loss in preload is reflected in a decreased LV dP/dt_{max} and stroke volume.

OPTIMAL AV DELAY

At optimal AV delay, the end of diastolic LV filling resulting from atrial contraction (represented by the end of the A wave on pulsed-wave Doppler imaging of transmitral flow) coincides with the onset of rise in LV pressure (isovolumic contraction with mitral valve closure). In this scenario, late diastolic filling by atrial contraction is complete in the absence of diastolic mitral regurgitation; diastolic filling is maximized, resulting in maximum cardiac output and stroke volume (Figure 11.3). In other words, there is maximum time for 'passive' LV filling without impairment of active filling by the LA. As a rule of thumb, one should program the shortest AV delay that does not compromise the transmitral Doppler A wave.

INVASIVE AND NON-INVASIVE DETERMINATION OF LV dP/dt_{max}

The maximal or peak rate of increase of intraventricular pressure during isovolumetric contraction (dP/dt_{max}) is one of the most sensitive indices of LV contractility.[1,3,6,17–20] This index has stood the test of time and is reproducible. It is measured during cardiac catheterization (Figure 11.2), but it can also be estimated non-invasively in patients with mitral regurgitation from the continuous-wave Doppler-derived mitral regurgitation velocity profile[21] (Figure 11.4). Invasive testing at the time of CRT implantation can be used to guide AV delay programming by measuring LV dP/dt_{max} or aortic pulse pressure, but non-invasive methods are preferable.

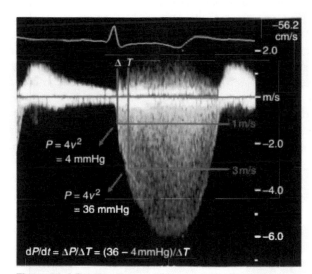

Figure 11.4 Doppler-derived dP/dt determined by measuring the time difference (Δ*T*) between two points on the continuous-wave mitral regurgitation spectral signal corresponding, as indicated, to 1 m/s and 3 m/s. These points correspond to pressure gradients between the LV and LA of 4 and 36 mmHg according to the modified Bernoulli equation (ΔP=4v²). dP/dt is determined by this change in pressure (32 mmHg) divided by the time difference. *P*, pressure; *T*, time; *v*, velocity.

A recent report described a newly developed non-invasive technique to provide a speedy and simple alternative method of measuring dP/dt_{max} by accurately measuring the ascending limb of the central arterial pressure with equipment placed over the brachial artery.[22]

ECHOCARDIOGRAPHY

Limitations of the Ritter method in CRT patients

AV delay optimization is commonly performed by evaluating the transmitral flow velocity profile in patients with conventional and CRT devices by the Ritter method.[23,24] Measurements are made at two AV delay settings (short and long AV delay). The method is based on the premise that LV diastolic filling is optimized when mitral valve closure due to LV systole coincides with the end of the Doppler A wave (Figure 11.5). This approach provides the longest diastolic filling time and allows completion of atrial systole prior to ventricular contraction. The method does not assess forward output. Previous investigations have evaluated the Ritter method in patients with normal LV ejection fraction (LVEF) and dual-chamber pacemakers for AV block. In CRT patients with a normal or short PR interval (< 150 ms), the second part of the Ritter method protocol cannot ensure biventricular pacing with a long AV delay due to intact intrinsic conduction. Furthermore, it is difficult to determine whether or not the A wave is abbreviated, as the increased LVEDP in CHF promotes mitral valve closure immediately following the A wave. The Ritter method is difficult to carry out at high rates. Finally, there is evidence that it may not represent the maximum achievable hemodynamic benefit.[6]

Doppler-derived stroke volume, cardiac output, and velocity–time integral

Stroke volume and cardiac output can be determined using Doppler echocardiography. Most commonly, the method uses two-dimensional (2D) echocardiography (in the parasternal long-axis view) to measure the diameter of the LVOT and pulsed-wave Doppler interrogation of the

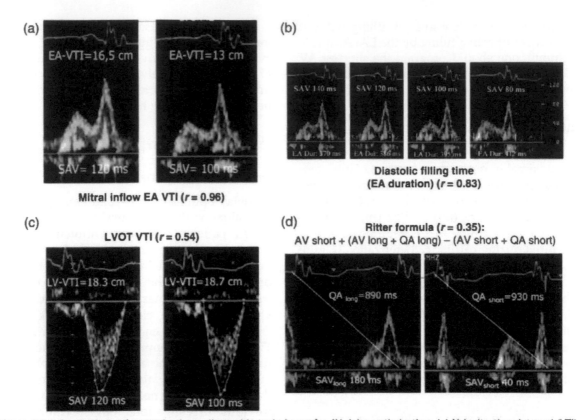

Figure 11.5 Comparison of several echocardiographic techniques for AV delay optimization. (a) Velocity–time integral (VTI) of transmitral flow (EA VTI) at two consecutive sensed AV delays (SAV). The values are the average of four heartbeats. Note the clear difference in EA VTI value with change in the sensed AV delay. (b) EA duration of four different sensed AV delays (SAV). Shortening of the sensed AV delay increased the EA duration by progressively separating the E and A waves. At 80 ms, the A wave is abbreviated; therefore, the optimal AV delay by EA duration is 100 ms. This example illustrates the difficulty in judging A-wave abbreviation. (c) Example of the VTI of the left ventricular outflow tract (LV VTI) at two adjacent sensed AV delays (SAV). The LV VTI is averaged from four beats. Note that the left and right panels in (c) represent, respectively, long and short sensed AV delays (SAV). The corresponding QA time (time from the onset of electrical activation until the end of the A wave) is measured and there is a small difference in outcome. (d) The Ritter formula for optimizing AV delay: the left optimal AV delay is calculated as AV short + (AV long + QA long) − (AV short + QA short). In this example, the derived optimal AV delay is 140 ms. (Reprinted with permission from Am J Cardiol Vol 97(4) Jansen AH, Bracke FA, van Dantzig JM, et al. Correlation of Echo-Doppler Optimization of Atrioventricular Delay in Cardiac Resynchronization Therapy With Invasive Hemodynamics In patients With Heart Failure Secondary to Ischemic or Idiopathic Dilated Cardiomyopathy:552–557; (2006). With permission from Elsevier.[6])

LVOT (in apical five-chamber view) to obtain its blood flow velocity profile, which is traced to yield the velocity–time integral (VTI) of blood flow. Measuring the diameter of the LVOT allows calculation of its cross-sectional area by assuming it to be circular. The product of the cross-sectional area and the VTI determines the Doppler-derived stroke volume. AV delay optimization with Doppler echocardiography is often done by assessing the VTI without measuring the stroke volume and cardiac output.[5,6,25–30]

The optimal AV delay is associated with the largest average LVOT VTI, which is directly proportional to stroke volume and correlates well with invasive hemodynamic data. Obtaining LVOT VTI measures under different AV delays requires a skilled operator, maintenance of constant position of the transducer and Doppler interrogation site, a cooperative patient for a long study, and quantification of the Doppler VTI by tracing numerous blood flow velocity envelopes. Small changes in the angle of incidence between the outflow jet and the ultrasound transducer or a small miscalculation of the LVOT dimension can introduce significant error into the calculation of LV stroke volume. Sonographers should be thoroughly trained in the technique to maintain consistency in methodology.

The LVOT or diastolic transmitral VTI (in the absence of significant mitral or aortic regurgitation) is directly proportional to the stroke volume. LVOT VTI data are used more often than the mitral VTI data. Transmitral E and A waves are usually obtained by pulsed-wave Doppler interrogation from the apical four-chamber view, sampling at the tip of the mitral valve leaflets – a site from which the stroke volume cannot be derived.

AV optimization. Echocardiographically guided programming with aortic VTI versus empiric programming of a fixed AV delay: correlation with clinical outcomes

A randomized, prospective, single-blind clinical trial was conducted to compare two methods of AV delay programming in 40 patients who received CRT for severe CHF.[31] Patients were randomized to either an optimized AV delay determined by Doppler echocardiography (group 1, $n = 20$) or an empiric AV delay of 120 ms (group 2, $n = 20$), with both groups being programmed in the biventricular VDD mode. The optimal AV delay was defined in terms of the largest aortic VTI at one of eight tested AV intervals (60–200 ms). New York Heart Association (NYHA) functional classification and quality-of-life (QOL) score were compared 3 months after randomization. Immediately after CRT initiation with AV delay programming, VTI improved by 4.0 ± 1.7 cm versus 1.8 ± 3.6 cm ($p < 0.02$), and LVEF increased by $7.8 \pm 6.2\%$ versus $3.4 \pm 4.4\%$ ($p < 0.02$) in group 1 versus group 2, respectively. After 3 months, NYHA classification improved by 1.0 ± 0.5 versus 0.4 ± 0.6 class points ($p < 0.01$), and QOL score improved by 23 ± 13 versus 13 ± 11 points ($p < 0.03$) for group 1 versus group 2, respectively at 3 months compared with an empiric AV delay program of 120 ms.

Aortic Doppler VTI versus mitral inflow (Ritter) method

Forty consecutive CRT patients (age 59 ± 12 years) with severe CHF were studied using 2D Doppler echocardiography, comparing the acute improvement in stroke volume in response to two methods of AV delay optimization according to (i) the largest increase in the aortic VTI derived from continuous-wave Doppler (aortic VTI method) versus (ii) the mitral inflow method, where the optimal AV delay was obtained by the Ritter method and then the determined optimal AV delay was used to measure the corresponding aortic VTI.[32] The optimized AV delay determined by the aortic VTI method resulted in an increase in aortic VTI of $19 \pm 13\%$, compared with an increase of $12 \pm 12\%$ by the mitral inflow Ritter method ($p < 0.001$). The optimized AV delay by the aortic VTI method was significantly longer than the optimized AV delay calculated from the Ritter method (119 ± 34 ms vs 95 ± 24 ms; $p < 0.001$).

AV delay optimization guided by LV dP/dt determination

LV dP/dt can be measured non-invasively from continuous-wave spectral Doppler recordings of mitral regurgitation. The methodology involves measuring the time for the mitral regurgitant velocity to increase from 1 m/s to 3 m/s, dP/dt is equal to 32 divided by this time difference (Figure 11.4). Morales et al[21] assessed whether an optimal AV delay, defined as the highest echo-Doppler-derived dP/dt_{max}, could provide clinical and functional benefits in CRT patients. They evaluated 38 consecutive patients. In 23 patients, echo-Doppler recordings were obtained at AV delays of 60, 80, 100, 120, 140, 160, and 180 ms (group I). In 15 patients, an empiric AV delay of 120 ms was chosen (group II). There were no clinical differences between the two groups. Devices in both groups were programmed to atriosynchronous pacing mode, with simultaneous interventricular stimulation, and the patients were followed for 6 months. None died. In group I, optimal AV delay was 60 ms in one patient, 80 ms in six, 100 ms in six, 120 ms in eight, and 140 ms in two. At 6 months' follow-up, group I showed a significantly lower NYHA class (2.1 ± 0.1 vs 3 ± 0.2; $p < 0.01$) and higher LVEF (32.1 ± 1% vs 27.5 ± 1.6%; $p < 0.05$), as compared with group II programmed with an empiric AV delay. The data also showed that the maximal difference among dP/dt values in each patient during the entire sequence of AV delays ranged from 27% to 100%.

WHAT IS THE BEST ECHOCARDIOGRAPHIC METHOD TO OPTIMIZE AV DELAY?

Jansen et al[6] recently investigated the optimal echocardiographic indices to determine the most hemodynamically appropriate AV delay in 30 CHF patients less than 24 hours after CRT device implantation. Doppler echocardiographic optimization of AV delay was correlated with the optimal sensed AV delay determined by LV dP/dt_{max} measured with a sensor-tipped pressure guidewire (Figure 11.5). The Doppler echocardiographic methods included the VTI of the diastolic transmitral flow (EA VTI), diastolic filling time (EA duration), the VTI of the LVOT or aorta, and the Ritter formula. The optimal

AV delay with the EA VTI method was concordant with LV dP/dt_{max} in 29 of 30 patients ($r = 0.96$), with EA duration in 20 of 30 patients ($r = 0.83$), with LV VTI in 13 patients ($r = 0.54$), and with the Ritter formula in none of the patients ($r = 0.35$). Measurement of the maximal VTI of mitral inflow was found to be the most accurate method compared with the invasive LV dP/dt_{max} index (Figure 11.6).

ALTERNATIVE TECHNIQUES TO ECHOCARDIOGRAPHY

Limited but promising non-invasive techniques other than echocardiography are becoming available, allowing simpler and faster ways to optimize the AV delay

Plethysmography

Several encouraging studies have shown that plethysmography can easily optimize the AV delay.[13-15] The results are important, because this technique is easily and quickly done by continuous finger photoplethysmography to detect the

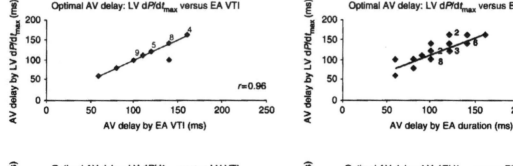
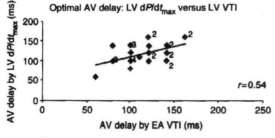
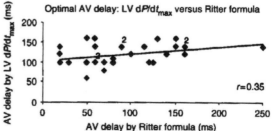

Figure 11.6 Correlation of different modes of Doppler echocardiographic optimization of the AV delay with invasive LV dP/dt_{max} according to the methods shown in Figure 11.5. The number of patients is indicated for each point if > 1. (Reproduced from Jansen AH et al. Am J Cardiol 2006;97:552–7.[6])

hemodynamic response directly during adjustment of the AV delay, compared with echocardiography, which requires skilled operators.

Butter et al[13] compared measurements obtained by finger photoplethysmography with those recorded by invasive aortic pressure collected simultaneously from 57 CHF patients during intrinsic rhythm alternating with very brief periods of pacing at 4–5 AV delays. Plethysmography correctly identified positive aortic pulse pressure responses with 71% sensitivity and 90% specificity, and negative aortic pulse pressure responses with 57% sensitivity and 96% specificity. The magnitude of plethysmography changes were strongly correlated with positive aortic pulse pressure changes ($r^2 = 0.73$; $p < 0.0001$), but less well correlated with negative aortic pulse pressure changes ($r^2 = 0.43$; $p < 0.001$). Plethysmography selected 78% of the patients having positive aortic pulse pressure changes to CRT and identified the AV delay giving maximum aortic pulse pressure change in all selected patients. Accordingly, plethysmography can provide a simple non-invasive method for identifying significant changes in aortic pulse pressure in CRT patients and the optimal AV delay giving the maximum aortic pulse pressure.

Whinnett et al[14,15] demonstrated that even small changes in AV delay from its hemodynamic peak value produce a significant effect on blood pressure (BP) (Figure 11.7). Twelve patients were studied, with six re-attending for reproducibility assessment. At each AV delay, systolic blood pressure (SBP) relative to a reference AV delay of 120 ms was calculated. These workers found that at higher heart rates, altering the AV delay had a more pronounced effect on BP (average range of SBP 17.4 mmHg) compared with resting rates (average range of SBP 6.5 mmHg; $p < 0.0001$). The optimal AV delay differed between patients (minimum 120 ms, maximum 200 ms). Small changes in AV delay had significant BP effects: programming AV delay 40 ms below the optimal AV delay reduced SBP by 4.9 mmHg ($p < 0.003$); having it 40 ms above the peak decreased systolic BP by 4.4 mmHg ($p < 0.0005$). The mean absolute difference between the photoplethysmographic method and the LVOT VTI method was 23 ± 7 ms, while

between the photoplethysmographic method and the Ritter method, the difference was 35 ± 6 ms. Finally, the peak AV delay was highly reproducible both on the same day and at 3 months.

Impedance cardiography

Thoracic electrical bioimpedance (TEB) is a rapid, accurate, cost-effective technique that has been used for some time as a useful alternative to Doppler echocardiography to optimize the AV interval during standard dual-chamber pacing with permanent RV stimulation. In addition to measurements of cardiac output, TEB provides other hemodynamic indices. Thoracic electrical bioimpedance claims to non-invasively measure the cardiac output by monitoring the change in impedance of an alternating current applied across the thorax, and takes only minutes to perform. Tse et al[11] examined the value of the impedance cardiography method of cardiac measurement to optimize the AV interval in five men and one woman (mean age 72 ± 11 years) during permanent LV pacing. Simultaneous measurements of cardiac output by impedance cardiography and echocardiography (aortic VTI × cross-sectional area of LVOT × heart rate) were performed at AV intervals of 50, 80, 110, 150, 180, and 225 ms during DDD pacing at 85 bpm. The optimal AV interval varied between 110 and 180 ms. In five of six patients (83%), the optimal AV interval by echocardiography and impedance cardiography was identical. While cardiac output measurements were higher with impedance cardiography than with echocardiography (6.1 ± 0.4 l/min vs 4.7 ± 0.3 l/min; $p < 0.05$), the cardiac output measurements by two methods were closely correlated ($r = 0.67$; $p < 0.001$).

Braun et al[12] also compared impedance cardiography with echocardiography for AV delay optimization in CRT patients. Twenty-four patients (64 ± 8 years) were evaluated at baseline and 1 month after implantation of a CRT device. The optimal AV interval was defined by impedance cardiography and subsequently by Doppler echocardiography as the interval corresponding to the highest cardiac output measured at different AV intervals, varying from

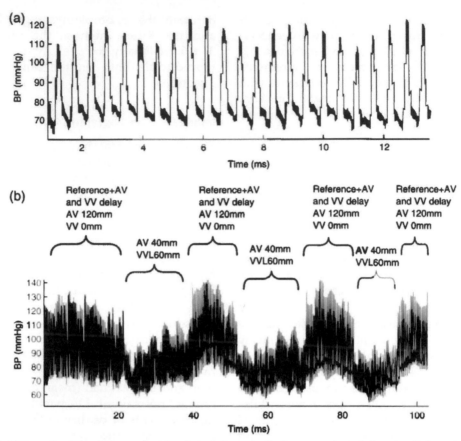

Figure 11.7 (a,b) Example of the data acquired by photoplathymography for measuring relative change in systolic blood pressure for tested atrioventricular (AV) and interventricular (VV) delays. Each tested AV and VV delay was compared with the reference AV and VV delays (AV 120 ms and VV 0 ms) in (a). The recording was returned to this reference delay between each tested delay. The relative change in systolic blood pressure was calculated as the mean of 10 beats prior to a change and the 10 beats immediately after a change. The mean was established for at least six replicate transitions. (Reproduced from Whinnett ZI et al. Heart 2006;92:1628–34.[14])

60 to 200 ms (with 20 ms increments). For standardization and comparison of both techniques, a fixed atriobiventricular pacing rate of 90 bpm was used. Absolute values of the maximum cardiac output were higher by impedance echocardiography (5.8 ± 0.9 l/min) compared with Doppler echocardiography (4.6 ± 0.9 l/min; $p < 0.01$). The optimal AV interval as determined by impedance cardiography varied interindividually from 80 to 180 ms (mean 121 ± 18 ms). In Doppler echocardiography, the range was also 80–180 ms, with a mean optimal AV interval of 128 ± 23 ms. Thus, there was a strong correlation for AV-interval optimization in CRT patients between both methods ($r = 0.74$; $p < 0.001$).

AV OPTIMIZATION DURING ACTIVITY

Exercise testing in CRT patients is technically difficult and inconvenient. There is preliminary evidence in acute studies suggesting that the short AV delay at rest should be prolonged during exercise to achieve optimal LV systolic performance.[33] This is in contrast to the proven benefit of programming rate-adaptive shortening of the AV delay in patients with conventional DDDR pacemakers. The dynamic changes of LV dyssynchrony on exercise may partially explain what appears to be paradoxical behavior of the AV delay on exercise in CRT patients.[34] If confirmed by other studies, it would be desirable to provide CRT devices with dynamic lengthening of the AV delay on exercise. In the meantime, it might be wise to program CRT devices without dynamic shortening of the AV delay in patients with normal sinus node function. At present, there are no chronic data available that provide insight regarding the optimal AV interval during activity states. In future, it might be possible to predict the optimal AV delay on exercise from the value of the optimal resting AV delay.[35]

In CRT patients with severe chronotropic incompetence (defined by the failure to achieve 85% of the age-predicted heart rate determined as 220 – the patient's age), rate-adaptive pacing DDDR with a rate-adaptive AV delay may provide incremental benefit on exercise capacity.[36] Therefore, an exercise test would be desirable to demonstrate the effect of a rate-adaptive AV delay if atrial pacing is likely to occur on exercise. Further studies are required to determine how to program the sensed and paced AV delay offset during exercise.

LONG-TERM EVALUATION OF AV DELAY

The optimal follow-up and long-term programming of the AV delay are uncertain. It is unknown if the acute AV interval programmed by whatever method at implantation or before hospital discharge remains optimal during follow-up. Biventricular stimulation will change the sequence of ventricular activation, and the end-diastolic and end-systolic LV volumes will decrease over time. Consequently, LV diastolic and systolic pressures will also change along with LV filling. Such reverse remodeling may take several months to produce maximum improvement in LV function. The status of AV delay optimization should be assessed periodically. Further studies are needed to determine how often the AV delay needs to be optimized.

There is only one study about this issue, and it suggests that the optimal AV delay changes with time.[37] Before, during, and at specified intervals over 9 months after implantation, 40 recipients of CRT devices were studied with echocardiography. There was a trend toward an increase in the AV delay during follow-up.

The mean AV delay at implantation was 115 ms, versus 137 ms at 9 months. Individual changes could not be accurately predicted.

FUSION WITH SPONTANEOUS VENTRICULAR ACTIVATION: BENEFICIAL OR HARMFUL?

van Gelder et al[38] have investigated the effect of intrinsic conduction over the right bundle branch (causing fusion with the LV-paced complex) on the LV dP/dt_{max} index. LV pacing (biventricular activation with LV monochamber pacing) was compared with biventricular pacing in 34 patients with NYHA class III or IV, sinus rhythm with normal AV conduction, left bundle branch block (LBBB), QRS >130 ms, and optimal medical therapy. LV dP/dt_{max} was measured invasively during LV and simultaneous biventricular pacing. The AV interval (AVI) was varied in four steps starting with an AVI 40 ms shorter than the intrinsic PQ time, and decreased with 25% for each step with ventricular fusion caused by intrinsic activation. LV dP/dt_{max} was higher with LV pacing than with biventricular pacing, provided that LV pacing was associated with ventricular fusion caused by intrinsic activation via the right bundle branch.

The clinical implications of the study by van Gelder et al[38] are unclear. It is impossible to obtain LV stimulation with a sustained degree of stable fusion with right bundle branch depolarization because of variability of the PR interval related to autonomic factors. As present, it is probably best to program the AV delay to avoid all forms of ventricular fusion with spontaneous ventricular activity until more data are available, and a reliable way is found to synchronize right bundle branch activity (unpaced RV) with LV stimulation. Programming an AV delay that permits fusion with right bundle branch activity should not be contraindicated, since it may provide the best resting hemodynamics in occasional patients if the PR interval is normal.

INTRA- AND INTERATRIAL CONDUCTION DELAY

This is characterized by a wide and notched P wave (>120 ms) traditionally in ECG lead II, associated with a wide terminal negativity in lead V_1. The latter is commonly labeled LA enlargement, although it reflects LA conduction disease. Interatrial conduction time is also measured as the activation time from the high RA activation to distal coronary sinus (60–85 ms).[39] In the presence of interatrial conduction delay with late LA activation, LA systole occurs late – even during LV systole. Consequently, the need to program a long AV delay to overcome delayed LA systole can preclude ventricular resynchronization, because the lack of AV conduction disease permits the emergence of a conducted QRS complex. The incidence of interatrial conduction delay in patients who are candidates for CRT is unknown. In this respect, Daubert et al[39] have suggested that it might be about 20%. When the ECG suggests interatrial conduction delay, it would be wise to look for delayed LA activation at the time of CRT implantation by showing that the conduction time from the RA to the LA is longer than the conduction time from the RA to the QRS complex.[40] In the presence of interatrial conduction delay, one should consider placing the atrial lead in the interatrial septum, where pacing produces a more homogeneous activation of both atria and abbreviates the total atrial conduction time

judged by a decrease of P-wave duration.[41,42] In the presence of established CRT with an atrial lead in the RA appendage, restoration of mechanical left-sided AV synchrony requires simultaneous biatrial pacing performed by the implantation of a second atrial lead either in the proximal coronary sinus or in the low RA near the coronary sinus to preempt LA systole.[43,44] Difficult cases can be managed by AV nodal ablation to permit extension of the AV delay to promote mechanical left-sided AV synchrony although biventricular ICDs may limit the maximum programmable AV delay.

LATE ATRIAL SENSING (INTRAATRIAL CONDUCTION DELAY)

In some patients with right intraatrial conduction delay, conduction from the sinus node to the RA appendage (the site of atrial sensing) is delayed without significant conduction delay to the LA. In this situation, LA activation may take place or may even be completed by the time the device senses the RA electrogram (Figure 11.8). In these circumstances it may be difficult or impossible to program an optimal delay with

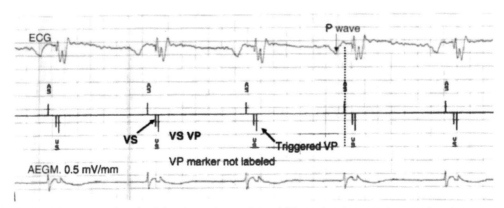

Figure 11.8 Marked shortening of the AV delay due to late or delayed RA sensing. Intraatrial conduction delay causes impaired conduction from the sinus node to the electrode in the RA appendage, where atrial sensing occurs. The ECG is on top, the marker channel in the middle, and the atrial electrogram (AEGM) at the bottom. The timing of the atrial electrogram is so delayed that the device senses atrial activity beyond the P wave on the surface ECG. The ventricular marker channel displays a ventricular sensing event (first downward deflection, VS), followed by a second, larger, deflection representing triggered biventricular stimulation, which the marker channel does not label as a ventricular paced event (VP) because it is too close to the preceding marker. The pacemaker sees an AS–VS interval of 60 ms. This problem was solved by allowing biventricular triggering within 4 ms of a sensed ventricular event within the programmed AV delay. The patient's hemodynamic status improved – presumably because of a well-timed important contribution by LV pacing, which cannot always be guaranteed with this arrangement. In difficult cases AV nodal ablation is required to ensure cardiac resynchronisation. The paper speed was 50 mm/s.

CRT in the absence of ventricular fusion. A trial of ventricular-triggered biventricular pacing upon sensing the spontaneous QRS complex may be worthwhile provided it can be shown to be hemodynamically effective. In difficult cases, ablation of the fast pathway of the AV node or the AV node itself can be performed.

EFFECT OF RATE SMOOTHING ON AV DELAY

Rate smoothing is a programmable feature in some devices designed to prevent the pacing rate from changing by more than a programmable percentage from one cycle to the next.[45] This algorithm may be useful in patients with supraventricular tachyarrhythmias. The pacemaker stores in memory the most recent R–R interval – either intrinsic or paced. Based on this R–R interval, and the rate smoothing value or percentage, the device determines the duration of the next pacing cycle involving atrium and ventricle. Figure 11.9 illustrates how inappropriately programmed rate smoothing can promote spontaneous AV conduction by delaying the emission of biventricular pacing according to

the rate smoothing algorithm. Rate smoothing should be used cautiously in CRT patients by using a rate smoothing value with a high percentage (e.g., 25%) to prevent the response shown in Figure 11.9.

DEVICE-BASED AUTOMATIC OPTIMIZATION OF AV DELAY

St Jude Medical has designed a simple device-based way to calculate and optimize the AV delay (Figure 11.10). The system measures the duration of the activation–recovery interval on the atrial electrogram (which represents the sum of the RA and far-field LA electrograms) and utilizes this value to optimize the paced and sensed delay via a proprietary formula.[46]

AV OPTIMIZATION IN MAJOR TRIALS

There is no universally accepted gold standard method for optimizing the AV delay. This is evidenced by the variable use of different techniques in major CRT trials as outlined below. The question therefore arises as to whether

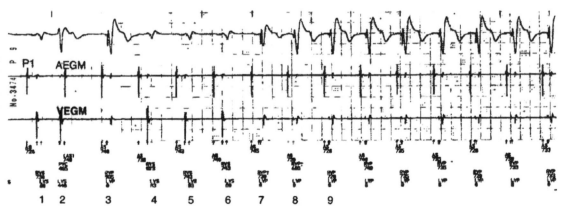

Figure 11.9 Impact of rate smoothing on AV delay and CRT. The second ventricular beat is a premature ventricular complex (PVC). The ventricular cycle between V2 and V3 is relatively long and is governed by the ongoing rate smoothing factor (6%). Accordingly, the subsequent ventricular cycle ending with a ventricular paced beat should measure 6% less than the preceding V2–V3 cycle. This means that the device would have to deliver the next ventricular stimulus at a time beyond the fourth ventricular beat (if this spontaneous ventricular beat had not occurred). However, the spontaneous ventricular beat was sensed by the pacemaker earlier than the expected ventricular stimulus. As a result, a P wave is sensed and conducted the ventricle with a PR interval longer than the programmed AV delay. This disrupts CRT for several beats until the rate smoothing function restores CRT by providing progressively a shorter ventricular pacing cycle dependent on the rate smoothing factor. A rate smoothing factor of 25% might have prevented loss of CRT. AS, atrial sensed event; (AS), atrial event sensed in the pacemaker atrial refractory period; RVS, sensed RV event; RVP, paced RV event; LVS, sensed LV event; LVP, paced LV event.

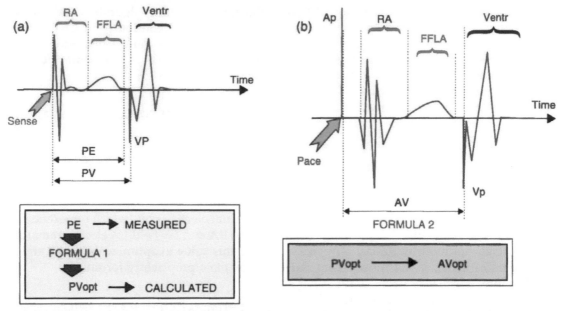

Figure 11.10 (a) Diagrammatic representation of the St Jude Medical system for optimizing the sensed AV delay. The device senses the entire atrial electrogram: right atrial (RA) and far-field left atrial electrogram (FFLA). The atrial electrogram duration (PE) is equal to RA + FFLA. PV is the interval from the atrial sensed event to the ventricular (Ventr) event (Vp). The device calculates the optimal AV delay (PVopt) according to a proprietary formula. (b) Diagrammatic representation of the St Jude Medical system for optimizing the paced AV delay. Abbreviations are as in (a) Ap is the atrial-paced event. The device calculates the optimal AV delay according to a proprietary formula.

patients in the trials would have improved further, had the AV delay been optimized using more current techniques.

PATH-CHF: Pacing Therapies in Congestive Heart Failure

The PATH-CHF and PATH II European trials of CRT evaluated the hemodynamic impact of acute AV optimization in two studies that clearly demonstrated the importance of AV optimization in maximizing cardiac output.[1,3] The initial study involved 20 patients with QRS 180 ± 22 ms and PR ≥ 150 ms.[1] The effect of different programmed AV delays was studied (five different AV delays, ranging from 0 ms to close to intrinsic PR intervals) during RV, LV and biventricular pacing (Figure 11.2). The optimal AV interval was assessed by aortic pulse pressure and dP/dt determinations and varied widely among CRT patients. Using LV dP/dt_{max} determined invasively as well as the pulse pressure as an endpoint, the optimal programmed AV interval for

LV and biventricular pacing was at the middle of the AV setting [$0.5 \times (PR - 30\,ms)$]. The initial study also included another five CRT patients ('non-responders') with a narrower QRS (128 ± 12 ms) in whom AV testing at various durations produced no improvement.[1]

The second PATH-CHF study involved 39 CRT patients.[3] The 'responder' subgroup (27 patients) displayed an increase in pulse pressure with respect to their intrinsic baseline by more than 5% for LV and biventricular pacing, and AV delay combination, while the remaining patients were placed in a 'non-responder' subgroup (12 patients) (Figure 11.2). The label 'non-responder' in this study refers only to the lack of response with AV delay manipulation, and not to CRT itself. The results for LV and biventricular pacing were similar to those in the first study. For all patients, the maximum increases in pulse pressure and dP/dt_{max} occurred at 43% of the intrinsic AV interval (Figure 11.2). Shortening the AV delay (from 43% to 0%) decreased pulse pressure and dP/dt_{max}, and the LVEDP fell.

The 'responder' subgroup showed the same changes as the group of all patients, but, due to its definition, the increases in pulse pressure were larger.[3] The 'non-responder' subgroup showed a decrease in pulse pressure when the AV delay was shortened. This decrease occurred with no significant decrease in LVEDP until AV delays were shorter than 43% of the intrinsic AV interval, whereupon LVEDP fell.

MUSTIC: Multisite Stimulation in Cardiomyopathy

AV delay optimization in the MUSTIC trial used the Ritter method.[23,24,47]

MIRACLE: Multicenter InSync Randomized Clinical Evaluation

Optimization in the AV delay optimization in the MIRACLE trial of CRT was performed in the VDD mode using the Ritter formula.[48] Patients underwent AV interval optimization at pre-discharge and at 3 and 6 months of follow-up. An AV delay averaging 100 ms was optimized in the majority of patients and remained stable over time.[49]

COMPANION: Comparison of Medical Therapy, Pacing and Defibrillation in Heart Failure

In the COMPANION trial, the optimal AV delay was calculated from a proprietary algorithm based on measures of the intrinsic PR interval, the QRS interval, and the sensed AV interval (derived from intracardiac electrograms) at the time of implantation.[50] This was based on the method of Auricchio et al,[51] who demonstrated that the AV delay providing optimum dP/dt_{max} can be reliably predicted from the intrinsic AV interval:

$$AVD = 0.7 \times \text{intrinsic AV interval} - 55 \text{ ms}$$
$$\text{if QRS} > 150 \text{ ms}$$

$$AVD = 0.7 \times \text{intrinsic AV interval}$$
$$\text{if } 120 \text{ ms} \leqslant \text{QRS} \leqslant 150 \text{ ms}$$

The intrinsic AV interval was measured from the atrial sense marker to the first ventricular sense marker.

CONTAK CD

In the CONTAK CD trial of CRT, the AV interval was programmed short enough to ensure complete biventricular capture on treadmill testing, but these values were not correlated with echocardiographic measures.[52]

CARE-HF: Cardiac Resynchronization–Heart Failure

There was little variability of the optimal AV delay over time in the CARE-HF trial. AV optimization was performed using Doppler echocardiography of transmitral flow to provide the maximum LV filling time without compromising cardiac resynchronization and the LA contribution to LV filling.[53] The AV delay was set at a value that provided maximum separation of the E and A waves, representing passive ventricular filling and atrial contraction, respectively.

InSync III

In the InSync III CRT study, which evaluated the benefit of sequential biventricular pacing, RV and LV timing offsets were also studied according to the Ritter method prior to V–V optimization and then retained.[54] Alterations of V–V timing were performed and forward flow, or stroke volume was assessed. The InSync III trial is described in Chapter 12.

POTENTIAL FOR DEVICE-BASED AUTOMATIC OPTIMIZATION OF AV INTERVAL

Echocardiographic techniques for AV (and V–V) optimization require experienced personnel and are time-consuming. Furthermore, CRT optimization by echocardiography is sensitive to intra- and interobserver variability. The ideal tool would be a pacemaker-based system with a specific sensor-based system capable of recording and monitoring cardiac function independently of the variable 'human touch'. Such a sensor-based system would continually optimize CRT hemodynamic parameters, and avoid many outpatient visits. A number of sensors are presently being assessed by pacemaker companies. Peak Endocardial Acceleration (PEA; SORIN Group,

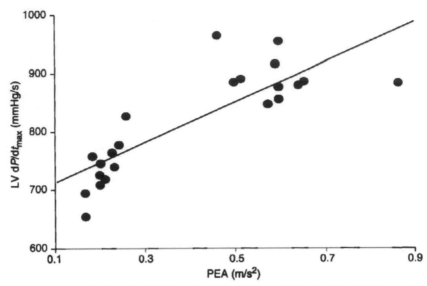

Figure 11.11 Correlation between variations of LV dP/dt_{max} and Peak Endocardial Acceleration (PEA) in a patient with severe heart failure (LVEF 28%) in whom 22 combinations of acute sequential CRT (3 minutes for each combination) at different LV and RV pacing sites were assessed hemodynamically. (Reproduced from Garrigue S. Optimization of cardiac resynchronization therapy: the role of echocardiography in atrioventricular, interventricular and intraventricular delay optimization. In: Yu CM, Hayes DL, Auricchio A, eds. Cardiac Resynchronization Therapy. Malden, MA: Blackwell–Futura, 2006: 310–28. Reprinted with permission from Blackwell publishing).

Milan, Italy), which has been evaluated for over 10 years, consists of a microaccelerator inserted in the tip of an endocardial RV lead. Signals measured by the sensor are based on the amplitude of first heart sound vibrations. Nothing is implanted on the left side of the heart. A number of studies suggest that the PEA data recorded by this sensor can be highly correlated with the dP/dt_{max} index of LV function[16,55–57] (Figure 11.11).

Implantable hemodynamic monitors have been implanted in a few CRT patients.[58] These devices monitor the filling pressures of the heart by recording RV systolic and diastolic pressure and estimate the pulmonary arterial diastolic pressure. It is conceivable that future CRT devices will incorporate such hemodynamic monitors for long-term recording so as to optimize AV and V–V intervals automatically.

REFERENCES

1. Auricchio A, Stellbrink C, Block M, et al. Effect of pacing chamber and atrioventricular delay on acute systolic function of paced patients with congestive heart failure. The Pacing Therapies for Congestive Heart Failure Study Group. The Guidant Congestive Heart Failure Research Group. Circulation 1999;99:2993–3001.

2. Kass DA, Chen CH, Curry C, et al. Improved left ventricular mechanics from acute VDD pacing in patients with dilated cardiomyopathy and ventricular conduction delay. Circulation 1999;99:1567–73.

3. Auricchio A, Ding J, Spinelli JC, et al. Cardiac resynchronization therapy restores optimal atrioventricular mechanical timing in heart failure patients with ventricular conduction delay. J Am Coll Cardiol 2002;39:1163–9.

4. Panidis I P, Ross J, Munley B, Nestico P, Mintz GS. Diastolic mitral regurgitation in patients with atrioventricular conduction abnormalities: a common finding by Doppler echocardiography. J Am Coll Cardiol 1986;7:768–74.

5. Bax JJ, Abraham T, Barold SS, et al. Cardiac resynchronization therapy: Part 2 – Issues during and after device implantation and unresolved questions. J Am Coll Cardiol 2005;46:2168–82.

6. Jansen AH, Bracke FA, van Dantzig JM, et al. Correlation of echo-Doppler optimization of atrioventricular delay in cardiac resynchronization therapy with invasive hemodynamics in patients with heart failure secondary to ischemic or idiopathic dilated cardiomyopathy. Am J Cardiol 2006;97:552–7.

7. Bax JJ, Ansalone G, Breithardt OA, et al. Echocardiographic evaluation of cardiac resynchronization therapy: ready

for routine clinical use? A critical appraisal. J Am Coll Cardiol. 2004;44:1–9.

8. Breithardt OA, Stellbrink C, Franke A, et al. Pacing Therapies for Congestive Heart Failure Study Group; Guidant Congestive Heart Failure Research Group. Acute effects of cardiac resynchronization therapy on left ventricular Doppler indices in patients with congestive heart failure. Am Heart J 2002;143:34–44.

9. Breithardt OA. Conventional echocardiography. In: Yu CM, Hayes DL, Auricchio A, eds. Cardiac Resynchronization Therapy. Malden, MA: Blackwell-Futura, 2006:76–88.

10. Burri H, Sunthorn H, Somsen A, Zaza S, et al. Optimizing sequential biventricular pacing using radionuclide ventriculography. Heart Rhythm 2005;2:960–5.

11. Tse HF, Yu C, Park E, Lau CP. Impedance cardiography for atrioventricular interval optimization during permanent left ventricular pacing. Pacing Clin Electrophysiol 2003;26:189–91.

12. Braun MU, Schnabel A, Rauwolf T, Schulze M, Strasser RH. Impedance cardiography as a noninvasive technique for atrioventricular interval optimization in cardiac resynchronization therapy. J Interv Card Electrophysiol 2005;13:223–9.

13. Butter C, Stellbrink C, Belalcazar A, et al. Cardiac resynchronization therapy optimization by finger plethysmography. Heart Rhythm 2004;1:568–75.

14. Whinnett ZI, Davies JE, Willson K, et al. Haemodynamic effects of changes in atrioventricular and interventricular delay in cardiac resynchronisation therapy show a consistent pattern: analysis of shape, magnitude and relative importance of atrioventricular and interventricular delay. Heart 2006;92:1628–34.

15. Whinnett ZI, Davies JE, Willson K, et al. Determination of optimal atrioventricular delay for cardiac resynchronization therapy using acute non-invasive blood pressure. Europace 2006;8:358–66.

16. Dupuis JM, Kobeissi A, Vitali L, et al. Programming optimal atrioventricular delay in dual chamber pacing using peak endocardial acceleration: comparison with a standard echocardiographic procedure. Pacing Clin Electrophysiol 2003;26:210–13.

17. Hay I, Melenovsky V, Fetics BJ, et al. Short-term effects of right–left heart sequential cardiac resynchronization in patients with heart failure, chronic atrial fibrillation, and atrioventricular nodal block. Circulation 2004;110:3404–10.

18. Perego GB, Chianca R, Facchini M, et al. Simultaneous vs. sequential biventricular pacing in dilated cardiomyopathy: an acute hemodynamic study. Eur J Heart Fail 2003;5:305–13.

19. Kurzidim K, Reinke H, Sperzel J, et al. Invasive optimization of cardiac resynchronization therapy: role of sequential ventricular and left ventricular pacing. Pacing Clin Electrophysiol 2005;28:754–61.

20. van Gelder BM, Bracke FA, Meijer A, et al. Effect of optimizing the VV interval on left ventricular contractility in cardiac resynchronization therapy. Am J Cardiol 2004;93:1500–3.

21. Morales MA, Startari U, Panchetti L, Rossi A, Piacenti M. Atrioventricular delay optimization by Doppler-derived left ventricular dP/dt improves 6-month outcome of resynchronized patients. Pacing Clin Electrophysiol 2006;29:564–8.

22. Gorenberg M, Marmor A, Rotstein H. Detection of chest pain of non-cardiac origin at the emergency room by a new non-invasive device avoiding unnecessary admission to hospital. Emerg Med J 2005;22:486–9.

23. Ritter P, Dib JC, Mahaux V, et al. New method for determining the optimal atrio-ventricular delay in patients paced in DDD mode for complete atrioventricular block. Pacing Clin Electrophysiol 1995;18:237 (abst).

24. Kindermann M, Frolhig G, Doerr T, Schieffer H. Optimizing the AV delay in DDD pacemaker patients with high degree AV block: mitral valve Doppler versus impedance cardiography. Pacing Clin Electrophysiol 1997;20:2453–62.

25. Porciani MC, Dondina C, Macioce R, et al. Echocardiographic examination of atrioventricular and interventricular delay optimization in cardiac resynchronization therapy. Am J Cardiol 2005;95:1108–10.

26. Riedlbauchova L, Kautzner J, Fridl P. Influence of different atrioventricular and interventricular delays on cardiac output during cardiac resynchronization therapy. Pacing Clin Electrophysiol 2005;28(Suppl 1):S19–23.

27. Bordachar P, Lafitte S, Reuter S, et al. Echocardiographic parameters of ventricular dyssynchrony validation in patients with heart failure using sequential biventricular pacing. J Am Coll Cardiol 2004;44:2157–65.

28. Mortensen PT, Sogaard P, Mansour H, et al. Sequential biventricular pacing: evaluation of safety and efficacy. Pacing Clin Electrophysiol 2004;27:339–45.

29. Vanderheyden M, De Backer T, Rivero-Ayerza M, et al. Tailored echocardiographic interventricular delay programming further optimizes left ventricular performance after cardiac resynchronization therapy. Heart Rhythm 2005;2:1066–72.

30. Boriani G, Muller CP, Seidl KH, et al. Resynchronization for the HemodYnamic Treatment for Heart Failure Management II Investigators. Randomized comparison of simultaneous biventricular stimulation versus optimized interventricular delay in cardiac resynchronization therapy. The Resynchronization for the HemodYnamic Treatment for Heart Failure Management II Implantable Cardioverter Defibrillator (RHYTHM II ICD) study. Am Heart J 2006;151:1050–8.

31. Sawhney NS, Waggoner AD, Garhwal S, et al. Randomized prospective trial of atrioventricular delay programming for cardiac resynchronization therapy. Heart Rhythm 2004;1:562–7.

32. Kerlan JE, Sawhney NS, Waggoner AD, et al. Prospective comparison of echocardiographic atrioventricular delay optimization methods for cardiac resynchronization therapy. Heart Rhythm 2006;3: 148–54.

33. Scharf C, Li P, Muntwyler J, et al. Rate-dependent AV delay optimization in cardiac resynchronization therapy. Pacing Clin Electrophysiol 2005;28:279–84.

34. Bordachar P, Lafitte S, Reuter S, et al. Echocardiographic assessment during exercise of heart failure patients with cardiac resynchronization therapy. Am J Cardiol 2006;97:1622–5.

35. Whinnett ZI, Davies JE, Briscoe CA, et al. Optimal haemodynamic AV delay during exercise can be predicted by performing optimization at rest with an elevated pacing rate. Heart Rhythm 2006;3(Suppl): S249.

36. Tse HF, Siu CW, Lee KL, et al. The incremental benefit of rate-adaptive pacing on exercise performance during cardiac resynchronization therapy. J Am Coll Cardiol. 2005;46:2292–7.

37. O'Donnell D, Nadurata V, Hamer A, Kertes P, Mohammed W. Long-term variations in optimal programming of cardiac resynchronization therapy devices. Pacing Clin Electrophysiol 2005;28(Suppl 1): S24–6.

38. van Gelder BM, Bracke FA, Meijer A, Pijls NH. The hemodynamic effect of intrinsic conduction during left ventricular pacing as compared to biventricular pacing. J Am Coll Cardiol 2005;46:2305–10.

39. Daubert JC, Pavin D, Jauvert G, Mabo P. Intra- and interatrial conduction delay: implications for cardiac pacing. Pacing Clin Electrophysiol 2004;27:507–25.

40. Worley SJ, Gohn DC, Coles Jr. JA. Optimize the AV delay before it's too late. Heart Rhythm 2006;3(Suppl):S77 (abst).

41. Porciani MC, Sabini A, Colella A, et al. Interatrial septum pacing avoids the adverse effect of interatrial delay in biventricular pacing: an echo-Doppler evaluation. Europace 2002;4:317–24.

42. Di Pede F, Gasparini G, De Piccoli B, et al. Hemodynamic effects of atrial septal pacing in cardiac resynchronization therapy patients. J Cardiovasc Electrophysiol 2005;16:1273–8.

43. Doi A, Takagi M, Toda I, et al. Acute hemodynamic benefits of bi-atrial atrioventricular sequential pacing with the optimal atrioventricular delay. J Am Coll Cardiol 2005;46:320–6.

44. Doi A, Takagi M, Toda I, et al. Acute haemodynamic benefits of biatrial atrioventricular sequential pacing: comparison with single atrial atrioventricular sequential pacing. Heart 2004;90:411–18.

45. Van Mechelen R, Ruiter J, de Boer H, Hagemeijer F. Pacemaker electrocardiography of rate smoothing during DDD pacing. Pacing Clin Electrophysiol 1985; 8:684–90.

46. Analysis of QuickOpt™ Timing Cycle Optimization. An IEGM Method to Optimize AV, PV, and VV Delays. Sylmar, CA: St Jude Medical, 2006.

47. Cazeau S, Leclercq C, Lavergne T, et al. Multisite Stimulation in Cardiomyopathies (MUSTIC) Study Investigators. Effect of multisite biventricular pacing in patients with heart failure and intraventricular conduction delay. N Engl J Med 2001;344:873–80.

48. Abraham WT, Fisher WG, Smith AL, et al. MIRACLE Study Group. Multicenter InSync Randomized Clinical Evaluation. Cardiac resynchronization in chronic heart failure. N Engl J Med 2002;346:1845–53.

49. Steinberg JS, Maniar PB, Higgins SL, et al. Noninvasive assessment of the biventricular pacing system. Ann Noninvasive Electrocardiol 2004;9:58–70.

50. Bristow MR, Saxon LA, Boehmer J, et al. Comparison of Medical Therapy, Pacing, and Defibrillation in Heart Failure (COMPANION) Investigators. Cardiac resynchronization therapy with or without an implantable defibrillator in advanced chronic heart failure. N Engl J Med 2004;350:2140–50.

51. Auricchio A, Kramer A, Spinelli JC, et al. PATH CHF I and II Investigator Groups. Can the optimum dosage of resynchronization therapy be derived from the intracardiac electrogram? J Am Coll Cardiol 2002; 39(Suppl A):124A (abst).

52. Higgins SL, Hummel JD, Niazi IK, et al. Cardiac resynchronization therapy for the treatment of heart failure in patients with intraventricular conduction delay and malignant ventricular tachyarrhythmias. J Am Coll Cardiol 2003;42:1454–9.

53. Cleland JG, Daubert JC, Erdmann E, et al. Cardiac Resynchronization–Heart Failure (CARE-HF) Study Investigators. The effect of cardiac resynchronization on morbidity and mortality in heart failure. N Engl J Med. 2005;352:1539–49.

54. Leon AR, Abraham WT, Brozena S, et al. InSync III Clinical Study Investigators. Cardiac resynchronization with sequential biventricular pacing for the treatment of moderate-to-severe heart failure. J Am Coll Cardiol 2005;46:2298–304.

55. Garrigue S, Bordachar P, Reuter S, et al. Comparison of permanent left ventricular and biventricular pacing in patients with heart failure and chronic atrial fibrillation: prospective haemodynamic study. Heart 2002;87: 529–34.

56. Delnoy PP, Oudeluttikhuis H, Nicastia D, et al. Validation of a new cardiac resynchronization therapy

optimization algorithm based on peak endocardial acceleration: first clinical results. Heart Rhythm 2006;3(Suppl):S248 (abst).

57. Ritter P, Padeletti L, Delnoy PP, et al. Device based AV delay optimization by peak endocardial acceleration in cardiac resynchronization therapy. Heart Rhythm 2004;1:120 (abst).

58. Braunschweig F, Bruns HJ, ErsgÂrd D, Reiters P, Linde C. AV-delay optimization in cardiac resynchronization therapy using an implanted hemodynamic monitor. Heart Rhythm 2006;3(Suppl):S165 (abst).

12

Optimization of the interventricular (V–V) interval during cardiac resynchronization therapy

S Serge Barold, Arzu Ilercil, Stéphane Garrigue, and Bengt Herweg

Programmability of the interventricular interval • Pathophysiologic basis for programming the V–V interval • Clinical studies of V–V interval programming • General considerations • Effect of V–V timing on the ECG of biventricular pacemakers • Automatic device-based optimization of the V–V delay

PROGRAMMABILITY OF THE INTERVENTRICULAR INTERVAL

The methods for atrioventricular (AV) optimization in patients receiving cardiac resynchronization therapy (CRT) are almost universally used for programming the optimal interventricular (V–V) delay.[1-6] Conventional M-mode echocardiography for the measurement of left ventricular (LV) dyssynchrony using septal-to-posterior wall motion delay may be unreliable and poorly reproducible.[7] Determination of the extent of residual LV dyssynchrony after V–V programming requires more sophisticated echocardiographic techniques such as tissue Doppler techniques (peak velocity time difference, delayed longitudinal contraction score, etc.), three-dimensional (3D) echocardiography, and automatic endocardial border detection.[8-12]

Contemporary biventricular devices permit programming of the V–V interval usually in steps from +80 ms (LV first) to −80 ms (right ventricle (RV) first) to optimize LV hemodynamics. This design was the result of cogent pathophysiologic considerations that simultaneous activation of the two ventricles for CRT was illogical.[13]

PATHOPHYSIOLOGIC BASIS FOR PROGRAMMING THE V–V INTERVAL

Perego et al[13] advanced arguments that the best mechanical efficiency in CRT is not necessarily achieved by simultaneous pacing of the two ventricles (hence the importance of programmability of the V–V interval) (Figure 12.1):

1. In normal hearts, activation of the two ventricles does not occur simultaneously, i.e., epicardial RV depolarization starts a few milliseconds earlier than LV depolarisation.[14,15]
2. In CRT, epicardial LV pacing delays transmission of activation that is normally supposed to reach the subendocardial conduction system before it spreads to the remaining ventricle.
3. In advanced cardiomyopathy, RV-to-LV interactions can be different from those in normal hearts.
4. Myocardial disease is associated with different locations and sizes of scars, and heterogeneity of conduction disturbances. The baseline ventricular conduction defect differs considerably from case to case, especially in patients with a QRS duration >150 ms.[16] Theoretically, slow conduction in

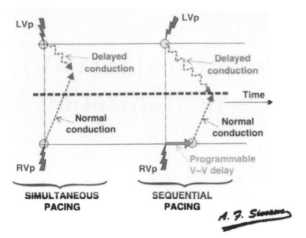

Figure 12.1 Diagrammatic representation of left ventricular (LV) conduction delay interfering with synchronous activation of the two ventricles at the broken horizontal line. Programmability of the interventricular (V–V) interval permits pre-activation of the LV to compensate for the LV conduction delay. In this way, both ventricles are activated synchronously at the broken horizontal line. LVp, LV pacing event; RVp, right ventricular pacing event.

the presence of scar tissue in ischemic cardiomyopathy would necessitate more LV pre-excitation. Conduction delay may be caused not only by isolated left bundle branch block (LBBB), but also by more global anisotropic disturbances of the conduction system and/or myocardial scars, latency of LV stimulation, and delayed global depolarization.[17-20] Despite similar QRS morphology, congestive heart failure (CHF) patients with LBBB, and LV dyssynchrony exhibit different locations and patterns of dyssynchrony.[21]

5. The ventricular leads (particularly the LV leads) are placed in quite different anatomic positions, depending on the operator's choice and coronary sinus anatomy, producing paced ventricular activation patterns that differ from patient to patient. V–V programmability may compensate for less than optimal LV lead position by tailoring ventricular timing to correct for individual heterogeneous ventricular activation patterns commonly found in patients with LV dysfunction and CHF.

6. The presence and varying degree of fusion with the spontaneous QRS complex and possibly with right bundle branch activation alter QRS configuration and hemodynamics.

On the basis of the above arguments, it is therefore not surprising that V–V programmability in the reported studies has shown a heterogeneous response, with great variability of the optimal V–V delay from patient to patient, so that adjustment of the V–V delay, like the AV delay, must be individualized (Figures 12.1 and 12.2). In addition, assessment of the role of V–V programmability is compounded by the varied cut-off QRS duration for inclusion in the various studies, the different testing procedures to determine the optimum V–V delay, and whether AV delay optimization was performed before testing the V–V response.

CLINICAL STUDIES OF V–V INTERVAL PROGRAMMING

Although V-V programmability produces a rather limited improvement in stroke volume, the response is important in patients with a less than desirable response to CRT. It is presently unknown whether AV and/or V–V interval optimization can actually decrease the percentage of non-responders to CRT.

Sogaard et al[21] performed one of the first studies evaluating the role of V–V delay in CRT patients, and convincingly demonstrated that the site and degree of mechanical asynchrony can vary from patient to patient and are influenced by the underlying etiology of disease, whether ischemic or non-ischemic. They defined a new parameter that they called the extent of delayed LV longitudinal contraction (DLC) (Figure 12.3). This is calculated using tissue Doppler imaging (TDI) coupled with strain rate analysis. A segment was considered to have DLC if the strain rate analysis demonstrated motion reflecting true contraction and if the end of the segmental contraction occurred after aortic valve closure. Sogaard et al[21] found that the extent of myocardium with DLC predicted improvement of LV systolic performance and reversion of LV remodeling during short- and long-term CRT. Their observations indicated that DLC represented mechanical LV asynchrony and thus a contractile reserve, which could be recruited by CRT (Figure 12.3).

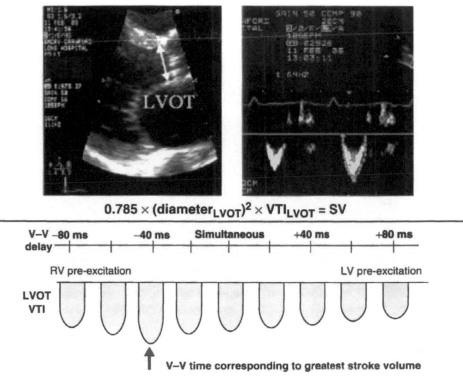

$$0.785 \times (\text{diameter}_{\text{LVOT}})^2 \times \text{VTI}_{\text{LVOT}} = \text{SV}$$

Figure 12.2 Interventricular V–V interval delay using left ventricular outflow tract (LVOT) measurements of blood flow velocities for estimation of stroke volume (SV). SV is exponentially related to the LVOT diameter and directly to the velocity–time integral (VTI) of the LVOT. Variation of the V–V interval affects the SV, as evidenced by varying VTI measurements that can serve as surrogate markers for resynchronization. The optimal V–V interval in this example is derived from pacing the right ventricle (RV) 40 ms before the left ventricle (LV). The optimal AV delay becomes equal to optimal AS-LVP minus the 40 ms V–V interval. LVP, monochamber LV pacing. (Reproduced from Gassis S, Leon AR. Cardiac resynchronization therapy: strategies for device programming, troubleshooting and follow-up. J Interv Card Electrophysiol 2005;13:209–22.)

However, the location of myocardium displaying DLC is variable in patients with heart failure and ventricular conduction disturbances. It was hypothesized that individually tailored pre-activation of myocardium displaying DLCs could further improve the overall response to CRT.

Sogaard et al,[21] using Doppler imaging techniques, studied 21 patients with LBBB, QRS > 130 ms, and New York Heart Association (NYHA) functional class III or IV heart failure, specifically before and after CRT (Figure 12.4). Post-implantation studies were performed during simultaneous CRT and at 12, 20, 40, 60, and 80 ms V–V delay intervals, with either LV or RV pre-excitation. The study population consisted of 11 patients with ischemic cardiomyopathy and 9 patients with idiopathic dilated cardiomyopathy.

As noted in prior studies, DLC in patients with idiopathic dilated cardiomyopathy was identified in the lateral and posterior LV walls. In contrast, ischemic cardiomyopathy exhibited DLC more frequently in the septal and inferior walls. Echocardiographic parameters improved during sequential CRT, with LV pre-activation being superior in 9 patients and RV pre-activation being superior in 11 patients (Figure 12.4). Compared with simultaneous CRT, tailored sequential CRT reduced the extent of segments with DLC in the base from 23 ± 13% to 11 ± 7% ($p<0.05$). The LV ejection fraction (LVEF) increased from 29.7 ± 5% to 33.9 ± 6% ($p<0.01$). After 3 months of sequential CRT the LVEF improved further from 33.6 ± 6% to 38.6 ± 7% ($p<0.01$). Sogaard et al[21] observed that despite

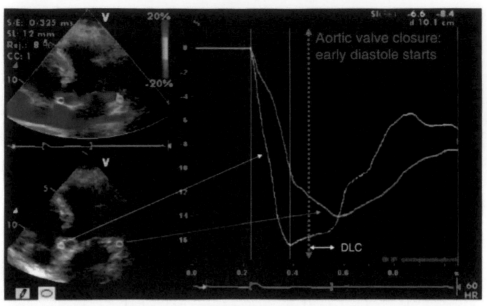

Figure 12.3 Tissue Doppler imaging showing left ventricular (LV) dyssynchrony. Apical long-axis view in a patient with a dilated cardiomyopathy and left bundle branch block. One Doppler sample (yellow) is positioned at base of the septal LV wall, and another (green) is at the base of the lateral wall. In each of the two points, strain rate analysis is carried out in a range of 10 mm around the cursor center. The first vertical line (right) shows the onset of negative strain rate (yellow curve), indicating active contraction in systole. The second vertical line indicates cessation of septal systole, where the strain rate (yellow curve) becomes positive. The third vertical line (red) represents aortic valve closure: note the still-negative strain rate in the lateral wall (green curve); this phenomenon persists, indicating active shortening in early diastole until the strain rate becomes positive (i.e., delayed longitudinal contraction, (DLC). (Reproduced from Garrigue S. Optimization of cardiac resynchronisation therapy: the role of echocardiography in atrioventricular, interventricular and intraventricular delay optimisation. In: Yu CM, Hayes DL, Auricchio A, (eds.) Cardiac Resynchronization Therapy. Malden, MA, Blackwell-Futura, 2006:310–28. With permission from Blackwell Publishing.)

comparable LBBB patterns, the location of DLC differed between the two groups of patients. Additionally, the diastolic filling time increased even without any AV delay optimization. Finally, they concluded that the location of DLC predicted the optimal sequential CRT as posterior lateral wall DLC was associated with optimal sequential CRT via LV pre-activation, while septal and inferior wall-DLC was associated with optimal sequential CRT via RV pre-activation. The optimal V–V delay ranged between 12 and 20 ms.

InSync III study

The InSync III clinical study was a landmark large-scale investigation that firmly established the importance of V–V timing in CRT patients. It used a multicenter, prospective, non-randomized design to evaluate the clinical effectiveness of sequential biventricular CRT.[22] All patients (359 with sequential devices and 216 with simultaneous CRT devices) underwent reassessment of quality of life, follow-up 6-minute hall walk test, and estimation of NYHA functional class before hospital discharge and at 1, 3, and 6 months after implant. At follow-up, optimization of the AV and V–V stimulation intervals was carried out. Echo Doppler interrogation first determined the optimal AV interval that maximized transmitral filling using the Ritter method. The right atrium (RA) to LV interval was kept constant at the optimal setting while varying the LV–RV interval in random sequence –80 ms (RV first) to +80 ms (LV first) to identify the V–V offset producing the greatest LV stroke volume. The Doppler-derived stroke volume at each V–V setting was determined by LV outflow tract

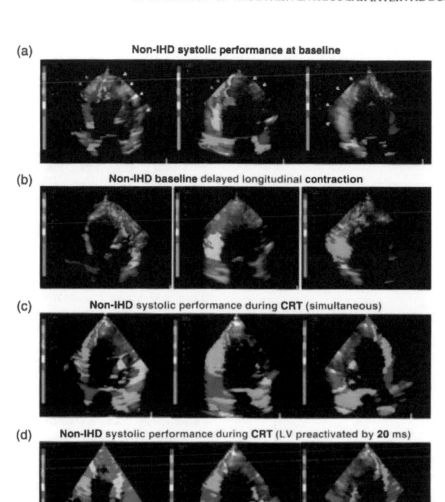

Figure 12.4 Effect of sequential biventricular pacing. (a) Transthoracic tissue tracking echocardiographic images in apical four-chamber view in systole in a patient with idiopathic dilated cardiomyopathy before implantation of a CRT device. Most of the lateral wall, the posterior wall, and distal parts of the anterior wall are gray, indicating lack of systolic motion toward the apex (white arrows). Color-coded scaling on the left side of each image indicates regional motion amplitude. Mechanical function of the interventricular septum and inferior walls is abnormal, with greater motion amplitude in segments adjacent to the apex (green arrows). (b) Extent of myocardium (colored segments) with delayed longitudinal contraction (DLC) in diastole (mitral valve open) shown in the lateral wall. Note that the remaining part of the left ventricle (LV) is gray, indicating no motion (the rest of the LV entered the relaxation phase). (c) The same patient with simultaneous CRT, resulting in contraction of a larger proportion of the lateral wall. In addition, each segment shows improved systolic shortening as judged from color coding. Moreover, abnormal distribution of myocardial motion in the interventricular septum has been normalized. (d) Impact of sequential CRT with the LV activated by 20 ms before the right ventricle (RV). Compared with simultaneous CRT, sequential CRT yields further improvement in the overall proportion of contracting myocardium in the lateral wall. In addition, each segment shows further improvement in systolic shortening amplitude. (Adapted from Sogaard P et al. Circulation 2002; 106:2078–84.[21])

(LVOT) VTI multiplied by the LVOT cross-sectional area. The improvement in stroke volume was defined as the difference between the stroke volume at the optimal V–V setting and that at the nominal, or simultaneous, V–V setting (Figure 12.5).

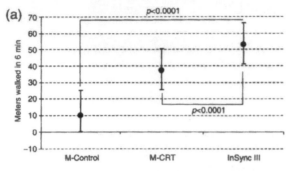

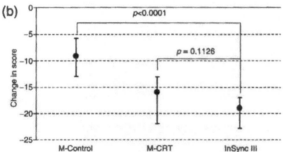

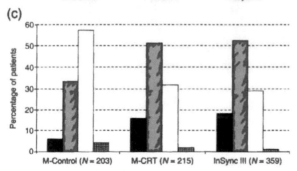

Figure 12.5 InSync III study comparing simultaneous biventricular pacing with sequential biventricular pacing: changes in 6-minute hall walk (a), quality-of-life score (b), and changes in NYHA functional class (c) after 6 months. In (c): black bars, improved ⩾2; diagonally lined bars, improved; white bars, no change; dotted bars, worsened. M, Multicenter InSync Randomized Clinical Evaluation (MIRACLE); M-CRT, MIRACLE Cardiac Resynchronization Therapy trial. (Reprinted from J Am Coll Cardiol. Vol 46. Leon AR, Abraham WT, Brozena S, et al; Insync III Clinical Study Investigators. Cardiac resynchronization with sequential biventricular pacing for the treatment of moderate-to-severe heart failure. Pages 2298–304. (2005). With permission from the American College of Cardiology Foundation.[22])

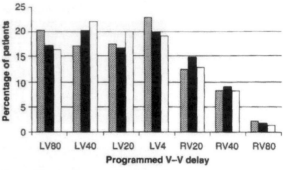

Figure 12.6 Optimal V–V timing settings in the InSync III trial (simultaneous vs sequential biventricular pacing) at pre-hospital discharge and at 3 and 6 months. LV80, LV lead pre-excitation 80 ms, etc.; RV20, RV lead pre-excitation 20 ms, etc. Diagonally lined bars, pre-hospital discharge; black bars, 3 months; white bars, 6 months. (Reproduced with permission from Leon AR et al. J Am Coll Cardiol 2005;46:2298–304.[22])

Figure 12.6 illustrates the distribution of the optimal LV–RV settings in the InSync III study prior to hospital discharge and at 3 and 6 months of follow-up. More than 75% of patients at each assessment had an optimal LV–RV setting between –40 ms and +40 ms.[22] The majority of patients had an optimal V–V setting delivering LV stimulation first (55%, 54%, and 58% at hospital discharge and 3- and 6-month visits, respectively). The proportion of patients with a simultaneous optimal V–V setting remained fairly stable over time (23%, 20%, and 19% at hospital discharge and 3- and 6-month visits, respectively). The proportion of patients with an optimal V–V setting delivering RV stimulation first also remained consistent at the three follow-up visits (23%, 26%, and 23%, respectively) (Figure 12.6). Individual patient changes during follow-up were not performed. Increased stroke volume was found in 81% of the V–V patients at 6 months. Stroke volume improved (optimal vs simultaneous V–V setting) by 8.6% (median percentage) prior to hospital discharge, by 8.4% at 3 months, and by 7.3% at 6 months. Sixty-four patients (17%) prior to hospital discharge, 49 patients (14%) at 3 months, and 49 patients (14%) at 6 months experienced an improvement in stroke volume of 20% or more during sequential pacing. Patients with a history of myocardial infarction were identified as experiencing statistically significant more improvement in stroke volume (p = 0.03) during optimal V–V programming versus the nominal V–V setting. The improvement in stroke volume at the optimal V–V interval continued throughout all follow-up intervals (prior to hospital discharge and at 3 and 6 months). This suggests that the ability to vary V–V timing compensated for infarct-related conduction block. Increase in stroke volume in NYHA functional class IV patients with an optimized V–V setting was not statistically significant (p = 0.1344), yet it was consistent across all follow-up intervals (prior to hospital discharge, and at 3 and 6 months).

There was no significant difference in the effect of optimized sequential and simultaneous CRT on NYHA functional class or quality-of-life score and functional capacity.[22] However, the V–V group experienced a greater improvement in 6-minute hall walk from baseline to 6 months compared with the simultaneous CRT group (p = 0.0015). There was no correlation between improvement in stroke volume and improved exercise capacity.

Overview of small-scale studies

Table 12.1 outlines data from studies involving a relatively small number of patients, as well as the large InSync III trial.[2, 22–31] The overall results of the smaller studies are basically similar to those of the larger InSync III study.

GENERAL CONSIDERATIONS

The optimal V–V delay should decrease LV dyssynchrony and provide a more homogeneous LV activation with faster LV emptying and improved and longer diastolic filling. V–V programmability may increase LVEF and other indices of LV function, and may also reduce mitral regurgitation in some patients,[30] but overall improvement is only moderate. V–V programming may be particularly helpful in compensating for less than optimal LV lead position, by tailoring ventricular timing to correct for individual heterogeneous ventricular activation patterns. The benefit of V–V programming is additive to AV delay optimization. The optimal V–V delay cannot be identified clinically in the majority of patients (Table 12.1).

The range of optimal V–V delays is relatively narrow and most commonly involves LV pre-excitation by 20 ms. LV pre-excitation is required in most patients. RV pre-excitation should be used cautiously, because advancing RV activation may cause a decline in LV function. Consequently, RV pre-excitation should be reserved for patients with dyssynchrony in the septal and inferior segments, provided there is hemodynamic proof of benefit.[21] Patients with ischemic cardiomyopathy (with slower-conducting scars) may require more pre-excitation than those with idiopathic dilated cardiomyopathy.[24] V–V programming is of particular benefit in patients with a previous myocardial infarction.[22]

V–V programming in patients with permanent atrial fibrillation

Most of the studies listed in Table 12.1 excluded patients with atrial fibrillation. The study by van Gelder et al[24] suggests that V–V programming is also beneficial in CRT patients with atrial fibrillation and continual biventricular pacing, but further work is required to confirm these results.[23]

Order of AV and V–V programming

The order in which CRT systems are hemodynamically optimized is important. Ideally, the optimal left-sided AV delay should be determined before each V–V setting. This may be accomplished by determining the optimal AV delay from the time of sensing in the RA to the LV stimulus (AS–LV delay) during monochamber LV pacing. This AV delay remains optimized if the RV is not pre-excited, simply because the LV is activated at the end of the programmed AV delay. RV pre-excitation should be used cautiously, because it may impair the optimal AV delay by delaying the left-sided AV delay. With RV pre-excitation, the optimal AV delay becomes equal to the optimal AS–LV delay minus the programmed V–V interval[32] (Figure 12.2). The timing of the AV delay in Guidant devices is RV-based. Consequently, the programmed AV delay for LV pre-excitation is equal to the optimal AV delay plus the V–V interval.

Table 12.1 Studies of sequential biventricular pacing

Ref	Year	No. of pts	QRS (ms)	Parameter	Results[a]
21	2002	20	>130	TDI and 3D echocardiography	LV_1 9, RV_1, 11 pts
13	2003	12	≥150	Invasive dP/dt_{max}	LV_1 9, BiV_0 3 pts
23	2004	9 AF	152 ± 44 (7 LBBB, 1 RBBB, 1 normal)	Invasive dP/dt_{max}	BiV_0 > RV_1, LV_1 minimal effect
24	2004	53:41 SR, 12 AF	>150	Invasive LV dP/dt_{max}	LV_1 44 (84%), BiV_0 6, and RV_1 3 pts. Mean V–V interval was greater for ischemic than idiopathic cardiomyopathy
25	2004	34	≥130 (≥180 in PM dependent pts)	Echo Doppler determination of stroke volume	LV_1 62%
26	2005	22	>130	Invasive LV dP/dt_{max}	Sequential pacing 41% pts, with only 1 RV_1 pt. Others BiV_0 equivalent
2	2005	27	>120	Radionuclide angiography (LVEF)	LV_1 45%, BiV_0 33%, RV_1 22%
27	2005	21	>130	Echocardiography MPI	LV_1 48%, RV_1 48%, BiV_0 4%
28	2005	19	≥150	Echo Doppler determination of cardiac output	LV_1 best in most pts, RV_1 best in 2 pts
29	2005	20	≥130	LVOT VTI	LV_1 12, RV_1 5, BiV_0 3 pts
22	2005	207 BiV_0, 359 sequential	≥130	Echo Doppler determination of stroke volume	At 6 months: LV_1 58%, BiV_0 19%, RV_1 23%,
30	2006	23	>120	Aortic VTI	LV_1 60, BiV_0 22%, RV_1 18%
31	2006	86	>150	Echo Doppler determination of stroke volume	LV_1 36%, RV_1 35%, BiV_0 29%

3D, 3-dimensional; AF, atrial fibrillation; BiV_0, simultaneous biventricular pacing; LBBB, left bundle branch block; LV, left ventricle; LV_1, LV pre-activation; LVEF, LV ejection fraction; LVOT, LV outflow tract; MPI, myocardial performance index. PM, pacemaker; pts, patients; RBBB, right bundle branch block; RV, right ventricle; RV_1, RV pre-activation; SR, sinus rhythm; TDI, tissue Doppler imaging; VTI, velocity–time integral.
[a]The results indicate the distribution of the optimal V–V delay according to its corresponding pacing mode: LV_1, RV_1, and BiV_0 in terms of the number of patients or percentage. All patients were in sinus rhythm unless indicated otherwise (AF).

Long-term stability of the optimal V–V interval and clinical response

The optimal V–V delay may change with the passage of time, and individual changes cannot be accurately predicted. Detailed, regular re-evaluations and reprogramming of optimal parameters seem appropriate.

Boriani et al[31] reported disappointing results at the 6-month follow-up after V–V optimization. They selected patients at random and compared the results of CRT with simultaneous biventricular pacing (*n* = 23) versus V–V optimized devices (*n* = 72) after a follow-up of

6 months. There were no differences in symptoms, quality of life, or functional capacity between the two groups. These results are difficult to explain, but they may be related to the selection of sicker patients (QRS ≥150 ms), the lack of AV optimization after programming the V–V interval, a change in the optimal V–V interval after 6 months, or progression of disease. In this respect, O'Donnell et al[33] studied 40 recipients of CRT devices. Optimized V–V delays were determined according to echocardiographic criteria. There was a trend toward reduction in the LV predominance of the optimal

V–V delay during follow-up. The mean optimal V–V delay at implantation was 22 ms (range −12 to +32 ms) with the LV activated first, versus 12 ms (range −16 to +32 ms) at 9 months. These observations are partially supported by the data of Mortensen et al,[25] who found that the optimal V–V interval changed in 56% of CRT patients at the 3-month follow-up.

V–V interval optimization on exercise

A recent study assessed the impact of sequential biventricular pacing during exercise.[30] Simultaneous biventricular pacing was optimal during exercise in only about 25% of patients (Figure 12.7). Most of the improvement was observed with short V–V delays, ranging from 12 to 20 ms. Optimized sequential biventricular pacing offered substantial additional benefit when considering the aortic VTI and mitral regurgitation. Differences between resting and exercise optimization were observed in more than half of the patients. With future technological advances, separate automatic programming between resting and exercise for V–V delay may become possible by means of sensors or other ways to control hemodynamics at rest and with activity. Recent data from the same group suggest that the degree of LV dyssynchrony varies with exercise and may diminish in some patients.

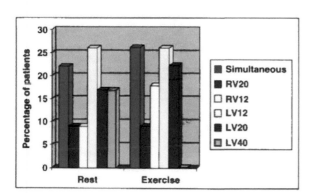

Figure 12.7 Optimal V–V delay at rest and during exercise. RV20, RV lead pre-excitation 20 ms, etc.; LV12, LV lead pre-excitation 12 ms, etc. (Reproduced from Bordachar P et al. Am J Cardiol 2006;97:1622–5.[30])

EFFECT OF V–V TIMING ON THE ECG OF BIVENTRICULAR PACEMAKERS

The electrocardiographic (ECG) consequences of temporally different RV and LV activation with programmable V–V timing in the latest biventricular devices have not yet been studied in detail. In the absence of anodal stimulation, increasing the V–V interval gradually to 80 ms (LV first) will progressively increase the duration of the paced QRS complex and alter its morphology, with a larger R wave in lead V_1, indicating more dominant LV depolarization.[34] The varying QRS configuration in lead V_1 with different V–V intervals has not been correlated with the hemodynamic response. Consequently, at this, juncture it is unwise to attempt programming the optimal V–V interval according to the height of the paced R wave in lead V_1.

Anodal stimulation

RV anodal stimulation during biventricular pacing interferes with a programmed V–V delay (often programmed with the LV preceding the RV) aimed at optimizing cardiac resynchronization. This interference occurs because RV anodal capture causes simultaneous RV and LV activation (the V–V interval becomes zero). In the presence of anodal stimulation, the ECG morphology and its duration will not change if the device is programmed with V–V intervals of 80, 60, and 40 ms (LV before RV). The delayed RV cathodal output (80, 60, and 40 ms) then falls in the myocardial refractory period initiated by the preceding anodal stimulation. At V–V intervals ≤ 20 ms, the paced QRS may change because the short LV–RV interval prevents propagation of activation from the site of RV anodal capture in time to render the cathodal site refractory.[34] Thus, the cathode also captures the RV and contributes to RV depolarization, which then takes place from two sites: RV anode and RV cathode.[34]

AUTOMATIC DEVICE-BASED OPTIMIZATION OF THE V–V DELAY

St Jude Medical have recently introduced a method whereby the programmer itself can

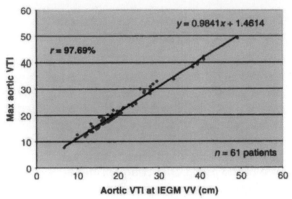

Figure 12.8 Comparison of the aortic velocity–time integral with the corresponding value obtained from analysis of intracardiac electrograms (IEGM). (Reprinted from Heart Rhythm; 3(Suppl.)) Meine M, Min X, Paris M, et al. An intracardiac EGM method for VV optimization during cardiac resynchronization (Abstract). Pages S63–S64 (2006).[36]

determine and then program the V–V delay automatically.[35] This design was based on a study involving 61 patients who received a St Jude

EPIC HF device, which used the ventricular electrogram (IEGM) to obtain the optimal V–V interval.[36] Optimal V–V delays based on the IEGM algorithm were compared with the optimal V–V interval obtained by the maximum aortic VTI over seven V–V delays (20, 40, and 80 ms), with both RV and LV leads pre-activated and simultaneous biventricular pacing (Figure 12.8). The maximum aortic VTI (22.1 ± 8.2 cm) was equivalent to the IEGM aortic VTI values (20.9 ± 8.3 cm) (concordance $r = 0.98$ and a 95% confidence lower limit of 97%; $p < 0.0001$). In 36 patients, the differences between the IEGM V–V delays and echo-optimal V–V delays were within 20 ms.

The St Jude system consists of a sensed followed by a paced determination (Figure 12.9):

1. *Intrinsic depolarization delay (sensing).* For optimization of the V–V delay, the algorithm first measures the intrinsic interventricular depolarization delay (Δ) between the RV and LV during atrial pacing or sensing (Figure 12.8). From there, it assumes that the

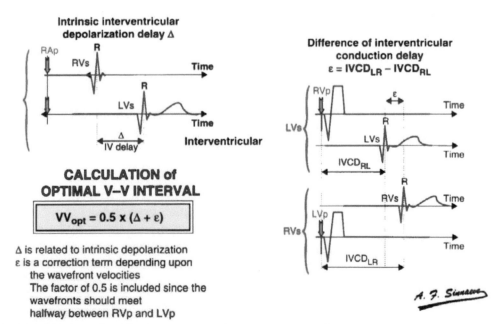

Figure 12.9 Diagrammatic representation of the St Jude Medical system for optimizing the V–V interval. RAp, right atrial pacing event; RVs, right ventricular sensed event; RVp, right ventricular paced event; LVs, left ventricular sensed event; LVp, left ventricular paced event; IVCD$_{RL}$, right-to-left interventricular conduction delay; IVCD$_{LR}$, left-to-right interventricular conduction delay; Δ, interventricular delay. See the text for details.

ventricle that is detected latest will have to be stimulated first (which makes sense). Internally, the device assigns a 'sign' to the measured Δ (positive if LV has to be paced first and negative in the case of RV first).

2. *Interventricular conduction delays (pacing)*. After measurement of the intrinsic depolarization, the algorithm determines the RV-to-LV and LV-to-RV conduction delays ($IVCD_{RL}$ and $IVCD_{LR}$, respectively) by pacing one ventricle and looking to the response in the opposite ventricle. The difference between the left-to-right and right-to-left interventricular conduction delays is denoted by ε:

$$\varepsilon = IVCD_{LR} - IVCD_{RL}$$

As ε is used as a correction term depending on the wavefront velocity, its sign (plus or minus) is important. Thus, if the conduction is slower from the LV lead, ε will be positive.

3. *Calculation of optimal V–V delay*. Finally the optimal V–V delay is determined as half the sum of the intrinsic depolarization delay and the interventricular conduction delay:

$$VV_{opt} = 0.5 \times (\Delta + \varepsilon)$$

- If Δ is positive and ε positive, the sum is positive and LV is first.
- If Δ is negative and ε negative, the sum is negative and RV is first
- If Δ is positive and ε negative (or vice versa), the sum can either be positive or negative, depending on the relative values of Δ and ε. But, in any case, if the sum is positive, LV will be first. If the sum is negative, RV will be first.

The device knows what chamber to stimulate first, because it takes the signs into account for the calculation. It only expresses the results using absolute values and mentioning what chamber is paced first.

REFERENCES

1. Whinnett ZI, Davies JE, Willson K, et al. Haemodynamic effects of changes in atrioventricular and interventricular delay in cardiac resynchronisation therapy show a consistent pattern: analysis of shape, magnitude and relative importance of atrioventricular and interventricular delay. Heart 2006;92:1628–34.

2. Burri H, Sunthorn H, Somsen A, et al. Optimizing sequential biventricular pacing using radionuclide ventriculography. Heart Rhythm 2005;2:960–5.

3. Bax JJ, Abraham T, Barold SS, et al. Cardiac resynchronization therapy: Part 2 – Issues during and after device implantation and unresolved questions. J Am Coll Cardiol. 2005;46:2168–82.

4. Jansen AH, Bracke FA, van Dantzig JM, et al. Correlation of echo-Doppler optimization of atrioventricular delay in cardiac resynchronization therapy with invasive hemodynamics in patients with heart failure secondary to ischemic or idiopathic dilated cardiomyopathy. Am J Cardiol 2006;97:552–7.

5. Bax JJ, Ansalone G, Breithardt OA, et al. Echocardiographic evaluation of cardiac resynchronization therapy: ready for routine clinical use? A critical appraisal. J Am Coll Cardiol 2004;44:1–9.

6. Breithardt OA, Stellbrink C, Franke A, et al. Pacing Therapies for Congestive Heart Failure Study Group; Guidant Congestive Heart Failure Research Group. Acute effects of cardiac resynchronization therapy on left ventricular Doppler indices in patients with congestive heart failure. Am Heart J 2002;143:34–44.

7. Marcus GM, Rose E, Viloria EM, et al. VENTAK CHF/CONTAK-CD Biventricular Pacing Study Investigators. Septal to posterior wall motion delay fails to predict reverse remodeling or clinical improvement in patients undergoing cardiac resynchronization therapy. J Am Coll Cardiol 2005;46:2208–14.

8. Yu CM, Zhang Q, Chan YS, et al. Tissue Doppler velocity is superior to displacement and strain mapping in predicting left ventricular reverse remodelling response after cardiac resynchronisation therapy. Heart 2006; 92:1452–6.

9. Yu CM, Wing-Hong Fung J, Zhang Q, Sanderson JE. Understanding nonresponders of cardiac resynchronization therapy – current and future perspectives. J Cardiovasc Electrophysiol 2005;16:1117–24.

10. Delfino JG, Bhasin M, Cole R, et al. Comparison of myocardial velocities obtained with magnetic resonance phase velocity mapping and tissue Doppler imaging in normal subjects and patients with left ventricular dyssynchrony. J Magn Reson Imaging 2006; 24:304–11.

11. Burri H, Lerch R. Echocardiography and patient selection for cardiac resynchronization therapy: a critical appraisal. Heart Rhythm 2006;3:474–9.

12. Notabartolo D, Merlino JD, Smith AL, et al. Usefulness of the peak velocity difference by tissue Doppler imaging technique as an effective predictor of response to cardiac resynchronization therapy. Am J Cardiol 2004;94:817–20.

13. Perego GB, Chianca R, Facchini M, et al. Simultaneous vs. sequential biventricular pacing in dilated cardiomyopathy: an acute hemodynamic study. Eur J Heart Fail 2003;5:305–13.

14. Ramanathan C, Jia P, Ghanem R, Ryu K, Rudy Y. Activation and repolarization of the normal human heart under complete physiological conditions. Proc Natl Acad Sci USA 2006;103:6309–14.

15. Wyndham CR, Meeran MK, Smith T, et al. Epicardial activation of the intact human heart without conduction defect. Circulation 1979;59:161–8.

16. Nelson GS, Curry CW, Wyman BT, et al. Predictors of systolic augmentation from left ventricular preexcitation in patients with dilated cardiomyopathy and intraventricular conduction delay. Circulation 2000;101: 2703–9.

17. Rodriguez LM, Timmermans C, Nabar A, Beatty G, Wellens HJ. Variable patterns of septal activation in patients with left bundle branch block and heart failure. J Cardiovasc Electrophysiol 2003;14:135–41.

18. Fung JW, Yu CM, Yip G, et al. Variable left ventricular activation pattern in patients with heart failure and left bundle branch block. Heart 2004;90:17–19.

19. Auricchio A, Fantoni C, Regoli F, et al. Characterization of left ventricular activation in patients with heart failure and left bundle-branch block. Circulation 2004;109: 1133–9.

20. Herweg B, Ilercil A, Madramootoo C, et al. Latency during left ventricular pacing from the lateral cardiac veins: a cause of ineffectual biventricular pacing. Pacing Clin Electrophysiol 2006;29:574–81.

21. Sogaard P, Egeblad H, Pedersen AK, et al. Sequential versus simultaneous biventricular resynchronization for severe heart failure: evaluation by tissue Doppler imaging. Circulation 2002;106:2078–84.

22. Leon AR, Abraham WT, Brozena S, et al. InSync III Clinical Study Investigators. Cardiac resynchronization with sequential biventricular pacing for the treatment of moderate-to-severe heart failure. J Am Coll Cardiol 2005;46:2298–304.

23. Hay I, Melenovsky V, Fetics BJ, et al. Short-term effects of right-left heart sequential cardiac resynchronization in patients with heart failure, chronic atrial fibrillation, and atrioventricular nodal block. Circulation 2004;110: 3404–10.

24. van Gelder BM, Bracke FA, Meijer A, Lakerveld LJ, Pijls NH. Effect of optimizing the VV interval on left ventricular contractility in cardiac resynchronization therapy. Am J Cardiol 2004;93:1500–3.

25. Mortensen PT, Sogaard P, Mansour H, et al. Sequential biventricular pacing: evaluation of safety and efficacy. Pacing Clin Electrophysiol 2004;27:339–45.

26. Kurzidim K, Reinke H, Sperzel J, et al. Invasive optimization of cardiac resynchronization therapy: role of sequential ventricular and left ventricular pacing. Pacing Clin Electrophysiol 2005;28:754–61.

27. Porciani MC, Dondina C, Macioce R, et al. Echocardiographic examination of atrioventricular and interventricular delay optimization in cardiac resynchronization therapy. Am J Cardiol 2005;95:1108–10.

28. Riedlbauchova L, Kautzner J, Fridl P. Influence of different atrioventricular and interventricular delays on cardiac output during cardiac resynchronization therapy. Pacing Clin Electrophysiol 2005;28(Suppl 1): S19–23.

29. Vanderheyden M, De Backer T, Rivero-Ayerza M, et al. Tailored echocardiographic interventricular delay programming further optimizes left ventricular performance after cardiac resynchronization therapy. Heart Rhythm 2005;2:1066–72.

30. Bordachar P, Lafitte S, Reuter S, et al. Echocardiographic assessment during exercise of heart failure patients with cardiac resynchronization therapy. Am J Cardiol 2006;97:1622–5.

31. Boriani G, Muller CP, Seidl KH, et al. Resynchronization for the HemodYnamic Treatment for Heart Failure Management II Investigators. Randomized comparison of simultaneous biventricular stimulation versus optimized interventricular delay in cardiac resynchronization therapy. The Resynchronization for the HemodYnamic Treatment for Heart Failure Management II Implantable Cardioverter Defibrillator (RHYTHM II ICD) study. Am Heart J 2006;151:1050–8.

32. Kay GN. Troubleshooting and programming of cardiac resynchronization therapy. In: Ellenbogen KA, Kay GN, Wilkoff BL, eds. Device Therapy for Congestive Heart Failure. Philadelphia: WB Saunders, 2004:232–93.

33. O'Donnell D, Nadurata V, Hamer A, Kertes P, Mohammed W. Long-term variations in optimal programming of cardiac resynchronization therapy devices. Pacing Clin Electrophysiol 2005;28(Suppl 1):S24–6.

34. van Gelder BM, Bracke FA, Meijer A. The effect of anodal stimulation on V–V timing at varying V–V intervals. Pacing Clin Electrophysiol 2005;28:771–6.

35. Analysis of QuickOpt™ Timing Cycle Optimization. An IEGM Method to Optimize AV, PV, and VV delays. Sylmar, CA: St Jude Medical, 2006.

36. Meine M, Min X, Paris M, Park E. An intracardiac EGM method for VV optimization during cardiac resynchronization. Heart Rhythm 2006;3(Suppl): S63–4 (abst).

13

Complications of cardiac resynchronization therapy

Christoph Stellbrink

Introduction • Complications associated with the implantation procedure • Complications during chronic CRT • Summary

INTRODUCTION

With the increased use of cardiac resynchronization therapy (CRT) as a routine approach in the management of patients with moderate to advanced heart failure and ventricular conduction delay, this therapy has spread from few investigational centers with long-term experience, high implant volumes, and state-of-the art equipment to smaller units that may have started implementing CRT only recently. One has to bear in mind that the requirements for CRT are much higher than for a regular pacemaker or implantable cardioverter–defibrillator (ICD) service. This concerns the implantation setting as well as follow-up procedures. Therefore, it is wise to be aware of the potential complications and pitfalls of CRT before setting up such a program at a specific center. This chapter aims to give an overview of the available data on CRT complications, combined with some comments from individual experience.

The complications of CRT can be roughly divided into those associated with the implantation procedure and those arising during chronic therapy.

COMPLICATIONS ASSOCIATED WITH THE IMPLANTATION PROCEDURE

General remarks

The risks associated with the implantation procedure may be classified as the general risks, i.e., those associated with anesthesia, device implantation (pacemaker or ICD), right-sided lead placement, and defibrillation threshold testing, and the specific risks of CRT, i.e., those associated with left ventricular (LV) lead implantation. A summary of the different risks is shown in Table 13.1.

A complete discussion of the general risks of the CRT implantation procedure lies beyond the scope of this chapter. Although it has to be taken into consideration that patients undergoing implantation of a CRT device generally have a higher perioperative risk than those undergoing regular pacemaker or ICD implantation due to the higher morbidity of the heart failure population, data from large series are reassuring that the actual incidence of perioperative adverse events is acceptable. In the largest published series,[1] the overall incidence of perioperative complications was 13.8%, but only about half of these could be attributed to coronary sinus intubation, LV lead implantation, or heart failure decompensation, which may be regarded as specific complications of CRT. The perioperative mortality rate in this series was only 0.4% and the 30-day mortality rate 1.6%. Most patients died from either sudden cardiac death or progressive heart failure. In addition, these data include early experience from the MIRACLE, MIRACLE ICD, and Insync III trials. The analysis showed that the complication rate was already decreasing in the patients enrolled later in the studies. Thus, with the current increase in experience and the improved implantation tools

Table 13.1 Risks associated with CRT device implantation

General risks	Specific risks of CRT
Risks associated with anesthesia	Transvenous LV lead implantation:
Allergic reaction (contrast media)	Coronary sinus dissection/perforation
General surgical risks:	Complete heart block
Infection	Contrast-induced renal
Pneumothorax	failure
Bleeding	Epicardial lead implantation
Perforation	Pneumothorax
Risks associated with defibrillation threshold testing (only ICDs)	Need for thoracotomy

that are available, the actual complication rate may be considerably lower in large-volume centers. It has to be pointed out, though, that implantation of a resynchronization device requires a higher level of pre-, intra-, and postoperative preparation and care than either standard right-sided pacemaker or ICD implant procedures. Moreover, implantation should preferably be performed using optimal angiographic settings such as are usually available in cardiac catheterization laboratories, in order to improve the implant success rate and to reduce implant duration and radiation exposure to patients and implanting personnel.[2] The duration of the implantation procedure is still in the range of 2.5 hours, but may be considerably longer in some patients. The same applies to the fluoroscopy time, which is in the range of 20–30 minutes in most published series. It has to be considered that the radiation exposure associated with CRT device implantation is associated with a distinctly increased risk of fatal cancer.[3] However, many patients undergoing this procedure have a limited life-expectancy in spite of the implanted device, and thus the cancer risk may be a purely theoretical consideration in clinical routine.

Specific complications of CRT implantation: risks associated with LV lead placement

In principle, LV lead implantation may be performed via the coronary venous approach, the transseptal approach, or surgical epicardial implantation via a limited left lateral thoracotomy. In clinical routine, the coronary venous approach has become the preferred approach and thus will be discussed here in greater detail. The transseptal route cannot be recommended, despite its technical feasibility,[4] due to the potential long-term risk of systemic embolism associated with left endocardial leads.[5] The surgical approach, however, may be an alternative in the rare patient with difficult coronary venous anatomy or complete absence of a suitable venous branch. Thus, this approach will be briefly discussed at the end of this chapter.

Risks of coronary venous lead placement

There are risks associated with occlusion angiography of the coronary sinus. Coronary venous implantation can be performed using an 'over-the-wire' lead or a stylet-driven lead. Regardless of the lead used, it is advisable to perform a coronary sinus angiography before implantation in order to identify the most suitable vein for LV pacing. It is also useful in order to visualize different side-branches in case of problems with pacing threshold or phrenic nerve stimulation at the initially desired pacing site. Non-invasive imaging of the coronary sinus by multislice computed tomography (CT) has been proposed,[6] but this usually cannot replace coronary sinus angiography, which may be performed by a direct retrograde approach or an indirect approach using the venous phase after contrast injection into the left coronary artery.[7] Although indirect venography has the advantage that injury to the coronary sinus can be avoided, it requires arterial access and thus may be impractical in the operative setting. Moreover, in the author's view, direct retrograde coronary sinus angiography usually allows better opacification of the coronary venous vasculature, and thus has become the method of choice in most centers. It requires intubation of the coronary sinus with an angiography catheter. Contrast can be injected directly through the catheter; this may be associated with a lower incidence of coronary sinus dissection,[8] but has the disadvantage that the blood flow directed against the injection impedes optimal vessel visualization. Thus, the author prefers transient balloon occlusion angiography. This requires using a guiding catheter (usually 8 French) through which a balloon angiography catheter is entered into the posterior aspect of the coronary sinus. After brief occlusion of the vessel by inflating the balloon, contrast medium is injected into the vessel with gentle pressure, allowing visualization of the coronary venous vessels. This technique is superior to direct injection through the guiding catheter, especially in cases when different veins have to be tested and thus full visualization of all the different ventricular branches of the coronary sinus is important.

There are two major risks associated with coronary venous angiography: contrast-induced nephropathy and coronary venous dissection.

Many patients with heart failure have enlarged atria, which may make intubation of the coronary sinus with a guiding catheter sometimes difficult, requiring high amounts of contrast medium. At the same time, some pre-existing renal insufficiency is often present and patients may be dehydrated by treatment with diuretics. If too much contrast medium are used without adequate preparation of the patient, renal function may deteriorate or even acute renal failure may result. There are no published data on the incidence of renal failure after coronary sinus angiography. Nevertheless, it is advisable that patients should be adequately hydrated throughout the implantation procedure and possibly pretreated with acetylcysteine; renal function and urine output should be closely monitored after the operation if large amounts of contrast were necessary for LV lead deployment.

Introduction of the guiding catheter into the coronary sinus ostium is sometimes difficult, and too vigorous manipulation with the guiding catheter or the balloon catheter can cause venous dissection (Figure 13.1). This complication can also be caused by too vigorous contrast injection distal to the occluded balloon. Injury to the coronary sinus and its tributaries is much less commonly caused by the guidewire or the pacing lead itself. The incidence of venous dissection is in the range 2–3.5%.[9,10] Fortunately, coronary sinus dissection usually heals well and pericardial tamponade is a rare exception (its incidence

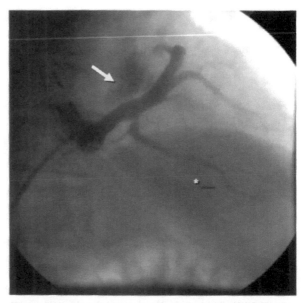

Figure 13.1 Coronary sinus angiography in the 30° anterior oblique view in a patient with ischemic cardiomyopathy and a previously implanted pacemaker lead (*). The vessel has been lacerated at the posterolateral aspect, and contrast injection into the proximal coronary sinus shows a contrast deposit adjacent to the vessel (arrow). The patient developed a minor pericardial effusion after the angiography, without any hemodynamic consequences. Upgrading of the pacemaker to a biventricular ICD could be performed successfully without complications 2 weeks later, after complete resolution of the pericardial effusion.

is 0.4–0.9%).[1,10] Nevertheless, it seems prudent to stop the implantation procedure if a severe coronary sinus dissection is noted and defer the procedure for 2–4 weeks, when the injury is usually healed. Echocardiographic monitoring is mandatory to exclude a hemodynamically relevant pericardial effusion.

Catheter or lead manipulation at the right ventricular (RV) septum can lead to transient mechanical right bundle branch block (RBBB). Since most CRT candidates have pre-existing left bundle branch block (LBBB), complete atrioventricular (AV) block may ensue. This complication occurs at an incidence of <1%,[10] but may occasionally lead to an emergency situation if no adequate escape rhythm is present. In the author's experience, complete AV block is most often induced during placement of the coronary sinus guiding catheter. It can thus be easily avoided by placing the RV lead before entering the coronary sinus, which allows immediate RV pacing should complete conduction block occur.

Risks of direct surgical epicardial implantation of the LV lead

Several approaches for direct epicardial lead implantation have been proposed, such as implantation by a limited left lateral thoracotomy,[11] thoracoscopic implantation,[12] or robotic assistance.[13] It is most important when using the surgical approach to realize that leads need to be placed in a lateral or even posterior position, as more anterior lead positions may lead to a suboptimal hemodynamic response to CRT.[14] The incidence of lead revisions is smaller than with the coronary venous approach, but the initial hospitalization is longer due to the prolonged recovery of the patient.[14] In addition, in about 7% of patients, the operative approach has to be extendend to a full thoracotomy because of an inability to place the leads in an adequate position with the limited surgical access.[15] Thus, epicardial lead implantation is usually reserved for those cases where coronary venous implantation is not feasible due to unsatisfactory coronary venous anatomy.

COMPLICATIONS DURING CHRONIC CRT

As for the perioperative risks, the chronic risks of CRT can be divided into the general risks of pacemaker/ICD therapy and those specific to CRT (Table 13.2). This chapter focuses on the specific complications that are caused by CRT itself or the potential influence of the triple-lead device on ICD detection or therapy delivery. The complications may be lead-related, device-related, or caused by patient-specific events such

as disease progression or arrhythmias. The overall incidence of chronic complications within the first 6 months after implantation in the largest published series was 10.6%.[1] Most complications were lead-related (7.9%), and of these, the majority concerned the LV lead.

Lead-related complications

Lead dislodgement

The incidence of coronary sinus lead dislodgement in large CRT series is in the range 4.0–13.6%.[1,16] Most dislodgements occur early (i.e., within the first weeks after implantation). With newer lead designs, which usually have some passive fixation mechanisms (Figure 13.2), the incidence may be lower, but long-term data on these leads are not yet available. A dislodged LV lead may potentially prolapse into the RV and cause ventricular arrhythmias, or induce atrial fibrillation if it is floating in the right atrium (RA). Moreover, due to the loss of synchronization, cardiac decompensation may be precipitated. Dislodged coronary sinus leads should be surgically removed and a new lead placed. Removal of coronary sinus leads is usually safe,[17] but surgical stand-by should be available.

Phrenic nerve stimulation

The left phrenic nerve can be located close to the (postero)lateral branch, which is usually the desired LV pacing site.[18] Therefore, the phrenic nerve threshold must always be tested during lead implantation, in addition to local sensing and ventricular pacing threshold. Every effort should be made to find a pacing site with an adequate LV pacing threshold (<2.0V) where the phrenic nerve is not captured at maximal device output. However, if this is not possible, the phrenic nerve threshold should at least be significantly higher than twice the LV pacing threshold. If the difference between the two thresholds is too small, diaphragmatic stimulation may make CRT deployment impossible. This is not a rare occurrence, since some chronic increase in ventricular pacing threshold is often observed and the phrenic nerve threshold may vary depending on the heart axis change with

---

Table 13.2 Risks associated with chronic CRT

General risks	Specific risks of CRT
Lead dislocation	Loss of LV lead pacing capture
Pocket or lead infection	Phrenic nerve stimulation
Arrhythmias	Heart failure decompensation

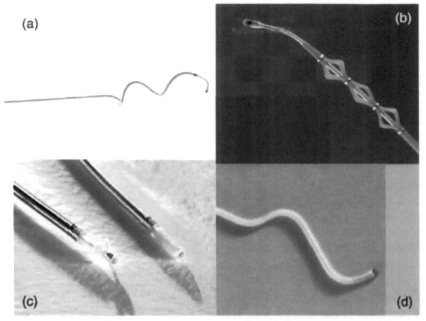

Figure 13.2 Coronary sinus leads with different fixation mechanisms. (a) Corox lead (BIOTRONIK, Berlin, Germany), using a helix for passive fixation. (b) Attain StarFix lead (Medtronic, Minneapolis, USA) with deployable lobes. (c) Endotak Reliance lead (Guidant, St Paul, USA) with active (screw) or passive (anchor) fixation. (d) Aescula lead (St Jude Medical, St Paul, USA), with a helix for passive fixation.

body position. The use of bipolar leads can be useful in reducing the incidence of phrenic nerve stimulation, as it offers the chance to test different pacing configurations, for example, bipolar stimulation between both coronary sinus poles or stimulation between the distal or proximal coronary sinus pole and a RV electrode. The incidence of diaphragmatic stimulation in larger series is 1.2–3%.[1,10] If it occurs after device implantation, it can sometimes be handled by reprogramming output or the pacing configuration, but lead revision is frequently necessary if the patient complains of intolerable hiccups.

Device-related complications

Device-related complications can be further classified into complications caused by delivery of resynchronization pacing therapy and those caused by inadequate tachycardia sensing or therapy. Apart from the well-known complications of pacemaker and defibrillator therapy, specific complications of biventricular devices

have been described in case reports. These include pacemaker-mediated tachycardia between the two ventricular electrodes[19] and double-sensing of RV and LV activation leading to inappropriate sensing of ventricular tachycardia and thus delivery of inadequate shocks.[20] The latter occurred only in first-generation devices – newer devices use only the RV signal for tachycardia detection. Loss of capture by the LV electrode may lead to lack of resynchronization and thus progressive heart failure. Loss of capture of the LV electrode may only be recognized by careful analysis of the paced QRS complex, for which specific algorithms have been proposed.[21]

Patient-related complications

Arrhythmia-related complications

Atrial fibrillation is common in patients with advanced heart failure. It may lead to precipitation of acute heart failure decompensation caused by three mechanisms: (1) loss of the atrial contribution to stroke volume; (2) impaired diastolic filling if rapid conduction to the ventricles occurs; (3) the irregularity in itself leading to variation in ventricular filling and contractility.[22] In CRT patients, a fourth very important pathophysiological mechanism is operative, namely, loss of the atrial-sensed event triggering the resynchronizing biventricular stimulus. This can lead to partial or complete inhibition of CRT delivery. Therefore, rapid clinical deterioration is common in CRT patients when atrial fibrillation occurs, and thus should be treated as an emergency. Cardioversion can be performed under conscious sedation either by applying a commanded device shock or by external cardioversion. Should the patient not be under adequate anticoagulation, transesophageal cardioversion can be used to rule out left atrial (LA) thrombi if the patient is hemodynamically stable and the arrhythmia is present for more than 48 hours.

Ventricular tachycardia (VT) or ventricular fibrillation clusters have been described in CRT patients.[23,24] An increased transmural dispersion of repolarization has been discussed as a potential mechanism for proarrhythmia.[25,26] Alternatively, increased occurrence of arrhythmia may simply reflect progression of a previously existing arrhythmogenic substrate. In these cases, antiarrhythmic drug treatment may reduce the incidence and rate of VT events. Amiodarone is preferred because of its efficacy and lack of negative inotropy, but sometimes even class I drugs may be necessary for rhythm stabilization. The negative inotropic effect of these drugs, however, limits their applicability, and they should never be used in a patient with a CRT device without defibrillation capability because of their proarrhythmic potential in heart failure. Radiofrequency ablation may be an attractive alternative, especially in the case of incessant monomorphic VT.

SUMMARY

CRT has emerged as an increasingly accepted approach to the treatment of advanced heart failure with ventricular dyssynchrony. This new therapy has not only broadened our understanding of the heart failure syndrome and added a completely new therapeutic option (i.e., electrical therapy) to the treatment of heart failure patients, but it has also introduced some new, specific complications that need the physician's consideration when implementing CRT in practice. Complications are mostly related to the implantation procedure and LV stimulation. Moreover, the high baseline morbidity of patients undergoing CRT has to be taken into account. Nevertheless, after adequate training and using an integrated approach involving the heart failure specialist, the electrophysiologist, and the cardiac surgeon, electrical therapy offers great benefit to those patients for whom it is indicated.

REFERENCES

1. Leon AR, Abraham WT, Curtis AB, et al. MIRACLE Study Program. Safety of transvenous cardiac resynchronization system implantation in patients with chronic heart failure: combined results of over 2000 patients from a multicenter study program. J Am Coll Cardiol 2005;46:2348–56.
2. Stellbrink C, Auricchio A, Lemke B, et al. Policy paper to the cardiac resynchronization therapy. Z Kardiol 2003;92:96–103.
3. Perisinakis K, Theocharopoulos N, Damilakis J, et al. Fluoroscopically guided implantation of modern cardiac resynchronization devices: radiation burden to the patient and associated risks. J Am Coll Cardiol 2005;46:2335–9.
4. Leclercq F, Hager FX, Macia JC, et al. Left ventricular lead insertion using a modified transseptal catheterization technique: a totally endocardial approach for permanent biventricular pacing in end-stage heart failure. Pacing Clin Electrophysiol 1999;22:1570–5.
5. Jais P, Takahashi A, Garrigue S, et al. Mid-term follow-up of endocardial biventricular pacing. Pacing Clin Electrophysiol 2000;23:1744–7.
6. Jongbloed MR, Lamb HJ, Bax JJ, et al. Noninvasive visualization of the cardiac venous system using multislice computed tomography. J Am Coll Cardiol 2005; 45:749–53.
7. Mischke K, Knackstedt C, Muhlenbruch G, et al. Imaging of the coronary venous system: retrograde coronary sinus angiography versus venous phase coronary angiograms. Int J Cardiol 2006 Oct 23; [Epub ahead of print].
8. De Martino G, Messano L, Santamaria M, et al. A randomized evaluation of different approaches to coronary sinus venography during biventricular pacemaker implants. Europace 2005;7:73–6.

9. Higgins SL, Hummel JD, Niazi IK, et al. Cardiac resynchronization therapy for the treatment of heart failure in patients with intraventricular conduction delay and malignant ventricular tachyarrhythmias. J Am Coll Cardiol 2003;42:1454–9.

10. Young JB, Abraham WT, Smith AL, et al. Multicenter InSync ICD Randomized Clinical Evaluation (MIRACLE ICD) Trial Investigators. Combined cardiac resynchronization and implantable cardioversion defibrillation in advanced chronic heart failure: the MIRACLE ICD trial. JAMA 2003;289:2685–94.

11. Izutani H, Quan KJ, Biblo LA, Gill IS. Biventricular pacing for congestive heart failure: early experience in surgical epicardial versus coronary sinus lead placement. Heart Surg Forum 2002;6:E1–6.

12. Gabor S, Prenner G, Wasler A, et al. A simplified technique for implantation of left ventricular epicardial leads for biventricular resynchronization using videoassisted thoracoscopy (VATS). Eur J Cardiothorac Surg 2005;28:797–800.

13. Derose JJ Jr, Belsley S, Swistel DG, Shaw R, Ashton RC Jr. Robotically assisted left ventricular epicardial lead implantation for biventricular pacing: the posterior approach. Ann Thorac Surg 2004;77:1472–4.

14. Koos R, Sinha AM, Markus K, et al. Comparison of left ventricular lead placement via the coronary venous approach versus lateral thoracotomy in patients receiving cardiac resynchronization therapy. Am J Cardiol 2004;94:59–63.

15. Mair H, Jansens JL, Lattouf OM, Reichart B, Dabritz S. Epicardial lead implantation techniques for biventricular pacing via left lateral mini-thoracotomy, videoassisted thoracoscopy, and robotic approach. Heart Surg Forum 2003;6:412–17.

16. Cazeau S, Leclercq C, Lavergne T, et al. Multisite Stimulation in Cardiomyopathies (MUSTIC) Study Investigators. Effects of multisite biventricular pacing in patients with heart failure and intraventricular conduction delay. N Engl J Med 2001;344:873–80.

17. De Martino G, Orazi S, Bisignani G, et al. Safety and feasibility of coronary sinus left ventricular leads extraction: a preliminary report. J Interv Card Electrophysiol 2005;13:35–8.

18. Butter C, Auricchio A, Stellbrink C, et al. Pacing Therapy for Chronic Heart Failure II Study Group. Effect of resynchronization therapy stimulation site on the systolic function of heart failure patients. Circulation 2001;104:3026–9.

19. Berruezo A, Mont L, Scalise A, Brugada J. Orthodromic pacemaker-mediated tachycardia in a biventricular system without an atrial electrode. J Cardiovasc Electrophysiol 2004;15:1100–2.

20. Schreieck J, Zrenner B, Kolb C, Ndrepepa G, Schmitt C. Inappropriate shock delivery due to ventricular double detection with a biventricular pacing implantable cardioverter defibrillator. Pacing Clin Electrophysiol 2001;24:1154–7.

21. Ammann P, Sticherling C, Kalusche D, et al. An electrocardiogram-based algorithm to detect loss of left ventricular capture during cardiac resynchronization therapy. Ann Intern Med 2005;142:968–73.

22. Melenovsky V, Hay I, Fetics BJ, et al. Functional impact of rate irregularity in patients with heart failure and atrial fibrillation receiving cardiac resynchronization therapy. Eur Heart J 2005;26:705–11.

23. Shukla G, Chaudhry GM, Orlov M, Hoffmeister P, Haffajee C. Potential proarrhythmic effect of biventricular pacing: fact or myth? Heart Rhythm 2005; 2:951–6.

24. Guerra J, Wu J, Miller J, Groh W. Increase in ventricular tachycardia frequency, after biventricular implantable cardioverter defibrillator upgrade. J Cardiovasc Electrophysiol 2003;14:1245–7.

25. Fish JM, Di Diego JM, Nesterenko V, Antzelevitch C. Epicardial activation of left ventricular wall prolongs QT interval and transmural dispersion of repolarization: implications for biventricular pacing. Circulation 2004;109:2136–42.

26. Medina-Ravell N, Lankipali R, Yan G, et al. Effect of epicardial or biventricular pacing to prolong QT interval and increase transmural dispersion of repolarization. Circulation 2003;7:740–6.

14

Non-responders and patient selection from an electrophysiological perspective

Ignacio García-Bolao and Alfonso Macías

Introduction • Inclusion criteria for CRT trials • Clinical significance of QRS duration in patients with heart failure • QRS duration and mechanical dyssynchrony • QRS duration and the response to CRT • Ventricular activation patterns in patients with LBBB and heart failure • Electrical and mechanical dyssynchrony • Conclusions

INTRODUCTION

Electrophysiological disturbances are a common finding in advanced heart failure.[1] In addition to abnormalities in cardiac muscle contraction (mainly dependent on the severity of the underlying myocardial disease), abnormal electrical conduction delays the timing of atrial contraction and generates discoordinate contraction of the left ventricle (LV), which further impairs the hemodynamic performance of the failing heart. Both abnormal electrophysiological timing and contractile discoordination can be offset by cardiac resynchronization therapy (CRT) through the use of atrial-synchronized biventricular pacing. Although QRS duration is not a direct marker of mechanical dyssynchrony, CRT has been shown to reduce morbidity and mortality in patients with ventricular dyssynchrony selected almost exclusively on the basis of a prolonged QRS width.[2-11]

As initially proposed, CRT is based on the original and logical (but probably oversimplified) theory that synchronous biventricular pacing and LV free-wall pre-excitation are able to reduce the interventricular delay caused by left bundle branch block (LBBB) and to counterbalance the delay of activation of the LV free wall. However, even the general assumption that biventricular or LV pacing is effective in removing the electrical component of the electromechanical delay is still under evaluation. Although the clinical results of CRT are promising – analysis of individual responses has revealed that almost 30% of patients do not exhibit any symptomatic or hemodynamic improvement: the so-called 'non-responders.' Current data indicate that the problem of non-response is multifactorial and not only related to the parameters of dyssynchrony (i.e., electrical vs mechanical) used for patient selection. However, and in order to improve clinical outcomes, investigators are seeking new markers of dyssynchrony that can prospectively identify the patients who are more likely to respond.[12,13]

This chapter aims at summarizing our understanding about the problem of non-response to CRT from an electrical perspective, to discuss the strengths and weakness of the QRS width as an index of dyssynchrony, and to go deeply into the relationship between electrical and mechanical dyssynchrony.

INCLUSION CRITERIA FOR CRT TRIALS

The weight of evidence supporting the beneficial effects of CRT in large prospective trials is now firmly established, with more than 4000 patients evaluated in randomized single- or double-blinded controlled trials. In these pivotal clinical trials,[2-11] CRT has been demonstrated unequivocally to improve functional status, quality of life and LV systolic performance and to reduce hospitalization and mortality. Patients were selected on the basis of three main well-known criteria: refractory heart failure with impaired functional status (New York Heart Association (NYHA) class III or IV), reduced LV ejection fraction (LVEF) (<0.36), and prolonged QRS duration (>130–150 ms) on the surface electrocardiogram (ECG) (Table 14.1). The last of these was considered a surrogate marker of underlying dyssynchrony. Only the CARE-HF (Cardiac Resynchronization in Heart Failure) study included echocardiographic enrolment criteria. In this study, 92 patients (11% of the total included population) with intermediate QRS (120–150 ms) and echocardiographic indicators of dyssynchrony were included.[11] However, the results of this subgroup analysis have not yet been published.

Based on the inclusion criteria of these landmark trials, recent international guidelines for the treatment of heart failure recommend CRT on the basis of a wide QRS complex as the key element for identifying the presence of a mechanical dyssynchrony potentially correctable by atrio-biventricular pacing.[14,15]

CLINICAL SIGNIFICANCE OF QRS DURATION IN PATIENTS WITH HEART FAILURE

In the general population, increasing ECG QRS duration is positively related to LV mass and dimensions and inversely associated with systolic performance.[1,16] Prolongation of QRS beyond 120 ms occurs in 20–47% of patients with heart failure.[17,18] Among the different forms of intraventricular conduction disturbances, typical LBBB is far more common than right bundle branch block (RBBB) in this population (25–36% vs 4–6%, respectively).[1] In heart failure patients, prolongation of QRS is a significant predictor of LV dysfunction, and an inverse correlation exists between QRS duration and LVEF.[19]

Not only the LVEF but also the clinical status shows a correlation with the width of the QRS complex. For example, in the Framingham cohort, longer ECG QRS was associated with an increased risk of developing congestive heart failure.[20] In another study,[21] the incidence of QRS prolongation increased from 10% to 53% when patients moved from NYHA functional class I to class III.

Patients with heart failure and QRS prolongation have a poorer prognosis than those with narrow QRS. Shamim et al[22] have shown that intraventricular conduction delay is the most powerful predictor amongst the simple ECG

Table 14.1 Dyssynchrony criteria of randomized controlled trials of cardiac resynchronization

Trial	Design	n	Dyssynchrony QRS criteria (ms)	Mean QRS at entry (ms)	LBBB (%)
MUSTIC[2]	Crossover	58	QRS >150	176±19	87
MUSTIC AF[3]	Intrapatient	41	QRS >200	207±17	NA
PATH CHF[4]	Crossover	41	QRS ⩾ 120	174±30	87
PATH CHF II[5]	Crossover	86	QRS ⩾ 120	163±25	88
MIRACLE[6]	Parallel	453	QRS ⩾ 130	165±20	ND
MIRACLE ICD[7]	Parallel	555	QRS ⩾ 130	162±22	77
CONTAK-CD[8]	Parallel	490	QRS ⩾ 120	164±27	54
MIRACLE ICD II[9]	Parallel	186	QRS ⩾ 130	165±23	90
COMPANION[10]	Parallel	1520	QRS ⩾ 120	160	70
CARE-HF[11]	Open-label, randomized	814	QRS 120–149 + Echo QRS > 150	160	ND

NA, not applicable; ND, no data.

parameters in patients with heart failure. They demonstrated that QRS <120 ms, QRS of 120–160 ms, and QRS >160 ms correlated with a mortality rate at 36 months of 20%, 36%, and 58% respectively. In a cohort of patients with heart failure it was estimated that the presence of LBBB was associated with a 60–70% higher risk of all-cause mortality.[23]

In summary, left-sided intraventricular conduction delay is unequivocally associated with more advanced myocardial disease, worse LV systolic performance, and poorer prognosis compared with a normal QRS complex. Whether QRS prolongation simply represents a marker of greater disease severity or there is a cause–effect relationship between the mechanical effects of intraventricular conduction defects and the severity and progression of heart failure remains to be elucidated.

QRS DURATION AND MECHANICAL DYSSYNCHRONY

CRT was originally conceived and developed on the basis of the premise that in patients with heart failure and disturbed electrical activation (particularly those with LBBB pattern and prolongation of the PR interval), depolarization of the LV free wall is significantly delayed compared with that of the right ventricle (RV) (interventricular dyssynchrony) and the interventricular septum (intraventricular dyssynchrony). These electrical disturbances result in discoordinate contraction, with paradoxical septal wall motion and reduction of LV contractility, which further impair the systolic function of an already spoiled ventricle. In addition, a prolonged atrioventricular (AV) delay can promote presystolic mitral regurgitation and inadequate LV filling. In this situation, synchronous atrio-biventricular pacing with LV free-wall pre-excitation should be able to reduce the interventricular delay caused by LBBB, to counterbalance the delay of activation of the LV free wall, and to correct the abnormal AV timing and hence to minimize their mechanical consequences.[24]

Observational echocardiographic studies have clearly demonstrated that the presence of left intraventricular mechanical dyssynchrony is the most important factor determining a positive response to CRT, while interventricular and AV dyssynchrony appear to be of less importance.[25] However, the correlation between QRS width and mechanical dyssynchrony is a long way from being exact.

Interventricular dyssynchrony and QRS prolongation

Some studies have shown that QRS duration is a more accurate reflection of interventricular (left–right) mechanical dyssynchrony than of intraventricular dyssynchrony. In fact, three studies[17,26,27] have demonstrated a good correlation between interventricular dyssynchrony and QRS duration (Table 14.2). These studies have

Table 14.2 Prevalence of dyssynchrony in heart failure patients according to QRS duration

Study	n	QRS<120 ms InterV	QRS<120 ms IntraV	QRS 120–150 ms InterV	QRS 120–150 ms IntraV	QRS>150 ms InterV	QRS>150 ms IntraV	Correlation with QRS InterV	Correlation with QRS IntraV
Bader et al[17]	104	12	56	34	84	46	89	r = 0.43; p<0.05	NS
Ghio et al[26]	158	13	30	52	57	72	71	r = 0.66; p<0.001	NS
Rouleau et al[27]	35	18	—	44	—	100	—	r = 0.86; p<0.001	—
Bleeker et al[28]	90	—	27	—	60	—	70	—	NS
Yu et al[29]	112	—	43–51	—	64–73	—	—	—	NS
Bleeker et al[30]	64	5	33	—	—	—	—	NS	NS

InterV, interventricular dyssynchrony; IntraV, intraventricular dyssynchrony; NS, not significant.

shown that the prevalence of interventricular dyssynchrony in heart failure patients with QRS > 150 ms ranges from 46%[17] to 100%,[26] while it is absent in more than three-quarters of patients with QRS < 120 ms. Bleeker et al[28] showed that while intraventricular dyssynchrony was present in 33% of patients with heart failure and QRS < 120 ms, the prevalence of interventricular dyssynchrony was only 5%.

This acceptable correlation between interventricular dyssynchrony and QRS duration is quite consistent with the electrical activation pattern of patients with LBBB and heart failure: as we will see later, the most constant (although not universal) activation pattern in this population is the preservation of RV activation coexisting with slow transseptal conduction.

Intraventricular dyssynchrony and QRS prolongation

Unlike interventricular dyssynchrony, mechanical intraventricular dyssynchrony seems to correlate poorly with QRS duration (Table 14.2) Bleeker et al[28] studied the relationship between LV dyssynchrony and QRS duration in 90 patients with advanced heart failure. Patients were categorized according to QRS width as narrow (QRS < 120 ms), intermediate (QRS 120–150 ms), and wide (QRS > 150 ms) QRS complex. The authors reported that 27% of patients with 'narrow' QRS showed significant LV dyssynchrony, while 30% of patients with 'wide' QRS (mainly LBBB) did not exhibit LV dyssynchrony. In this study, there was no significant relationship between QRS duration and intraventricular dyssynchrony in the whole group, while a weak relation was found between these two parameters in patients with idiopathic cardiomyopathy. Other authors,[17,26,28–30] using various echocardiographic parameters, have demonstrated that intraventricular dyssynchrony is absent in around one-third of patients with an intermediate or wide QRS, and conversely present in a relatively high percentage of patients (27–56%) with normal QRS duration.

Taken together, these studies suggest that there is a group of patients (around 30%) who meet conventional electrical dyssynchrony criteria (i.e., QRS width) but do not have mechanical dyssynchrony. However, the assumption that this 30% might partially explain the similar percentage of non-responders in the randomized trials has not been prospectively validated in randomized studies to date. Conversely, it is estimated that perhaps 20–30% of heart failure patients with QRS <130 ms have mechanical dyssynchrony. Again – and although this population is a potential target for CRT – extending the indication to patients with narrow QRS based on mechanical parameters of dyssynchrony is currently based only on data arising from observational and non-randomized studies.

QRS DURATION AND THE RESPONSE TO CRT

Baseline QRS duration

Although Kass et al[31] and Auricchio et al[32] found that a QRS > 150 ms was predictive of acute hemodynamic improvement, baseline QRS duration has consistently failed to predict a chronic clinical positive response to CRT. Only data from the PATH-CHF (Pacing Therapies in Congestive Heart Failure) II trial suggested that the clinical benefit of CRT, assessed by peak oxygen consumption, was more pronounced in (but not confined to) patients with QRS >150 ms when compared with patients with QRS of 120–150 ms.[5] In this study, 38% of individuals with QRS <150 ms had increased peak oxygen consumption by more than 1 ml/min/kg with LV pacing. However, other studies have consistently failed to demonstrate the value of the baseline QRS duration in predicting a positive response to CRT.[33–34]

These data suggest that there is a weak correlation between basal QRS duration and positive response, but with a very poor predictive value for identifying responders versus non-responders.

Change of QRS duration after CRT

One aspect that continues to be somewhat controversial is whether QRS narrowing after CRT can be used to indicate treatment efficacy. A hypothetical reduction in QRS duration produced by biventricular stimulation should represent the quality of electrical resynchronization and indirectly reflect the degree of correction of electromechanical abnormalities.

An acute echocardiographic study showed that the decrease in QRS duration was correlated with a decrease in systolic volume.[35] Shortening of QRS following CRT differs significantly between responders and non-responders in a number of chronic studies. For example, Molhoek et al[36] analyzed the value of QRS shortening as a marker of a positive clinical response to CRT. Their study included 61 patients, with a reported nonresponse of 26%. While baseline QRS duration was similar between responders and nonresponders, a significant shortening in QRS duration was observed only in responder patients after 6 months. A reduction in QRS >10 ms had a high sensitivity (73%), but a low specificity (44%) for the prediction of a positive response. Conversely, a reduction in QRS >50 ms showed a high specificity but with a low sensitivity (18%) to predict response to CRT (Figure 14.1). This finding was mirrored by a study reported by Lecoq et al,[37] which showed retrospectively that the degree of QRS shortening was the only independent predictor of positive response after multivariate adjustement in a series of 139 patients. At 6 months, the mean QRS shortening associated with CRT when compared with baseline was significantly greater ($p < 0.001$) among the responder patients (37 ms) when compared with nonresponders (11 ms). It should be noted that in this study, the RV implantation site was selected on a patient-to-patient basis, trying to reach the shortest QRS duration during biventricular pacing, which is not a routine implantation practice.

However, other studies did not replicate this finding, and reached different conclusions.[32,33,36,38] In daily practice, it is very common to see cases in which the QRS actually lengthens or remain unchanged despite substantial clinical improvement. Furthermore, with epicardial LV pacing, there is an obvious discrepancy between changes is QRS duration after CRT and hemodynamic and clinical improvement.

Nevertheless, it is important to point out that, as with any intra- or postoperative criteria, this parameter should not be considered as a *classical* predictor but rather as a marker of positive response.

VENTRICULAR ACTIVATION PATTERNS IN PATIENTS WITH LBBB AND HEART FAILURE

Correcting the mechanical problem arising from abnormal electrical conduction delays, particularly LBBB, by modifying electrical activation of the ventricles presupposes a good understanding of the propagation of electrical impulses in this condition.

While in the normal ventricle the spread of ventricular electrical activation is uniform and occurs within 40 ms through the Purkinje network, intraventricular conduction disturbances impair the velocity and direction of electrical propagation. In addition, abnormalities found in the damaged myocardium of heart failure patients, such as scar tissue, ischemia, or interstitial fibrosis with rearrangement of extracellular matrix and myocytes, can further alter the local activation and the specific pattern of LV activation.

Classically, it has been considered that electrical impulse propagation in patients with lone LBBB without heart disease starts in the RV, through the intact right bundle, and then proceeds to the LV, which is depolarized transseptally from

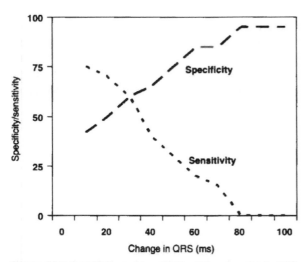

Figure 14.1 Specificity and sensitivity of the changes in QRS duration after CRT in predicting a positive response to CRT. (Adapted from Molhoek SG, Bax JJ, Van Erven L, et al. QRS duration and shortening to predict clinical response to cardiac resynchronization therapy in patients with end-stage heart failure. Pacing Clin Electrophysiol 2004;27:308–13.[36])

right to left. The two LV activation fronts – anterior and posterior – meet at the lateral apical region. However, some studies have shown that this 'classical' pattern is not so uniform in patients with heart failure and severe heart disease.[39,40]

Epicardial and endocardial mapping studies

Conventional epicardial mapping in patients with an LBBB pattern have consistently shown that while RV activation is preserved (although earlier within the QRS complex), transseptal conduction is slow. During LBBB, the location of the latest LV activation depends mainly on both the QRS axis and the underlying myocardial disease. Vassallo et al[40] nicely described how in patients with LBBB and QRS >140 ms and normal axis, the latest endocardial activation site was frequently at the base of the LV (in the A–V sulcus), just as it is with normal intraventricular conduction, while it was more variable in those with left axis deviation. In this study, the latest site of electrical endocardial activation in LBBB patients with QRS >140 ms and myocardial infarction was variable and frequently related to the site of prior infarction.

Thus, although a rapid delay of transseptal activation is a characteristic shared with most of the forms of LBBB, the nature of the underlying heart disease markedly influences the subsequent pattern, probably due to the different degree of integrity of the distal conduction system.[39] While patients with no heart disease or cardiomyopathy of non-ischemic origin appear to have a preserved distal conducting system, patients with large ischemic scars have a deterioration of the distal Purkinje system. In this situation, their endocardial activation is slowly completed via a cell-to-cell conduction. This interpretation is further supported by the finding of a greater LV activation time in patients with LBBB and prior myocardial infarction (219±77 ms: 113% of the total QRS duration) when compared with LBBB patients without heart disease or with cardiomyopathy of a non-ischemic origin (126±37 ms and 125±22 ms: approximately 80% of the QRS duration). From the electrophysiological point of view, these observations suggest that the bizarre nature of the QRS complex in patients with ischemic cardiomyopathy is more the reflection of a LV pathological condition than

of a primary conduction disturbance with a predictable activation pattern.[39,40]

Three-dimensional mapping studies

Most of the aforementioned observations are in accordance with recent data obtained with catheter-based three-dimensional (3D) nonfluoroscopic mapping systems, which permit in vivo reconstruction of the cardiac anatomy and assessment of the LV activation sequence more precisely. Using this technique, Peichl et al[41] elegantly showed that patients with cardiomyopathy of ischemic origin, heart failure, and QRS > 130 ms presented not only with variable activation patterns that reflected the location of the post-infarct scar, but also with longer LV activation time (corrected for the total QRS duration) when compared with non-ischemic patients. In contrast, patients with dilated cardiomyopathy of unknown origin had a homogeneous spread of the activation wavefront, with the latest activation located laterally (in typical LBBB) or anteriorly (in bifascicular block), and a shorter total LV activation time. Rodriguez et al[42] also documented different patterns of LV activation in heart failure patients with LBBB patterns according to the type of underlying heart disease. More recently, Auricchio et al[43] have demonstrated that patients with heart failure of different etiologies (mainly ischemic cardiomyopathy) and LBBB may have nearly normal transseptal conduction times and anterior, lateral, or inferior lines of block, independently of the duration of the QRS complex.

Electrical propagation in heart failure

Taken together, these data suggest that the different activation patterns of QRS prolongation with LBBB morphology in the setting of heart failure constitute a heterogeneous spectrum varying from cases with true LBBB and long interventricular conduction delay and only minor LV conduction problems to cases with nearly normal conduction via the left bundle and dominant intraventricular delays due to severely damaged and dilated LV.[41] Regarding the underlying etiology, on the one hand, patients with dilated cardiomyopathy tend to show a 'true' LBBB pattern with high interventricular delay but a subsequent homogeneous LV activation reflecting the integrity of the distal Purkinje system. On the other hand, patients with ischemic cardiomyopathy and old infarction scars present rather with non-specific intraventricular conduction disturbances or an LBBB-like pattern, with an endocardial activation characterized by nearly normal transseptal conduction with a major delay located within the LV and around the scar area.

ELECTRICAL AND MECHANICAL DYSSYNCHRONY

Several mechanisms have been proposed for explaining the discrepancy found in clinical and experimental studies between electrical and mechanical dyssynchrony.

Mechanical dyssynchrony without QRS prolongation

Delayed activation of the LV free wall despite short absolute conduction times as shown by a narrow QRS could be explained by the presence of discrete lines of functional block, especially in the lateral area of the LV, causing large areas of relative late endocardial activation and 'occult' electrical dyssynchrony.[43] Also, delayed electromechanical coupling due to myocardial fibrosis and heterogeneously dispersed scars or ischemic zones could be responsible for left intraventricular mechanical dyssynchrony in the absence of a significant electrical conduction delay. Both mechanisms could explain the presence of relatively large areas of late LV activation in narrow-QRS patients.

QRS prolongation without mechanical dyssynchrony

As we have seen, the concept that an electromechanical delay always exists in patients with LBBB is no longer supported. Fung et al[44] observed that electrical conduction delay could be absent in heart failure patients with LBBB. In this study, 3D non-contact mapping electrograms were recorded from seven patients with LBBB. Despite the prolongation of the QRS complex, three patients had a homogeneous propagation of the endocardial activation, like normal subjects. Not surprisingly, only the other four patients with electrical activation delay showed echocardiographic signs of mechanical delay. This finding is supported by the observation by Auricchio et al[43] in which about one-third of patients with heart failure and LBBB had normal transseptal activation time and a near-normal LV endocardial activation time.

Electromechanical resynchronization with CRT

Recently, it has been elegantly demonstrated that improvement in mechanical synchrony does not require electrical synchrony. Studying both LV and biventricular pacing in a dog model of heart failure associated with LBBB, Leclercq et al[45] showed how, in this experimental model, LV pacing alone actually increased electrical dispersion over that from LBBB or biventricular pacing, despite improving mechanical LV function and coordination just as effectively as biventricular pacing. The discordance between electrical activation and mechanical synchrony was further supported by the findings of a small observational study[46] in which both biventricular and LV pacing improved inter- and intraventricular mechanical synchrony in nine heart failure patients with normal QRS duration.

CONCLUSIONS

Growing experience with CRT has highlighted the limitations of a wide QRS complex as a surrogate for mechanical LV dyssynchrony. Prolongation of QRS in the setting of heart failure is a rather complex electrical disease resulting from conduction delay located at different anatomical levels of the activation sequence. The location and extent of specific ventricular delays are unpredictable with the surface ECG. Even patients with normal QRS duration may have occult electrical dyssynchrony causing mechanical disturbances. At best, QRS duration is an indirect correlate but not a direct reflection of mechanical synchrony, which is the real substrate that causes a decline in chamber function. However, QRS is the only index of dyssynchrony that has been prospectively validated to date in large randomized trials, and there are numerous other potential reasons for explaining the non-response phenomenon. The value of other parameters of dyssynchrony should be prospectively assessed before their application to clinical practice.

REFERENCES

1. Kashani A, Barold SS. Significance of QRS complex duration in patients with heart failure. J Am Coll Cardiol 2005; 46:2183–92.

2. Cazeau S, Leclercq C, Lavergne T, et al. Multisite Stimulation in Cardiomyopathies (MUSTIC) Study Investigators. Effects of multisite biventricular pacing in patients with heart failure and intraventricular conduction delay. N Engl J Med 2001;344:873–80.

3. Leclercq C, Walker S, Linde C, et al. Comparative effects of permanent biventricular and right-univentricular pacing in heart failure patients with chronic atrial fibrillation. Eur Heart J 2002;23:1780–7.

4. Auricchio A, Stellbrink C, Sack S, et al. Long-term clinical effect of hemodynamically optimized cardiac resynchronization therapy in patients with heart failure and ventricular conduction delay. J Am Coll Cardiol 2002;39:2026–33.

5. Auricchio A, Stellbrink C, Butter C, et al. Clinical efficacy of cardiac resynchronization therapy using left ventricular pacing in heart failure patients stratified by severity of ventricular conduction delay. J Am Coll Cardiol 2003;89:346–50.

6. Abraham WT, Fisher WG, Smith AL, et al. Cardiac resynchroniztion in chronic heart failure. N Engl J Med 2002;346:1845–53.

7. Young JB, Abraham WT, Smith AL, et al. Combined cardiac resynchronization and implantable cardioversion defibrillation in advanced chronic heart failure: the MIRACLE ICD trial. JAMA 2003;289:2685–94.

8. Higgins SL, Hummel JD, Niazi IK, et al. Cardiac resynchronization therapy for the treatment of heart failure in patients with intraventricular conduction delay and malignant ventricular tachyarrhythmias. J Am Coll Cardiol 2003;42:1454–9.

9. Abraham WT, Young B, Leon AR, et al. Effects of cardiac resynchronizaton on disease progression in patients with left ventricular systolic dysfunction, an indication for an implantable cardioverter defibrillator, and mildly symptomatic chronic heart failure. Circulation 2004;110:2864–8.

10. Bristow MR, Saxon LA, Boehmer J, et al. Cardiac-resynchronization therapy with or without an implantable defibrillator in advanced chronic heart failure. N Engl J Med 2004;350:2140–50.

11. Cleland JG, Daubert JC, Erdmann E, et al. The effect of cardiac resynchronization on morbidity and mortality in heart failure. N Engl J Med 2005;352:1539–49.

12. Hawkins NM, Petrie MC, MacDonald MR, Hogg KJ, McMurray JJV. Selecting patients for cardiac resynchronization therapy: electrical or mechanical dyssynchrony. Eur Heart J 2006;27:1270–81.

13. Birnie DH and Tang ASL. The problem of non-response to cardiac resynchronization therapy. Curr Opin Cardiol 2006;21:20–6.

14. Swedberg K, Cleland J, Dargie H, et al. Guidelines for the diagnosis and treatment of chronic heart failure: executive summary (update 2005). The Task Force for the Diagnosis and Treatment of Chronic Heart Failure of the European Society of Cardiology. Eur Heart J 2005;26:1115–40.

15. Hunt SA, Abraham WT, Chin MH et al. ACC/AHA Guideline Update for the Diagnosis and Treatment of Chronic Heart Failure in the Adult: Summary Article: a report of the American College of Cardiology/ American Heart Association Task Force on Practice Guidelines (Writting Committee to Update the 2001 Guidelines for the Evaluation and Management of Heart Failure). J Am Coll Cardiol 2005;46:1116–43.

16. Dhingra R, Ho Nam B, Benjamin EJ, et al. Cross-sectional relations of electrocardiographic QRS duration to left ventricular dimensions: the Framingham Heart Study. J Am Coll Cardiol 2005;45:685–9.

17. Bader H, Garrigue S, Lafitte S, et al. Intra-left ventricular electromechanical asynchrony. A new independent predictor of severe cardiac events in heart failure patients. J Am Coll Cardiol 2004;43:248–56.

18. Shen AY, Wang X, Doris J, Moore N. Proportion of patients with congestive heart failure management program meeting criteria for cardiac resynchronization therapy. Am J Cardiol 2004;94:673–6.

19. Iuliano S, Fisher SG, Karasik PE, Fletcher RD, Singh SN. QRS duration and mortality in patients with congestive heart failure. Am Heart J 2002;143:1085–91.

20. Dhingra R, Pencina MJ, Wang TJ, et al. Electrocardiographic QRS duration and the risk of congestive heart failure: the Framingham Heart Study. Hypertension 2006;47:861–7.

21. Stellbrink C, Auricchio A, Diem B, et al. Potential benefit of biventricular pacing in patients with congestive heart failure and ventricular tachyarrhythmia. Am J Cardiol 1999;83:143D–50D.

22. Shamim W, Francis DP, Yousufuddin M, et al. Intraventricular conduction delay: a prognostic marker in chronic heart failure. Int J Cardiol 1999;70:171–8.

23. Baldasseroni S, Opasich C, Gorini M, et al. Left bundle-branch block is associated with increased 1-year sudden and total mortality rate in 5517 outpatients with congestive heart failure: a report from the Italian

network on congestive heart failure. Am Heart J 2002; 143:398–405.

24. Leclercq C, Kass DA. Retiming the failing heart. Principles and current clinical status of cardiac resynchronization. J Am Coll Cardiol 2002;39:194–201.

25. Bax JJ, Ansalone G, Breithardt OA, et al. Echocardiographic evaluation of cardiac resynchronization therapy: ready for routine clinical use?. A critical appraisal. J Am Coll Cardiol 2004;44:1–9.

26. Ghio S, Constantin C, Klersy C, et al. Interventricular and intraventricular dyssynchrony are common in heart failure patients, regardless of QRS duration. Eur Heart J 2004;25:571–8.

27. Rouleau F, Merheb M, Geffroy S, et al. Echocardiographic assessment of the interventricular delay of activation and correlation to the QRS width in dilated cardiomyopathy. Pacing Clin Electrophysiol 2001;24:1500–6.

28. Bleeker GB, Schalij MJ, Molhoek SG, et al. Relationship between QRS duration and left ventricular dyssynchrony in patients with end-stage heart failure. J Cardiovasc Electrophysiol 2004;15:544–9.

29. Yu CM, Lin H, Zhang Q, Sanderson JE. High prevalence of left ventricular systolic and diastolic asynchrony in patients with congestive heart failure and normal QRS duration. Heart 2003;89:54–60.

30. Bleeker GB, Schalij MJ, Molhoek SG, et al. Frequency of left ventricular dyssynchrony in patients with heart failure and a narrow QRS complex. Am J Cardiol 2005;95:140–2.

31. Kass DA, Chen CH, Curry C, et al. Improved left ventricular mechanics from acute VDD pacing in patients with dilated cardiomyopathy and ventricular conduction delay. Circulation 1999;99:1567–73.

32. Auricchio A, Stellbrink C, Block M, et al. The effect of pacing chamber and atrioventricular delay on acute systolic function of paced patients with congestive heart failure. Circulation 1999;99:2993–3001.

33. Diaz-Infante E, Mont L, Leal J, et al. Predictors of lack of response to resynchronization therapy. Am J Cardiol 2005;95:1436–40.

34. Pitzalis MV, Iacoviello M, Romito R, et al. Cardiac resynchronization therapy tailored by echocardiographic evaluation of ventricular asynchrony. J Am Coll Cardiol 2002;40:1615–22.

35. Kim W, Sogaard P, Mortensen PT, et al. Three dimensional echocardiography documents haemodynamic improvement by biventricular pacing in patients with severe heart failure. Heart 2001;85:514–20.

36. Molhoek SG, Bax JJ, Van Erven L, et al. QRS duration and shortening to predict clinical response to cardiac resynchronization therapy in patients with end-stage heart failure. Pacing Clin Electrophysiol 2004;27:308–13.

37. Lecoq G, Leclercq C, Leray E, et al. Clinical and electrocardiographic predictors of a positive response to cardiac resynchronization therapy in advanced heart failure. Eur Heart J 2005;26:1094–100.

38. Reuter S, Garrigue S, Barold SS, et al. Comparison of characteristics in responders versus nonresponders with biventricular pacing for drug-resistant congestive heart failure. Am J Cardiol 2002;89:346–50.

39. Vassallo JA, Cassidy DM, Marchlinski FE, et al. Endocardial activation of left bundle branch block. Circulation 1984;69:914–23.

40. Vassallo JA, Cassidy DM, Miller JM, et al. Left ventricular endocardial activation during right ventricular pacing. Effect of underlying heart disease. J Am Coll Cardiol 1986;7:1228–33.

41. Peichl P, Kautzner J, Cihak R, Bytesnik J. The spectrum of inter- and intraventricular abnormalities in patients eligible for cardiac resynchronization therapy. Pacing Clin Electrophysiol 2004;27:1105–12.

42. Rodriguez LM, Timmermans C, Nabar A, Beatty G, Wellens HJJ. Variable patterns of septal activation in patients with left bundle branch block and heart failure. J Cardiovasc Electrophysiol 2003;14:135–41.

43. Auricchio A, Fantoni C, Regoli F, et al. Characterization of left ventricular activation in patients with heart failure and left-bundle branch block. Circulation 2004;109:1133–9.

44. Fung JW, Yu CM Yip G et al. Variable left ventricular activation pattern in patients with heart failure and left bundle-branch block. Heart 2004; 90:17–19.

45. Leclercq C, Faris O, Tunin R, et al. Systolic improvement and mechanical resynchronization does not require electrical synchrony in the dilated failing heart with left bundle-branch block. Circulation 2002; 106:1760–3.

46. Turner MS, Bleasdale RA, Vinereanu D, et al. Electrical and mechanical components of dyssynchrony in heart failure patients with normal QRS duration and left bundle-branch block. Impact of left and biventricular pacing. Circulation 2004;109:2544–9.

15

Asynchrony in coronary artery disease

Alison Duncan and Michael Henein

Introduction • Definition of asynchrony • Normal regional asynchrony • Asynchrony at rest in coronary artery disease • Ventricular asynchrony during acute ischemia • Conclusions

INTRODUCTION

Cardiac resynchronization therapy (CRT) has emerged as a method of reducing mortality and increasing ejection fraction in patients with severe left ventricular (LV) disease.[1-3] Treatment aimed at resynchronization clearly implies that asynchrony is present in the control state with associated deleterious physiological consequences. CRT was originally developed in patients whose LV disease was associated with severe disturbances of activation, referred to collectively as left bundle branch block (LBBB), in whom predictable relations with asynchrony had been demonstrated. More recently, the technique has been extended to patients in whom the QRS duration is normal[4,5] and in whom the basis for any asynchrony is less well defined. However, it has long been known that coronary artery disease (CAD) is frequently associated with disturbances of the timing of regional LV wall motion in the resting state, regardless of QRS duration. Since patients with ischemic heart disease are frequently considered for CRT, we have reviewed the nature of CAD-induced asynchrony and the effect of treatment. We also explore interrelations between QRS duration, pharmacological stress, and CAD, and their separate effects on regional wall motion in detail, since exploiting them may potentially enhance the performance of currently available CRT.

DEFINITION OF ASYNCHRONY

Ventricular asynchrony may usefully be defined as 'incoordinate ventricular wall motion that reduces the extent of energy transfer from myocardium to useful work on the circulation'. Its functional consequences are significant impairment of maximal cardiac function as a result of a reduction in the proportion of myocardial energy transmitted to the circulation (cycle efficiency). It also causes a fall in the peak rates of LV pressure rise and fall, which prolongs total isovolumic time (the duration within the cardiac cycle when the ventricle is neither ejecting nor filling: so-called 'wasted' time). It is rational to assume that the extent of overall cardiac dysfunction should also depend on the proportion of the ventricle that is asynchronous, as well as the degree of asynchrony itself. Technical consideration of the methods used to detect and measure asynchrony is therefore of paramount importance. Standard methods of describing regional LV function depend on determining regional amplitude of wall motion or extent of wall thickening, of which it is generally accepted that subjective analysis can give at least semiquantitative values. The term 'asyneresis' was introduced to describe a regional disturbance of timing by Cohen et al[6] in 1966, but was little used due to lack of objective methods to describe it. Techniques with frame rates higher than two-dimensional (2D) echocardio-graphy (contrast ventriculography, M-mode, and Doppler tissue velocity) have since evolved that can define it. When combined with continu-ous high-fidelity LV cavity pressure measure-ments, these techniques not only permit detection of asynchrony but also describe its nature and extent. Thus, they have the potential to deter-mine which patients would benefit most from resynchronization, and for monitoring response to resynchronization.

NORMAL REGIONAL ASYNCHRONY

One of the most striking features of normal con-traction is its symmetry and economy of motion. Nevertheless, it has long been recognized that normal regional wall motion is non-uniform. From ventricular base to apex, the extent of sys-tolic thickening normally increases (from 30% to 60%),[7] with little variation at the septum and almost no variation at the lateral wall; the thick-ening rate at the posterior wall increases (from 50% to 110%), while the extent of inward epicar-dial motion decreases.[8] Furthermore, the onset of inward motion may be delayed by up to 120 ms at anteroapical regions compared with regions of earliest motion at the base of the heart.[9] Similar non-uniformity occurs as a normal phenomenon during diastole; the anterior wall may move outward before other regions (segmental early relaxation phenomenon[10]), and the peak outward motion of the epicardium of the posterior wall may precede that of the endo-cardium by 20–30 ms.[8] In the normal heart, such regional non-uniformity correlates with myo-cardial fiber orientation in different regions. Indeed, maximal energy transfer from the myocardium to the circulation is dependent on the coordinate, but non-uniform, action of both circumferentially and longitudinally directed myocardial fibers.[11]

Normal LV timing and shape changes within the cardiac cycle

Following electrical activation of the LV, the ear-liest mechanical events are the onset of pressure rise followed by mitral valve closure. The inter-val between mitral valve closure and aortic valve opening (the isovolumic contraction time) has a mean duration of 25–35 ms. During this period of constant LV volume, shortening of the long axis begins before that of the minor axis (by approximately 25 ms), resulting in a more spherical LV cavity shape but with minimal change in wall thickness.[12] During ejection, the minor axis falls by 25% and the long axis short-ens by 10–12%,[13] producing a less spherical LV shape during systole, an increased change in volume per unit area of surrounding endo-cardium, and more effective ejection.[14] During isovolumic relaxation (the interval between aortic valve closure and mitral valve opening, normally ranging between 60 and 85 ms[15]), there is a minor change in LV shape to a more spheri-cal configuration as long-axis shortening contin-ues when circumferential fibers have begun lengthening.[14] After the mitral valve has opened and as the LV volume increases, the LV cavity reverts to a more spherical configuration by increasing its transverse dimension, thus reduc-ing the extent of myocardial distension per unit volume increase.[14] A detailed summary of normal non-uniform wall motion can be displayed using isometric plots derived from angiographic studies (Figure 15.1).

Neither the initial rise in LV pressure during isovolumic contraction nor the subsequent fall in LV pressure during isovolumic relaxation time are associated with significant changes in LV wall thickness. Thus, the initial upstroke of the pressure–wall thickness loop during isovolumic contraction and the downstroke during isovolu-mic relaxation are approximately vertical (Figure 15.2),[16] producing a rectangular-shaped loop when pressure and wall thickness are plot-ted against one another. The area of these loops has physical significance: it represents the exter-nal work done on the circulation by the region studied, which is greatest when the loop is rec-tangular. The maximum work that could have been done by the LV working over the same range of pressure and wall thickness is repre-sented by the product of the two (i.e., by the area that just encloses the loop). The ratio of the area of the loop to that of the rectangle is referred to in standard pump theory as cycle efficiency, and for any given myocardial segment, the cycle efficiency is normally >70%.

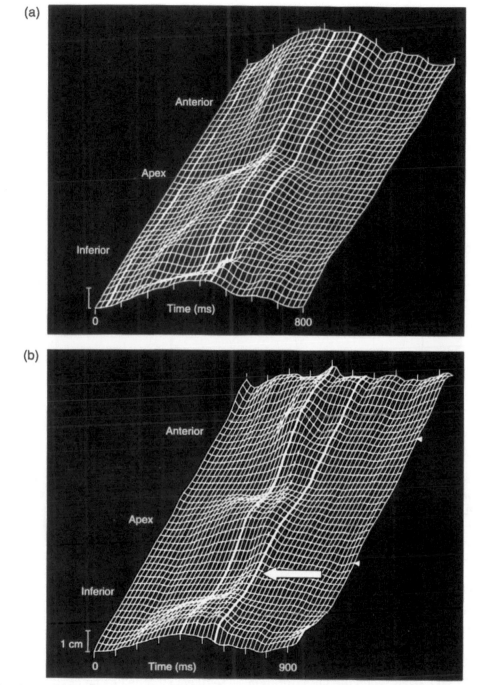

Figure 15.1 (a) Isometric plot of the left ventricular (LV) cavity showing endocardial motion from a normal subject. Diagonal lines represent simultaneous events; upward displacement represents inward motion, and accentuated lines represent aortic valve closure and mitral valve opening. The synchronous pattern of wall motion during ejection and filling is apparent. (b) Isometric plot in a patient with coronary artery disease. There is inferior hypokinesis during systole, with delayed inward wall motion during isovolumic relaxation (arrow). At the same time, there is early outward wall motion before mitral valve opening on the anterior wall.

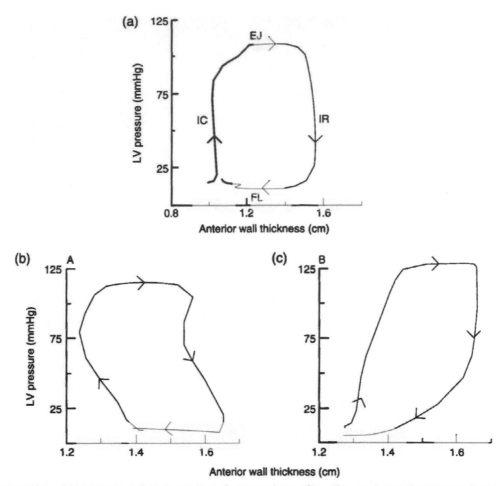

Figure 15.2 (a) Normal LV pressure–wall thickness loop. A rectangular configuration, as shown, denotes coordinate segmental wall motion, with anterior wall thickness remaining constant during isovolumic contraction (IC) and isovolumic relaxation (IR). EJ, ejection; FL, filling. (b) Primary asynchrony. Wall thinning during IC and thickening during IR causes the loop to lean to the left. (c) Secondary asynchrony. Wall thickening during IC and thinning during IR causes the loop to lean to the right. Cycle efficiency is reduced in both primary and secondary asynchrony. (Reprinted from Koh TW et al. Heart 1997;78:291–7 and 1999;81:285–91, with permission from BMJ Publishing Group Ltd.)

ASYNCHRONY AT REST IN CORONARY ARTERY DISEASE

Loss of normal regional uniformity and its consequence, LV asynchrony, is a major manifestation of CAD, even when the QRS duration is normal. It has long been recognized that patients with chronic stable angina have asynchronous wall motion at rest, even in the absence of chest pain or ischemic electrocardiographic (ECG) changes. Such asynchrony is most obvious during the isovolumic periods.

Early work based on contrast angiography demonstrated abnormal outward movement of endocardium (i.e., away from the cavity) during isovolumic contraction and abnormal inward movement during isovolumic relaxation in a segment supplied by an affected coronary artery in single-vessel coronary disease.[17] Moreover, since cavity volume remained constant, both these abnormalities were associated with reverse movements at distant segments of the ventricle[17–19] (Figure 15.1). More recent work has demonstrated abnormal long-axis function during the isovolumic periods. In patients with chronic stable CAD, the onset of long-axis shortening may be delayed by 25 ms or more during isovolumic contraction even at rest,[20,21] so that it frequently follows that of minor-axis shortening. Moreover, normal long-axis shortening may be replaced by abnormal lengthening during isovolumic contraction and early ejection. In early diastole, the combination of continued long-axis shortening after the aortic valve has closed, delayed onset of long-axis lengthening, and associated premature minor-axis lengthening results in a more spherical LV shape during isovolumic relaxation, rather than during early filling, which in turn suppresses early diastolic LV filling (E wave), with a corresponding increase in late diastolic LV filling (A wave).

Asynchrony during the isovolumic periods distorts the pressure–wall thickness loop in affected regions, reducing the ratio of observed external work to the maximum possible for a ventricle working over the same range of pressure and dimension and thereby reducing the cycle of that segment (Figure 15.2). Moreover, the nature of the distortion defines the exact nature of the asynchrony present in an individual segment. During coronary artery surgery, simultaneous intraoperative transesophageal echocardiography (TEE) and continuous high-fidelity LV cavity pressure measurement[22] has documented two distinct types of asynchrony: primary asynchrony shows wall thinning during isovolumic contraction due to local ischemia in the region subtended by a stenosed artery causing delay in the onset of thickening, while secondary asynchrony shows wall thickening in an otherwise normal segment, representing reciprocal changes of primary asynchrony elsewhere in the ventricle at a time of constant cavity volume and myocardial mass. The two types of asynchrony distort the pressure–wall thickness relation in different ways (Figure 15.2).

Primary and secondary types of asynchrony also have quite different connotations in terms of regional intrinsic myocardial systolic function. In primary asynchrony, peak myocardial power is approximately halved (from a normal

value of 35–40 mW/cm^2). Furthermore, the onset of local power production is delayed (by up to 155 ms after the onset of the QRS complex) and it persists beyond aortic closure (by 120 ms). Indeed, each 20 ms delay in the onset of power production reduces cycle efficiency by 10% (unpublished data). By contrast, intrinsic myocardial function is normal in regions of secondary asynchrony; the onset of power is 40 ms after the onset of the QRS complex, it ceases before aortic closure, and peak myocardial power is maintained (36 mW/cm^2). After revascularization, segmental wall motion becomes synchronous in areas of primary asynchrony within 30 minutes, and peak myocardial power and work return to normal.[22] Although secondary asynchrony promptly regresses with revascularization, neither wall thickening nor peak intrinsic power production change from their normal preoperative values.

Asynchrony in patients with CAD thus appears to be fundamentally different from normal ventricular asynchrony: primary asynchrony associated with CAD reduces useful work done on the circulation through the presence of segmental delay, while secondary asynchrony represents reciprocal change at a distal site with normal intrinsic myocardial function. Primary and secondary asynchrony coexist in patients with CAD: both are stable manifestations of CAD at rest, both occur in the absence of classical evidence of myocardial ischemia (chest pain or ST changes), and both are rapidly reversible after revascularization (thus excluding stunning and hibernation). Pressure–wall thickness loops can differentiate primary from secondary asynchrony. Clearly, segments demonstrating primary asynchrony are those most likely to respond to CRT.

VENTRICULAR ASYNCHRONY DURING ACUTE ISCHEMIA

Asynchrony present at rest in CAD is greatly exaggerated during provoked ischemia. Ischemia may be provoked either by reducing supply (during coronary occlusion) or by increasing demand (during atrial pacing or pharmacological stress).

Supply Ischemia

Coronary angioplasty

Early echocardiographic studies performed during percutaneous transluminal angioplasty showed that regional wall motion abnormalities appear rapidly, 15–20 seconds after coronary occlusion, often before or even in the absence of ECG changes.[23] These studies are limited when assessing asynchrony however, because they were based on semiquantitative detection of changes in wall motion, and did not directly measure differences in segmental delay. In contrast, long-axis segmental delay can be demonstrated objectively during angioplasty.[20,24] During balloon inflation, the onset of long-axis shortening becomes delayed (by 15–20 ms) and may be replaced by abnormal lengthening during isovolumic contraction and early ejection. The onset of long-axis lengthening in early diastole may also be delayed (Figure 15.3) – in extreme cases until the onset of atrial systole.[25] These abnormalities represent a shift in timing of segmental motion due to delay in the onset of long-axis shortening,[21] with local systole proceeding as normal thereafter.

Acute myocardial infarction

The most common wall motion disturbance early after myocardial infarction is ventricular asynchrony. During systole, the onset of inward motion may be delayed or even reversed because tension develops late or is inadequate to cause inward motion until late in ejection.[26] Moreover, the peak shortening velocity may be delayed by approximately 40 ms (from a normal value of 130 ms) in affected segments.[27] The degree of LV asynchrony is mainly determined by infarct size; the larger the infarct, the greater the dyssynchrony index.[27] These changes revert after successful thrombolysis.[28]

Coronary occlusion during beating heart surgery

During off-pump coronary artery bypass grafting (CABG), coronary arteries may be occluded rather than shunted while the graft to coronary anastomosis is performed to avoid local endothelial damage. Over this period, myocardium subtended by the occluded artery becomes ischemic for much longer periods than during coronary angioplasty, and the consequences can be measured using TEE with simultaneous high-fidelity pressure measurements. In areas of primary asynchrony, occlusion of the subtending coronary artery has two separate effects: further asynchrony develops (manifest as 60 ms delay in the onset of regional wall thickening)[29] and intrinsic myocardial work and power fall (manifest as reductions in segmental wall thickening (by 46%), regional work (by 56%), and cycle efficiency (by 38%)).[30] The extent of segmental delay is closely associated with wall thinning during isovolumic contraction, wall thickening during isovolumic relaxation, and reductions in effective work and cycle efficiency,[29] and results in a progressively left-leaning pressure–wall thickness loop during supply ischemia (Figure 15.4). Within 10 minutes of restoration of coronary flow, segmental wall motion returns to its preoperative level in areas of primary asynchrony, and normalizes completely by 30 minutes. Wall thickening and peak power increase, and levels of work and cycle efficiency return to levels consistently above baseline. Secondary asynchrony also promptly regresses with revascularization, but neither the extent nor the velocity of wall thickening, nor peak power production, increase from their previously normal values,[24] confirming the distinction between primary and secondary asynchrony.

Demand Ischemia

Atrial pacing

The nature of ventricular asynchrony produced during demand ischemia has been demonstrated using angiographic studies of rapid pacing,[31] and is similar to the asynchrony induced by coronary occlusion.[24] Timing disturbances at rest in patients with CAD become accentuated with pacing-induced ischemia, and result in delayed inward movement of the ischemic segment, segment lengthening during

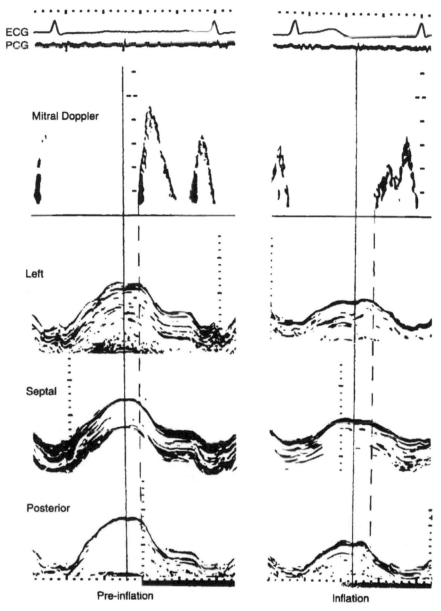

Figure 15.3 An M-mode example of the LV three long axes taken from a patient with left anterior descending coronary artery stenosis before (left) and during (right) balloon inflation (top: coinciding transmitral Doppler flow velocities). There is a significant reduction in total long-axis amplitude and delay in the onset of lengthening with respect to A2 (dotted line) during balloon inflation. At the same time, the transmitral E-wave velocity decreases and the transmitral A-wave velocity increases. (PCG, phonocardiogram).

isovolumic contraction, and premature inward movement of the normal segment. This asynchrony produces a leftward distortion of the LV pressure–wall thickness loops and a significant reduction in cycle efficiency.

Pharmacological stress

Dobutamine stress echocardiography is a practical non-invasive method of provoking demand ischemia. When high-frame-rate techniques (M-mode and tissue Doppler imaging) are used,

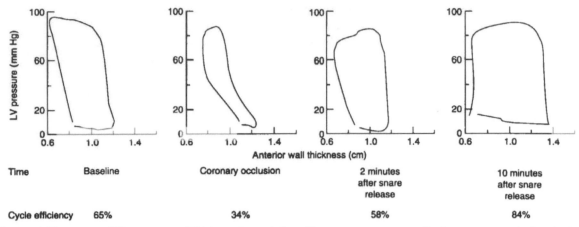

Figure 15.4 Sequence of LV pressure–wall thickness loops during off-pump coronary surgery. During coronary occlusion, the loop area falls and the loop itself leans further to the left. During reperfusion, segmental function becomes rapidly more synchronous, resulting in a more rectangular loop, with cycle efficiency greater than baseline at 10 minutes of reperfusion. (Reprinted from Koh TW et al. Heart 1999;81:285–91, with permission from BMJ Publishing Group Ltd.)

stress-induced asynchrony can be measured objectively with good reproducibility. Moreover, the complex relationship between electrical and mechanical asynchrony can be investigated in some detail. What is now apparent is that CAD is not only a cause of asynchrony at rest, but also modulates the response to stress of that due to LBBB.

Electromechanical response to stress in CAD

QRS duration is not static during pharmacological stress, but is highly labile. In normal subjects, it consistently shortens by 5–10 ms during stress, but broadens by 10–15 ms in patients with CAD.[32] These differences are very predictable. Furthermore, stress-induced changes in QRS duration significantly affect mechanical function. In normal individuals, shortening of the QRS duration is closely related to earlier onset of long-axis shortening and lengthening (by up to 50 ms compared with resting values) (Figure 15.5).[21] This earlier, coordinate, phase shift in segmental motion with stress results in an increase in overall long axis shortening during the time when the aortic valve is open (Figure 15.6). In contrast, QRS broadening in patients with CAD is closely associated with delayed long-axis shortening and lengthening (by up to 30 ms compared with resting values) (Figure 15.5).[21] The result

of stress-induced prolongation of activation in CAD is worsening asynchrony in the form of continued long-axis shortening after the aortic valve has closed and a reduction in the amount of long-axis shortening that actually occurs during ejection (Figure 15.6).

Changes in QRS duration and the resulting mechanical delay have important functional consequences on the pump function of the ventricle during stress, even in individuals with normal resting activation. When the components of the cardiac cycle are analyzed with respect to heart rate, total isovolumic time (t-IVT, the time, expressed in s/min, when the heart is neither ejecting nor filling) normally decreases with stress (from a normal value of 12 s/min to values of 5 s/min or less). Thus, as electromechanical delay normally shortens, the amount of wasted time in the cardiac cycle decreases. However, in CAD, QRS broadening and increasing long-axis asynchrony with stress is accompanied by prolongation of t-IVT (up to a mean value of 13 s/min)[33] (Figure 15.5), emphasizing the importance of the electrical component of the response to acute ischemia.

Interrelations between rest and stress, CAD, and LBBB

Acute changes in QRS duration and its mechanical associations have important implications

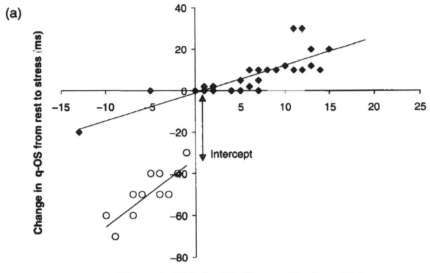

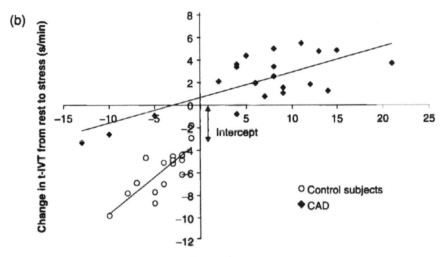

Figure 15.5 Association between changes in QRS duration, electromechanical delay, and total isovolumic time. In normal subjects, the extent of QRS shortening during pharmacological stress is associated with shortening of electromechanical delay (q wave of ECG to onset of long-axis shortening: q-OS) (a) and total isovolumic time (t-IVT) (b). Even with zero change in QRS duration, electromechanical delay and t-IVT shorten by 30 ms and 3 s/min, respectively, with stress. In CAD, however, QRS broadening is closely related to worsening electromechanical delay (a) and prolongation of t-IVT (b) during stress. Furthermore, the normal shortening of both electromechanical delay and t-IVT with zero change in QRS duration (i.e., the normal intercept) is lost during stress.

in the stress response of patients currently targeted for CRT. Both CAD and LBBB affect t-IVT, which is itself a major determinant of peak stress cardiac output,[34] exercise capacity,[35] and clinical response to CRT[36] in patients with heart failure (Figure 15.7). However, the mechanisms by which CAD and LBBB do this depend on resting or stress state. When activation is normal, t-IVT is normal at rest even when CAD is present, but is significantly prolonged if LBBB is present

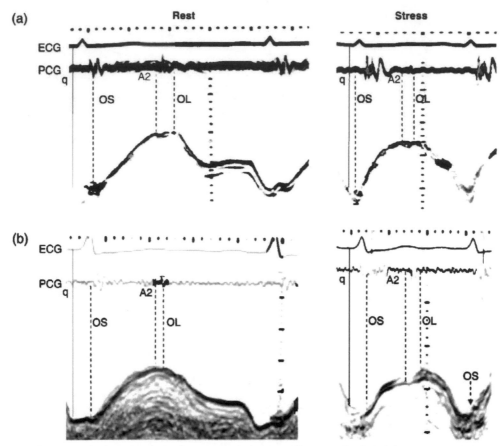

Figure 15.6 (a) Normal long-axis response to pharmacological stress. Electromechanical delay shortens during stress (q-OS, q wave to onset of long-axis shortening; A2-OL, aortic valve closure to onset of long-axis lengthening), so that there is an earlier, coordinate phase shift in segmental motion. In addition, total amplitude, systolic and lengthening velocities all increase. (b) Response to stress in CAD. Electromechanical delay lengthens during stress (both q-OS and A2-OL), so that motion of the entire segment is delayed. This results in continued shortening after aortic valve closure (A2) and reduces the amount of shortening occurring during ejection.

irrespective of CAD (Table 15.1). During stress, QRS duration, electromechanical delay, and t-IVT all shorten significantly in the absence of CAD, even if LBBB is present (Figures 15.8 and 15.9). However, when CAD and LBBB are both present, QRS duration, electromechanical delay, and t-IVT are all long at rest and all fail to shorten with stress (Figures 15.8 and 15.9). The close inverse relationship between t-IVT and cardiac output means that patients without either CAD or LBBB have the shortest values for t-IVT and the highest cardiac output at peak stress, while patients with both CAD and LBBB have the longest t-IVT and the lowest cardiac output at

peak stress (Figure 15.7). In extreme cases, the combination of CAD and LBBB may result in t-IVT lasting 20–25 s/min (i.e., more than a third of the cardiac cycle at peak stress), with corresponding values for peak cardiac output being 50% that of patients with neither CAD nor LBBB.

The electromechanical interrelations between CAD, LBBB, asynchrony, and t-IVT during pharmacological stress have potential practical implications during exercise in patients with heart failure.[35] Patients without either CAD or LBBB have the least asynchrony and shortest t-IVT during stress, and the highest values of peak VO$_2$

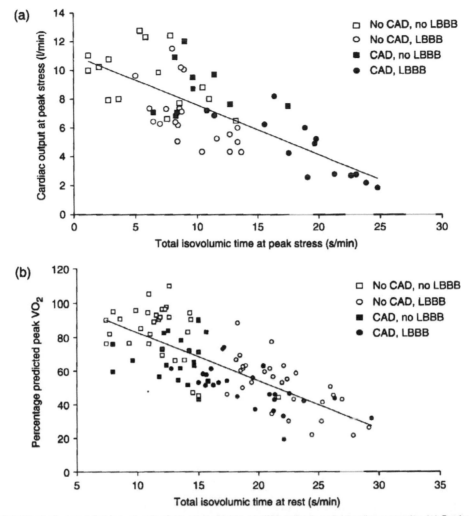

Figure 15.7 Relation between total isovolumic time, peak stress cardiac output, and exercise capacity. (a) During stress, there is a strong inverse correlation between peak total isovolumic time (t-IVT) and peak cardiac output. Patients with both left bundle branch block (LBBB) and coronary artery disease (CAD) have the longest t-IVT and lowest cardiac output. (b) During exercise, there is similar inverse relationship between t-IVT at rest and the percentage predicted peak oxygen consumption (VO_2). Patients with LBBB have the longest t-IVT and lowest percentage predicted VO_2, irrespective of concomitant CAD. (Part (a) reprinted from J Am Coll Cardiol Vol 41, Duncan AM et al. Limitation of cardiac output by total isovolumic time during pharmacologic stress in patients with dilated cardiomyopathy: activation-mediated effects of left bundle branch block and coronary artery disease, pages 121–8. Copyright 2003, with permission from the American College of Cardiology Foundation.[34] Part (b) reprinted from J Am Coll Cardiol Vol 43, Duncan AM et al. Limitation of exercise tolerance in chronic heart failure: distinct effects of left bundle branch block and coronary artery disease, pages 1524–31. Copyright 2004, with permission from the American College of Cardiology Foundation.[35])

on cardiopulmonary exercise testing. Patients with both CAD and LBBB have the most asynchrony and longest t-IVT during stress, and the lowest values for peak VO_2. CAD reduces peak VO_2 by 3.8 ml/kg/min (and percentage predicted peak VO_2 by 10%) compared with patients with no CAD, while LBBB reduces peak VO_2 by 8.8 ml/kg/min (and percentage predicted peak VO_2 by 28%) compared with patients with no LBBB, irrespective of concomitant CAD.

Table 15.1 Response to stress/exercise in dilated cardiomyopathy

During stress	No LBBB, no CAD (n=15)		CAD, no LBBB (n=20)		LBBB, no CAD (n=10)		LBBB and CAD (n=14)	
	Rest	Stress	Rest	Stress	Rest	Stress	Rest	Stress
QRS (ms)	99±8	95±14	96±12	102±12[a]	164±14	156±14[d]	150±14	152±22
q-OS (ms)	118±27	82±20	125±23	144±27[b]	156±31	103±20[d]	158±41	188±31
t-IVT (s/min)	13±3	6±5	11±3	9±3[b]	20±3	11±4[d]	20±4	19±5
CO (l/min)	4.6±1.8	9.3±3.2	5.4±2.3	6.7±2.3[b]	4.8±1.4	8.8±1.9[c]	3.3±1.3	4.9±2.4

During cardiopulmonary exercise testing	No LBBB, no CAD (n=30)	CAD, no LBBB (n=22)	LBBB, no CAD (n=30)	LBBB and CAD (n=29)
Peak VO$_2$ (ml/kg/min)	26±6	21±5[b]	16±5[d]	14±4
% predicted peak VO$_2$	85±15	71±17[a]	52±16[d]	50±13

[a]$p<0.01$; [b]$p<0.001$:CAD vs no CAD.
[c]$p<0.01$; [d]$p<0.001$:LBBB vs no LBBB.
CAD, coronary artery disease; CO, cardiac output; LBBB, left bundle branch block; q-OS, time from q wave to onset of long-axis shortening; t-IVT, total isovolumic time; VO$_2$, oxygen consumption.

Practical implications for CRT

Patients with the most pronounced segmental dyssynchrony and longest t-IVT are those most likely to respond clinically to CRT, although long total isovolumic time is somewhat superior to segmental markers of dyssynchrony in predicting clinical response to CRT.[36–38] The coexistence of CAD, however, also influences the clinical response to CRT: nearly twice as many non-responders to CRT have an ischemic etiology compared with non-ischemic etiology.[36] Addressing the differing hemodynamic responses to stress following CRT in patients with or without CAD may provide an explanation for this. Compared with native activation, optimal resynchronization shortens peak stress t-IVT by 15 s/min in patients with non-ischemic LBBB, whereas peak t-IVT only shortens by 5 s/min in patients with CAD and LBBB during resynchronization. Consequently, the percentage gain in peak stress cardiac output during resynchronization is significantly lower in patients with CAD (by 10%) than in those without (by 19%).[39] Similar changes could be expected during exercise, potentially reducing peak VO$_2$ in patients with CAD despite optimal resynchronization.

Given the close associations between t-IVT, peak stress cardiac output, and exercise capacity,

it would seem logical that the hemodynamic response to pharmacological stress should be studied in all individuals considered for, or undergoing, CRT. Disappointingly, most CRT studies have hitherto been set up and performed at rest, taking no account of important electromechanical interrelations at faster heart rates. This simplistic approach could explain some of the 30% non-response rate to resynchronization. For instance, it appears that the extent of remodeling with CRT is 2–3 times less in patients with CAD compared with those without.[37] Possible reasons for this difference include the presence of scar tissue in CAD, ongoing and repetitive episodes of ischemia, and loss of regional viable myocardium after implantation of CRT. What is clear is that much of the asynchrony present at rest in CAD is reversible after revascularization; indeed, after CABG, QRS duration shortens rather than lengthens with stress, and there is normalization of stress-induced segmental delay[40] (Figure 15.10). This surgical 'resynchronization' has the triple effect of normalizing t-IVT, peak stress cardiac output,[40] and regional intrinsic myocardial work.[29] Thus, investigations for the presence of viable myocardium, and revascularization whenever possible, should be performed before implementation of CRT. A second possible explanation for the non-response rate

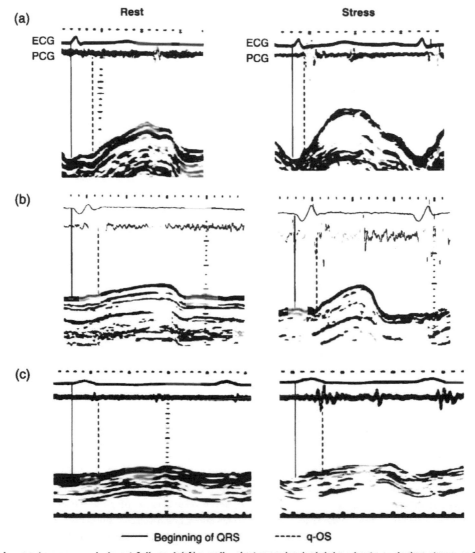

Figure 15.8 Long-axis response in heart failure. (a) Normally, electromechanical delay shortens during stress. q-OS, q wave to onset of long-axis shortening; A2-OL, aortic valve closure to onset of long axis lengthening. (b) In non-ischemic cardiomyopathy with LBBB, electromechanical delay is prolonged at rest but shortens normally with stress. (c) In ischemic cardiomyopathy with LBBB, electromechanical delay is prolonged at rest and fails to shorten during stress. A2, aortic valve closure, (Reprinted from Duncan AM et al. Circulation 2003;108:1214–20, with permission from Lippincott Williams and Wilkins.)

could be the introduction of iatrogenic asynchrony during CRT, in particular in patients with non-ischemic LBBB during stress. In this subgroup of patients, segmental asynchrony usually decreases and t-IVT shortens during stress; if such a patient receives CRT based on resting values alone, asynchrony may actually be induced during stress when electromechanical delay is already short. A final possible (and frequently under-considered) explanation for non-response could be compromised right ventricular (RV) function in CAD. Even after successful LV revascularization, RV long-axis asynchrony may persist during stress,[41] and may thus limit the full benefit of CRT during stress in patients with CAD.

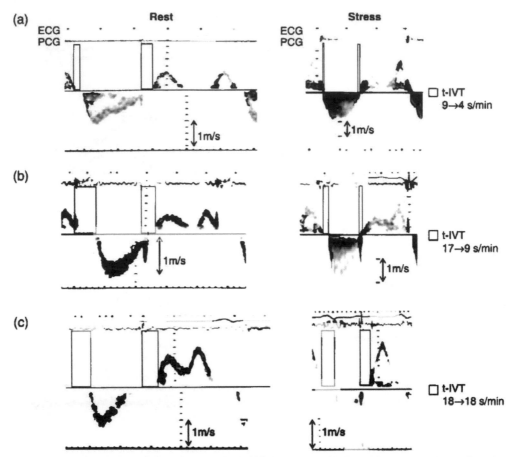

Figure 15.9 Doppler response in heart failure (aortic and mitral Doppler recordings have been superimposed). (a) Normally, the total isovolumic time (t-IVT) falls with stress. (b) In non-ischemic cardiomyopathy with LBBB, t-IVT is prolonged at rest, but shortens normally with stress. (c) In ischemic cardiomyopathy with LBBB, t-IVT is prolonged at rest and does not change during stress. Furthermore, systolic velocity fails to increase with stress. A2, aortic valve closure. (Reprinted from J Am Coll Cardiol Vol 41, Duncan AM et al. Limitation of cardiac output by total isovolumic time during pharmacologic stress in patients with dilated cardiomyopathy: activation-mediated effects of left bundle branch block and coronary artery disease, page 121–8. Copyright 2003, with permission from the American College of Cardiology Foundation.[34])

CONCLUSIONS

The aim of CRT is to correct ventricular asynchrony by advancing the activation of an abnormal LV segment with respect to the remainder of the LV using an additional electrode. If CRT is to be successful, the segmental delay should be significant compared with the rest of the LV, and, once activated, the time course of contraction in the affected segment should be normal. Such primary asynchrony is commonly found at rest in patients with chronic stable CAD or in those

with LBBB. Since primary asynchrony involves both isovolumic periods, it cannot exist in isolation but must be accompanied by secondary, reciprocal, changes elsewhere in the LV. Whatever its etiology, pathological asynchrony reduces the mechanical efficiency of energy transfer from myocardium to circulation, and prolongs isovolumic contraction and isovolumic relaxation times, with the result that t-IVT is increased. The effects of CRT can therefore be observed either from direct observation of regional wall

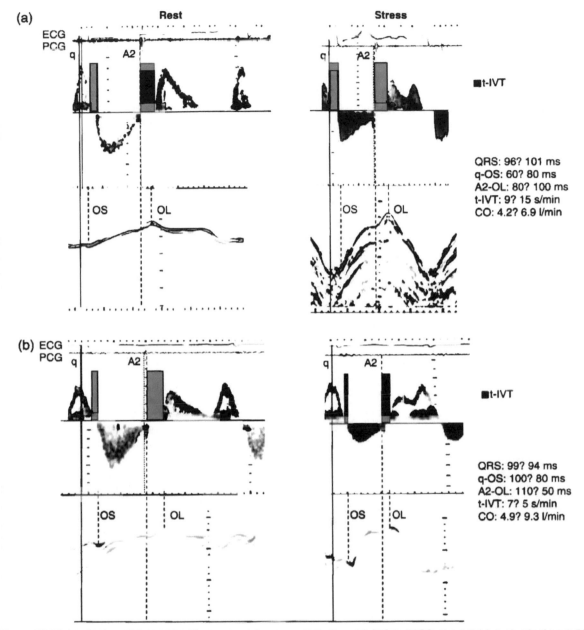

Figure 15.10 Long-axis and hemodynamic response to revascularization. (a) Before CABG, the total isovolumic time (t-IVT) increases as the electromechanical delay worsens during stress. (b) After coronary artery bypass grafting (CABG), t-IVT shortens as electromechanical delay shortens with stress, and the increment in cardiac output is augmented (95% after CABG vs 65% before CABG). A2, aortic valve closure; A2-OL, interval between aortic valve closure and onset of long-axis lengthening; q-OS, interval between q wave and onset of long-axis shortening.

motion to document regression of asynchrony or from a fall in t-IVT.[36] While CRT is the only means currently available for correcting asynchrony due to LBBB, asynchrony associated with CAD responds promptly to revascularization.

Clearly, segments showing secondary asynchrony are already advanced with respect to the remainder of the ventricle, so these would not be expected to respond to CRT: indeed, further asynchrony would be likely to be induced.

If CRT is to improve exercise tolerance, it should also be effective under conditions of stress, which cannot necessarily be predicted from those at rest. In normal subjects, pharmacological stress is associated with shortening of QRS duration and reductions in electromechanical delay and t-IVT. In patients with CAD without LBBB, these changes are reversed; QRS duration is prolonged and electromechanical delay and t-IVT are increased. In patients with isolated LBBB, stress is associated with consistent shortening of QRS duration, electromechanical delay, and t-IVT, so that stress values approach those in normal subjects, but in patients with CAD and LBBB, the effects of CAD during stress are superimposed on those of abnormal resting activation; thus, QRS duration, electromechanical delay, and t-IVT are all prolonged at rest and all fail to shorten with stress, with the result that peak cardiac output is greatly attenuated. CAD thus modulates the response of abnormal activation to stress. Indeed, its effects during stress are so large that LBBB with or without CAD can virtually be considered as two different conditions.

These observations have practical implications for the successful use of CRT. Not only will the technique be ineffective unless pacing is confined to delayed segments, but the function of secondarily asynchronous segments is likely to be aggravated by directly pacing them. The overall effects of changes in pacing mode can be monitored by simple measurement of t-IVT as well as by more extensive mapping of regional wall motion. Finally, the potential clinical significance of these complex interactions between stress and CAD may have been underestimated. There could thus be a case for pre-CRT stress testing, with individualized heart-rate-dependent pacemaker function depending on the result. It would also seem reasonable to screen all patients with resting asynchrony for CAD, regardless of QRS duration, and revascularize if at all possible. Although a 'one size fits all' approach to CRT has proven feasible in large controlled trials, a 30% failure rate persists. In part, this is due to the absence of control asynchrony. However, unlike drug treatment, CRT is much more susceptible to an individualized approach to initial non-responders, which could further enhance the applicability of this technique.

REFERENCES

1. Cazeau S, Leclercq M, Lavergne T, et al. for the MUltisite STimulation In Cardiomyopathies (MUSTIC) Study Investigators. Effects of multisite biventricular pacing in patients with heart failure and intraventricular conduction delay. N Engl J Med 2001;344:873–80.
2. Abraham WT, Fisher WG, Smith AL, et al. for the MIRACLE Study Group. Cardiac resynchronization in chronic heart failure. N Engl J Med 2002;346:1845–53.
3. Cleland JG, Daubert JC, Erdmann E, et al. Cardiac Resynchronization-Heart Failure (CARE-HF) Study Investigators. The effect of cardiac resynchronization on morbidity and mortality in heart failure. N Engl J Med 2005;352:1539–49.
4. Yu CM, Yang H, Lau CP, et al. Regional left ventricle mechanical asynchrony in patients with heart disease and normal QRS duration: implication for biventricular pacing therapy. Pacing Clin Electrophysiol 2003;26:562–70.
5. Turner MS, Bleasdale RA, Vinereanu D, et al. Electrical and mechanical components of dyssynchrony in heart failure patients with normal QRS duration and left bundle-branch block: impact of left and biventricular pacing. Circulation 2004;109:2544–9.
6. Cohen LS, Elliott WC, Klein MD, Gorlin R. Coronary heart disease. Clinical, cinearteriographic and metabolic correlations. Am J Cardiol 1966;17:153–68.
7. Haendchen RV, Wyatt HL, Maurer G, et al. Quantitation of regional cardiac function by two-dimensional echocardiography. I. Patterns of contraction in the normal left ventricle. Circulation 1983;67:1234–45.
8. Shapiro E, Marier DL, St John Sutton MG, Gibson DG. Regional non-uniformity of wall dynamics in normal left ventricle. Br Heart J 1981;45:264–70.
9. Hammermeister KE, Gibson DG, Hughes D. Regional variation in the timing and extent of left ventricular wall motion in normal subjects. Br Heart J 1986;56:226–35.
10. Altieri PI, Wilt SM, Leighton RF. Left ventricular wall motion during the isovolumic relaxation period. Circulation 1973;48:499–505.
11. Harvey W. An Anatomical Disputation Concerning the Movement of the Heart and Blood in Living Creatures (Whitteridge G, transl). Oxford: Blackwell Scientific, 1976:32–7.
12. Jones CJ, Raposo L, Gibson DG. Functional importance of the long axis dynamics of the human left ventricle. Br Heart J 1990;63:215–20.
13. Sandler H, Alderman E. Determination of left ventricular size and shape. Circ Res 1974;40:1–8.
14. Gibson DG, Brown DJ. Continuous assessment of left ventricular shape in man. Br Heart J 1975;37:904–10.
15. Wiggers CJ. Studies on the consecutive phases of the cardiac cycle. Am J Physiol 1921;56:415–59.

16. Gibson DG, Brown DJ. Assessment of left ventricular systolic function in man from simultaneous echocardiographic and pressure measurements. Br Heart J 1976; 38:8–17.

17. Gibson DG, Prewitt TA, Brown DJ. Analysis of left ventricular wall movement during isovolumic relaxation and its relation to coronary artery disease. Br Heart J 1976;38:1010–19.

18. Gibson DG, Doran JH, Traill TA, Brown DJ. Abnormal left ventricular wall movement during early systole in patients with angina pectoris. Br Heart J 1978;40:758–66.

19. Gaasch WH, Blaustein AS, Bing OH. Asynchronous (segmental early) relaxation of the left ventricle. J Am Coll Cardiol 1985;5:891–7.

20. Henein MY, Priestley K, Davarashvili T, Buller N, Gibson DG. Early changes in left ventricular subendocardial function after successful coronary angioplasty. Br Heart J 1993;69:501–6.

21. Duncan A, O'Sullivan C, Carr-White G, Gibson D, Henein M. Long axis electromechanics during dobutamine stress in patients with coronary artery disease and left ventricular dysfunction. Heart 2001;86:397–404.

22. Koh TW, Pepper JR, Gibson DG. Early changes in left ventricular anterior wall dynamics and coordination after coronary artery surgery. Heart 1997;78:291–7.

23. Alam M, Khaki F, Brymer J, Marzelli M, Golstein S. Echocardiographic evaluation of left ventricular function during coronary artery angioplasty. Am J Cardiol 1986;57:20–5.

24. Henein MY, O'Sullivan C, Davies SW, Sigwart U, Gibson DG. Effects of acute coronary occlusion and previous ischaemic injury on left ventricular wall motion in humans. Heart 1997;77:338–45.

25. Henein MY, Gibson DG. Suppression of left ventricular early diastolic filling by long axis asynchrony. Br Heart J 1995;73:151–7.

26. Gibson D, Mehmel H, Schwarz F, et al. Asynchronous left ventricular wall motion early after coronary thrombosis. Br Heart J 1986;55:4–13.

27. Zhang Y, Chan AK, Yu CM, et al. Left ventricular systolic asynchrony after acute myocardial infarction in patients with narrow QRS complexes. Am Heart J 2005;149:497–503.

28. Gibson D, Mehmel H, Schwarz F, Li K, Kubler W. Changes in left ventricular regional asynchrony after intracoronary thrombolysis in patients with impending myocardial infarction. Br Heart J 1986;56:121–30.

29. Carr-White GS, Lim E, Koh TW, et al. Regional ventricular dynamics during acute coronary occlusion: A comparison of invasive with non-invasive echocardiographic markers to detect and quantify myocardial ischaemia-observations made during off-pump coronary surgery. Int J Cardiol. 2006. Apr 25; [Epub ahead of print].

30. Koh TW, Carr-White GS, DeSouza AC, et al. Effect of coronary occlusion on left ventricular function with and without collateral supply during beating heart coronary artery surgery. Heart 1999;81:285–91.

31. Sasayama S, Nonogi H, Fujita M, et al. Analysis of asynchronous wall motion by regional pressure-length loops in patients with coronary artery disease. J Am Coll Cardiol 1984;4:259–67.

32. O'Sullivan CA, Henein MY, Sutton R, et al. Abnormal ventricular activation and repolarisation during dobutamine stress echocardiography in coronary artery disease. Heart 1998;79:468–73.

33. Duncan A, O'Sullivan C, Gibson D, Henein M. Electromechanical interrelations during dobutamine stress in normal subjects and patients with coronary disease: comparison of changes in activation and inotropic state. Heart 2001;85:411–16.

34. Duncan AM, Francis DP, Henein MY, Gibson DG. Limitation of cardiac output by total isovolumic time during pharmacologic stress in patients with dilated cardiomyopathy: activation-mediated effects of left bundle branch block and coronary artery disease. J Am Coll Cardiol 2003;41:121–8.

35. Duncan A, Francis D, Gibson D, Henein M. Limitation of exercise tolerance in chronic heart failure: distinct effects of left bundle branch block and coronary artery disease. J Am Coll Cardiol 2004;43:1524–31.

36. Duncan AM, Lim E, Clague J, Gibson D, Henein M. Comparison of segmental and global markers of dyssynchrony in predicting clinical response to cardiac resynchronization. Eur Heart J 2006;27:2426–32.

37. Duncan A, Wait D, Gibson D, Daubert JC: Left ventricular remodelling and haemodynamic effects of multisite biventricular pacing in patients with left ventricular systolic dysfunction and activation disturbances in sinus rhythm: sub-study of the MUSTIC (Multisite Stimulation in Cardiomyopathies) trial. Eur Heart J 2003;24:430–41.

38. Yu CM, Fung WH, Lin H, Zhang Q, Sanderson JE, Lau CP. Predictors of left ventricular reverse remodeling after cardiac resynchronization therapy for heart failure secondary to idiopathic dilated or ischemic cardiomyopathy. Am J Cardiol 2003;91:684–8.

39. Salukhe TV, Francis DP, Morgan M, et al. Mechanism of cardiac output gain from cardiac resynchronization therapy in patients with coronary artery disease or idiopathic dilated cardiomyopathy. Am J Cardiol 2006; 97:1358–64.

40. Duncan A, Lim E, Gibson D, Henein M. Electromechanical left ventricular resynchronisation by coronary artery bypass surgery. J Cardio-thorac Surg 2004;26:711–19.

41. Duncan A, Pepper J, Henein M. Persistence of right ventricular dysfunction during dobutamine stress following coronary artery bypass grafting. Euro J Echo 2006;7:Suppl I.865.

16

Assessment of left ventricular dyssynchrony for the prediction of response to CRT: The role of conventional echocardiography and 3D echocardiography

E Liodakis, Gabe B Bleeker, Jeroen J Bax, and Petros Nihoyannopoulos

Introduction • M-mode echocardiography • Two-dimensional echocardiography • Real-time 3D echocardiography in the assessment of LV dyssynchrony • Conclusions

INTRODUCTION

At present, cardiac resynchronization therapy (CRT) is considered a major breakthrough in the treatment of selected patients with drug-refractory heart failure.[1,2] In large randomized trials, CRT was able to improve heart failure symptoms and left ventricular (LV) function. In addition, CRT resulted in a significant reduction in the number of heart failure-related hospitalizations and an improvement in patient survival.[1,2] However, closer analysis of the results of these trials revealed that 20–30% of patients did not improve in clinical symptoms when patients were selected according to the established CRT selection (New York Heart Association (NYHA) class III and IV, LV ejection fraction (LVEF) <35%, and QRS complex width >120 ms).[3,4] This observation highlights the need for refinement of the current selection criteria in order to reduce the number of patients without response to CRT.

Mechanism of benefit from CRT

To better understand the mechanism of non-response to CRT, knowledge of the beneficial mechanisms of CRT is of utmost importance. The rationale behind CRT is the resynchronization of dyssynchronous activation (and consequent contractions) of the heart. Dyssynchronous contractions of the heart are a frequent observation in heart failure patients, and three levels of mechanical dyssynchrony can be identified:[4]

1. *Atrioventricular dyssynchrony* is the result of a delayed conduction over the AV node resulting in a decreased diastolic filling time, leading to a suboptimal ventricular filling.
2. *Interventricular dyssynchrony* is the result of premature activation of the right ventricle (RV) that mainly affects the intraventricular septum and causes an overall decrease in the systolic performance of the LV.
3. *Intra (LV) dyssynchrony* strongly affects LV pumping efficiency and is (usually) the result of an early-activated septum and a late-activated lateral wall, resulting in substantial blood volume shifts within the LV rather than blood being ejected into the aorta.

Recent studies have indicated that resynchronization of LV dyssynchrony is probably the key mechanism of response to CRT. Patients with substantial baseline LV dyssynchrony had a high likelihood of response to CRT, whereas patients without pre-implantation LV dyssynchrony were unlikely to respond to CRT. Since the observation that QRS duration is a weak marker of LV dyssynchrony, various echocardiographic techniques have been introduced for the detection of LV dyssynchrony in order to select those patients with the highest likelihood of response to CRT. In recent years, a number of parameters based both on conventional echocardiographic techniques (M-mode and two-dimensional echocardiography) and more advanced modalities (tissue Doppler imaging (TDI), strain rate, and 3D echocardiography) have been conceived and tested in patients undergoing CRT implantation.[1,2,5–18] This chapter will give an overview of the conventional echocardiographic techniques and 3D echocardiography for the detection of LV dyssynchrony for the prediction of response to CRT.

M-MODE ECHOCARDIOGRAPHY

A relatively simple and elegant echocardiographic technique for the detection of LV dyssynchrony has been developed by Pitzalis et al.[19,20] These authors used an M-mode recording through the parasternal short-axis view (at the papillary muscle level) to measure the delay between the systolic excursion of the (antero)septum and the posterior wall – the so-called septal-to-posterior wall motion delay (SPWMD)[19,20] (Figure 16.1). In an initial study, including 20 patients, responders to CRT had a significantly larger SPWMD as compared with non-responders. An optimal cut-off value in SPWMD of 130 ms was proposed, which yielded an accuracy of 85% (sensitivity 100% and specificity 63%) to predict response to CRT[19] (Figure 16.2). In a subsequent study,[20] the same authors evaluated another 60 patients undergoing CRT and demonstrated that the cut-off value of 130 ms was a strong predictor of cardiac events during long-term follow-up.

Recent data from Marcus et al,[21] however, revealed less favorable results (Figure 16.2). The SPWMD measurement was applied retrospectively in a large cohort (79 patients, 72% with ischemic cardiomyopathy) of heart failure patients who were included in the CONTAK-CD trial.

The authors reported difficulties in interpretation of M-mode recordings in more than 50% of patients (Figure 16.3). Similar findings were observed in two recent studies that also reported relatively high numbers (41–56%) of patients in whom the SPWMD could not be assessed, usually due to akinesia of the septal and/or posterior walls or poor acoustic windows.[22,23] In addition, the predictive value of the SPWMD for a positive response to CRT proved poor in these subsequent studies, with sensitivities ranging from 24% to 66% and with specificities from 50% to 66%.[21,22] Conversely, Bleeker et al[22] demonstrated that in patients without an interpretable SPWMD, color-coded tissue Doppler was still feasible in 90% of patients and was highly predictive for response to CRT (sensitivity 90% and specificity 82%)[22] (Figure 16.2).

TWO-DIMENSIONAL ECHOCARDIOGRAPHY

In patients with heart failure, severe LV dyssynchrony can sometimes be assessed visually from conventional two-dimensional (2D) echocardiography. It is displayed as a counterclockwise rotation of the LV in the apical four-chamber view or a delayed activation of the posterolateral LV segments. However, in the majority of cases, visual assessment alone is not precise enough to accurately characterize LV dyssynchrony. In addition, the presence of LV dyssynchrony will not be detected in patients with an intermediate extent of LV dyssynchrony, even in the hands of experienced sonographers.

Two more sophisticated echocardiographic approaches have recently been introduced that permit more accurate quantification of LV dyssynchrony from conventional 2D echocardiography. The first technique was introduced by Breithardt et al,[5] who used computer-generated regional wall movement curves compared by mathematical phase analysis based on Fourier transformation. This approach has been developed for more objective and standardized wall motion assessment and has proved to be highly reproducible in patients with coronary artery disease and Wolff–Parkinson–White (WPW) syndrome.[24,25] Breithardt et al[5] used this approach in 34 patients undergoing CRT implantation and studied the relationship between the wall motion

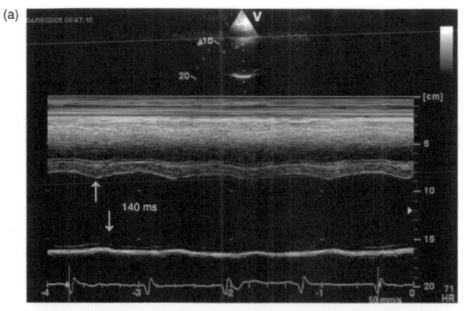

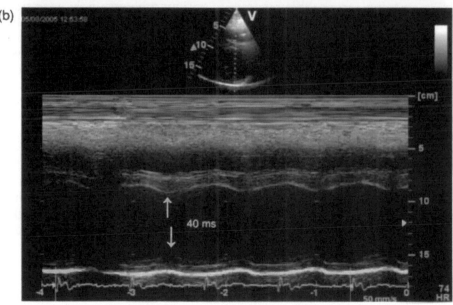

Figure 16.1 (a) Example of a heart failure patient with a significant septal-to-posterior wall motion delay (SPWMD: 140 ms) before CRT implantation. (b) Immediately after CRT implantation, the SPWMD is reduced to 40 ms. The SPWMD is obtained from an M-mode recording through the parasternal short-axis view (at the papillary muscle level), from which the delay between the systolic excursion of the (antero)septum and the posterior wall are measured (arrows indicate systolic excursion).

phase angles of the septum (ΦS) and lateral wall (ΦL) on the apical four-chamber views. Immediately following CRT, an acute reduction in ΦLS (where ΦLS = ΦL − ΦS) was observed: from 104° ± 41° to 66° ± 42°. In addition, a large baseline ΦLS was highly predictive of an immediate increase in dP/dt_{max} ($r = 0.74$, $p < 0.001$). In contrast, in patients with ΦLS $<$25°, improvement in dP/dt_{max} following CRT was unlikely.

An alternative approach for the use of 2D echocardiography for detection of LV dyssynchrony was introduced by Kawaguchi et al,[26]

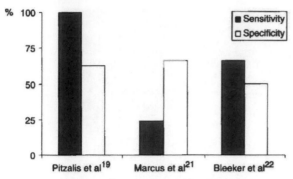

Figure 16.2 Sensitivity and specificity of the SPWMD for prediction of a positive response following CRT in three studies.[19,21,22]

who used contrast echocardiography to improve border delineation in 10 patients undergoing CRT. The contrast-enhanced images were processed using a technique known as cardiac variability imaging. An analysis program compared the regional fractional area change for a large number of 15° sectors in the four-chamber views. From this information, the dyssynchrony between the septum and lateral wall was calculated. Biventricular pacing increased septal inward motion from −20.4 ± 9.6% to −30.5 ± 14.0%, and the lateral wall motion occurred earlier in systole. Both the spatial and temporal dyssynchrony in the LV declined by nearly 40% with biventricular pacing ($p < 0.001$), and this reduction in LV dyssynchrony correlated with an increase in LVEF (from 31% to 39%; $p < 0.05$).[26] Despite these promising results, both techniques are restricted to the measurement of LV dyssynchrony in a single plane, while dyssynchrony in other planes (e.g., anterior and posterior walls) will be overlooked. Three-dimensional (3D) echocardiography, with its better spatial resolution, may potentially overcome this limitation and is discussed in the following section.

REAL-TIME 3D ECHOCARDIOGRAPHY IN THE ASSESSMENT OF LV DYSSYNCHRONY

The ability to provide an accurate evaluation of the dimensions and function of the LV is essential for patient's management, and echocardiography is the most widely used imaging modality for this purpose. Conventional echo modalities (M-mode and 2D) rely heavily on geometrical assumptions and have insufficient accuracy and inter- and intraobserver agreement, indicating the need for more objective quantification techniques.

Many studies that have sought to describe and create 3D models of the LV have been performed over the past two decades; however, widespread use of this technique was inherently limited by the time-consuming, copious data acquisition and the difficult offline reconstruction processes. Furthermore, the complicated analysis procedures applied to the 3D datasets rendered these early efforts subject to the same limitations as encountered with 2D techniques. Recent hardware and software advances, particularly the development of full matrix array transducers, have eliminated various problems in the acquisition and analysis processes, and offer significantly higher spatial resolution.[27]

Real-time 3D echocardiography (RT3DE), which is currently readily available from most of the major ultrasound manufacturers, permits rapid acquisition from a single apical acoustic window of four pyramidal subvolumes, which are then electronically reconstructed over four or five consecutive cardiac cycles. Several offline and online software packages offer extensive qualitative and quantitative features. The RT3DE LV volume dataset is then divided into several predetermined equi-angled longitudinal slices, and after the identification of anatomical landmarks (mitral and aortic valves and apex) and phases (end-systole and end-diastole) by the operator in all the views, a semi-automatic border-detection algorithm is then used to trace the endocardial borders throughout the cardiac cycle (Figure 16.4). The endocardial contours created by this process are then combined, and a dynamic 'cast' of the LV is obtained. This 3D model, as shown in Figure 16.5, simulates in real time the contraction and relaxation of the LV, and with the detection of hundreds of points over the LV surface, global and regional volumes as well as LVEF can be calculated, without the need for the geometrical assumptions encountered with 2D techniques.

(a)
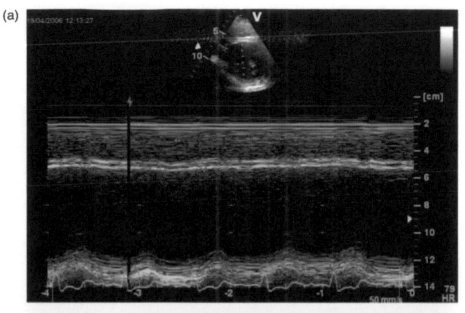

(b)
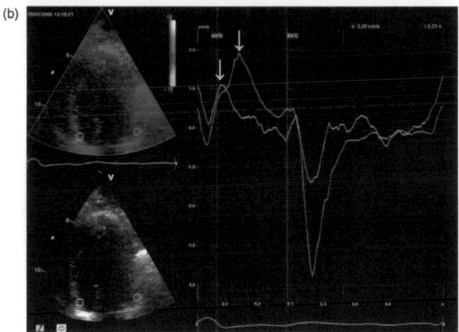

Figure 16.3 (a) Example of a patient in whom assessment of LV dyssynchrony using M-mode echocardiography was not feasible due to akinesia of the inter-ventricular septum. (b) LV dyssynchrony assessment using color-coded tissue Doppler imaging in the same patient as in (a). The sample volumes are placed in the basal parts of the septum and lateral wall, and tracings are derived. The delay in peak systolic velocity between the septum and the lateral wall is 70 ms. Yellow curve, septum; green curve, lateral wall; arrows, peak systolic velocity; AVO, aortic valve opening; AVC, aortic valve closure.

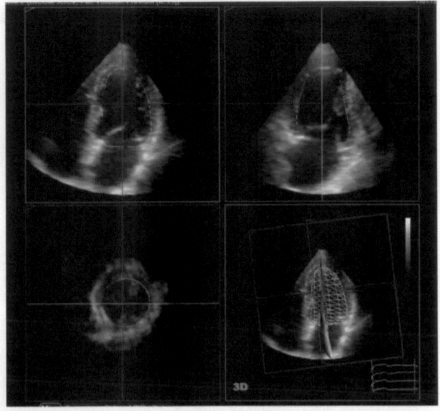

Figure 16.4 Example of real-time 3D analysis. A semi-automatic border-tracking technique is applied to obtain a dynamic 'cast' of the LV.

Evaluation of global and regional volumes and function

Many published studies have demonstrated a high degree of concordance between 3D echocardiography and magnetic resonance imaging (MRI) for the assessment of LV volumes and LVEF.[11,27–29] Furthermore, it has been shown that RT3DE is more reproducible and accurate in measuring LV volume, LVEF, and LV mass than conventional echocardiographic techniques, which can be used for serial follow-up of patients with cardiac disease.[28] The important role of RT3DE in the assessment of regional volumes and wall motion abnormalities has also been strongly supported by results of more recent studies.[30,31]

RT3DE and LV dyssynchrony assessment

In the context of LV dyssynchrony, the capability of analyzing the regional volumes and function

of the 16 or 17 segments according to the American Society of Echocardiography 'bull's-eye' model (Figure 16.5) provides a valuable tool for quantitative assessment of the synchronicity of LV contraction. A series of plots representing the change in volume in each of the 16 segments throughout a cardiac cycle can be obtained. With synchronous contraction (Figure 16.6a), all regions reach their minimum volumes at approximately the same time. Conversely, in the event of LV dyssynchrony (Figure 16.6b), a scattering of the minimum volume points is observed. From these time–volume curves, qualitative information such as the identification of the most delayed myocardial segments can be obtained, as well as a crude estimate of the degree of dispersion that exists between the timing of the minimum volume points of the LV segments.

From the time to minimal regional volume for each of the 16 segments, the systolic dyssynchrony index (SDI) can be derived as a marker of

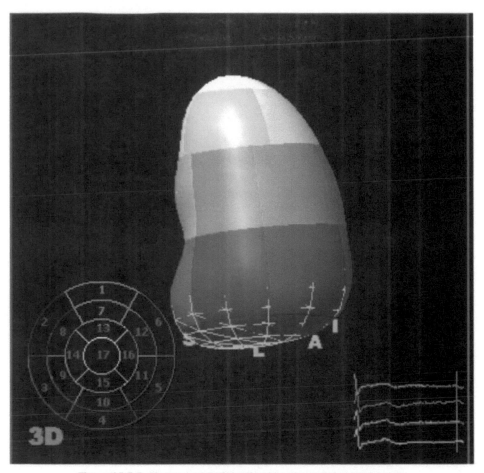

Figure 16.5 Bull's-eye model of the LV, with color-coded segmentation.

LV dyssynchrony: SDI is defined as the standard deviation of the time to minimum volume of all 16 segments. This parameter provides a comparison of all segments simultaneously during the same cardiac cycle, eliminating any variability caused by differences in the RR intervals, which are commonly observed in heart failure patients. This index was conceived with the same rationale as the TDI indices and has been shown to be simple, intuitive, and highly reproducible when used in the selection and follow-up of patients eligible for CRT.[11]

In particular, a strong inverse correlation has been noted between LVEF and the SDI, demonstrating that a larger extent of LV dyssynchrony is associated with a more severe impairment of systolic LV function. Conversely, the relationship between SDI and the electrical dyssynchrony as expressed by the QRS width appears much

weaker, with two outlier groups of particular interest with regard to CRT being identified in the regression analysis. The first group consists of heart failure patients who present with high mechanical dyssynchrony (high SDI) and a narrow QRS complex, which could represent a group that is not eligible to CRT according to the current selection criteria but could potentially benefit from CRT. At the other end of the spectrum, we can identify a group of patients who fit the current criteria, having a prolonged QRS duration, but who do not exhibit LV dyssynchrony (low SDI) and could represent the 20–30% of non-responders who have been found in several studies. Obviously, larger prospective studies are necessary to further validate these findings. To date, no optimal cut-off values have been developed for the SDI, and these have to be derived from future studies.

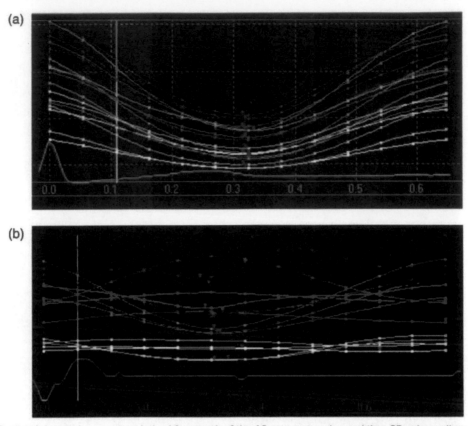

Figure 16.6 Regional time–volume curves derived from each of the 16 segments using real-time 3D echocardiographic (RT3DE) analysis. The systolic dyssynchrony index (SDI) is defined as the standard deviation of time to regional volume for each of the 16 segments. (a) Example of a patient in whom all regions reach their minimum volumes at approximately the same time, indicating the absence of LV dyssynchrony (SDI 1%). (b) Example of a patient with heart failure and dyssynchronous LV contraction (SDI 21%).

When compared with the TDI indices, which are currently considered the 'gold standard' for the evaluation of LV dyssynchrony, SDI presents a modest correlation particularly with the 12-segment Ts-SD (standard deviation of time to peak myocardial contraction of 12 LV segments). This could be explained by the fact that SDI is calculated using 16 rather than 12 segments, since it includes the 4 apical segments that have been shown to significantly contribute to intraventricular dyssynchrony – particularly in patients with ischemic cardiomyopathy. At the same time, although RT3DE offers a more extensive assessment of the LV, it is inherently limited by its inferior temporal resolution (20–25 Hz) when compared with TDI (>100 Hz).[11]

Novel approaches

A parametric display of the timing of the LV contraction derived from RT3DE has also been proposed as a novel technique to quantify LV dyssynchrony. Contraction front mapping is a technique based on the analysis of approximately 3000 points over the LV endocardial surface.[27] The pattern of contraction is presented with a special 'polar-map' display, and the different regions are coded with colors corresponding to the timing of the segmental contractions. This enables the observer to identify the most-delayed region and provide invaluable, noninvasive information before CRT implantation (Figure 16.7). Preliminary data suggest that color front mapping is a very sensitive technique that

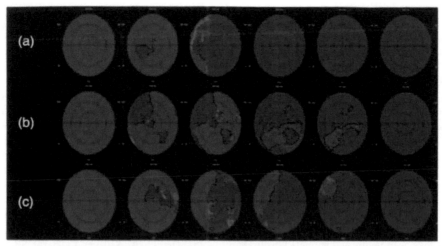

Figure 16.7 Contraction front mapping. The pattern of contraction is presented with a special 'polar-map' display, with the regions being coded with colors corresponding to the timing of their contraction (red representing early contraction and blue late contraction). This example shows (a) a normal individual, (b) a patient with heart failure and narrow QRS complex, and (c) a patient with heart failure and wide QRS complex. (Courtesy of Dr Monaghan, King's College London, UK.)

takes advantage of the excellent spatial resolution provided by RT3DE. Future larger studies will have to demonstrate the value of this technique in the identification of responders to CRT.

CONCLUSIONS

The presence of substantial LV dyssynchrony before CRT implantation proved to be the key predictor of response at mid-term follow-up. Since this observation, several echocardiographic techniques have been introduced for the quantification of LV dyssynchrony, ranging from simple M-mode and 2D echocardiography to more sophisticated techniques, such as RT3DE. Which technique is most optimal for prediction of response to CRT, and what extent of LV dyssynchrony is mandatory for response to CRT, are not yet defined and have to be established in future trials.

REFERENCES

1. Abraham WT, Fisher WG, Smith AL, et al. Cardiac resynchronization in chronic heart failure. N Engl J Med 2002;346:1845–53.
2. Abraham WT. Cardiac resynchronization therapy for heart failure: biventricular pacing and beyond. Curr Opin Cardiol 2002;17(4):346–52.
3. Leclercq C, Kass DA. Retiming the failing heart: principles and current clinical status of cardiac resynchronization. J Am Coll Cardiol 2002;39:194–201.
4. Kass DA. Ventricular resynchronization: pathophysiology and identification of responders. Rev Cardiovasc Med 2003;4(Suppl 2):S3–13.
5. Breithardt OA, Stellbrink C, Kramer AP, et al. Echocardiographic quantification of left ventricular asynchrony predicts an acute hemodynamic benefit of cardiac resynchronization therapy. J Am Coll Cardiol 2002;40:536–45.
6. Ansalone G, Giannantoni P, Ricci R, et al. Doppler myocardial imaging to evaluate the effectiveness of pacing sites in patients receiving biventricular pacing. J Am Coll Cardiol 2002;39:489–99.
7. Auricchio A, Stellbrink C, Sack S, et al. Long-term clinical effect of hemodynamically optimized cardiac resynchronization therapy in patients with heart failure and ventricular conduction delay. J Am Coll Cardiol 2002;39:2026–33.
8. Bax JJ, Molhoek SG, van Erven L, et al. Usefulness of myocardial tissue Doppler echocardiography to evaluate left ventricular dyssynchrony before and after biventricular pacing in patients with idiopathic dilated cardiomyopathy. Am J Cardiol 2003;91:94–7.
9. Bax JJ, Bleeker GB, Marwick T, et al. Left ventricular dyssynchrony predicts benefit of cardiac resynchronization therapy in patients with end-stage heart failure before pacemaker implantation. Am J Cardiol 2003;92:1238–40.
10. Bax JJ, Ansalone G, Breithardt OA, et al. Echocardiographic evaluation of cardiac resynchronization

therapy: ready for routine clinical use? A critical appraisal. J Am Coll Cardiol 2004;44:1–9.

11. Kapetanakis S, Kearney MT, Siva A, et al. Real-time three-dimensional echocardiography: a novel technique to quantify global left ventricular mechanical dyssynchrony. Circulation 2005;112:992–1000.

12. Sutherland GR, Kukulski T, Kvitting JE, et al. Quantitation of left-ventricular asynergy by cardiac ultrasound. Am J Cardiol 2000;86(4A):4G–9G.

13. Yu CM, Chau E, Sanderson JE, et al. Tissue Doppler echocardiographic evidence of reverse remodeling and improved synchronicity by simultaneously delaying regional contraction after biventricular pacing therapy in heart failure. Circulation 2002;105:438–45.

14. Yu CM, Lin H, Zhang Q, et al. High prevalence of left ventricular systolic and diastolic asynchrony in patients with congestive heart failure and normal QRS duration. Heart 2003;89:54–60.

15. Yu CM, Bax JJ, Monaghan M, et al. Echocardiographic evaluation of cardiac dyssynchrony for predicting a favourable response to cardiac resynchronisation therapy. Heart 2004;90(Suppl 6):vi17–22.

16. Yu CM, Fung JW, Zhang Q, et al. Tissue Doppler imaging is superior to strain rate imaging and postsystolic shortening on the prediction of reverse remodeling in both ischemic and nonischemic heart failure after cardiac resynchronization therapy. Circulation 2004;110:66–73.

17. Yu CM, Zhang Q, Fung JW, et al. A novel tool to assess systolic asynchrony and identify responders of cardiac resynchronization therapy by tissue synchronization imaging. J Am Coll Cardiol 2005;45:677–84.

18. Zhang Q, Yu CM, Fung JW, et al. Assessment of the effect of cardiac resynchronization therapy on intraventricular mechanical synchronicity by regional volumetric changes. Am J Cardiol 2005;95:126–9.

19. Pitzalis MV, Iacovello M, Romito R, et al. Ventricular asynchrony predicts a better outcome in patients with chronic heart failure receiving cardiac resynchronization therapy. J Am Coll Cardiol 2005;45:65–9.

20. Pitzalis MV, Iacovello M, Romito R, et al. Cardiac resynchronization therapy tailored by echocardiographic evaluation of ventricular asynchrony. J Am Coll Cardiol 2002;40:1615–22.

21. Marcus GM, Rose E, Viloria EM, et al. Septal to posterior wall motion delay fails to predict reverse remodeling or clinical improvement in patients undergoing cardiac resynchronization therapy. J Am Coll Cardiol 2005;46:2208–14.

22. Bleeker GB, Schalij MJ, Boersma E, et al. Relative merits of M-mode echocardiography and tissue Doppler imaging for prediction of response to cardiac resynchronization therapy in patients with heart failure secondary to ischemic or idiopathic dilated cardiomyopathy. Am J Cardiol 2006.

23. De Sutter J, Van de Veire NR, Muyldermans L, et al. Prevalence of mechanical dyssynchrony in patients with heart failure and preserved left ventricular function (a report from the Belgian Multicenter Registry on Dyssynchrony). Am J Cardiol 2005;96:1543–8.

24. Kuecherer HF, Abbott JA, Botvinick EH, et al. Two-dimensional echocardiographic phase analysis. Its potential for noninvasive localization of accessory pathways in patients with Wolff–Parkinson–White syndrome. Circulation 1992;85:130–42.

25. Hansen A, Krueger C, Hardt SE, et al. Echocardiographic quantification of left ventricular asynergy in coronary artery disease with Fourier phase imaging. Int J Cardiovasc Imaging 2001;17:81–8.

26. Kawaguchi M, Murabayashi T, Fetics BJ, et al. Quantitation of basal dyssynchrony and acute resynchronization from left or biventricular pacing by novel echo-contrast variability imaging. J Am Coll Cardiol 2002;39:2052–8.

27. Monaghan MJ. Role of real time 3D echocardiography in evaluating the left ventricle. Heart, 2006;92:131–6.

28. Kuhl HP, Schreckenberg M, Rulands D, et al. High-resolution transthoracic real-time three-dimensional echocardiography: quantitation of cardiac volumes and function using semi-automatic border detection and comparison with cardiac magnetic resonance imaging. J Am Coll Cardiol 2004;43:2083–90.

29. Jenkins C, Bricknell K, Hanekom L, et al. Reproducibility and accuracy of echocardiographic measurements of left ventricular parameters using real-time three-dimensional echocardiography. J Am Coll Cardiol 2004;44:878–86.

30. Corsi C, Lang RM, Veronesi F, et al. Volumetric quantification of global and regional left ventricular function from real-time three-dimensional echocardiographic images. Circulation 2005;112:1161–70.

31. Corsi C, Coon P, Goonewardena, et al. Quantification of regional left ventricular wall motion from real-time 3-dimensional echocardiography in patients with poor acoustic windows: effects of contrast enhancement tested against cardiac magnetic resonance. J Am Soc Echocardiogr 2006;19:886–93.

17

Left ventricular dyssynchrony in predicting response and patient selection

Cheuk-Man Yu, Qing Zhang, and Jeffrey Wing-Hong Fung

Introduction • Importance of early echocardiographic response after CRT • Role of myocardial imaging in identifying responders to CRT • Summary

INTRODUCTION

Identification of responders to cardiac resynchronization therapy (CRT) is important to establish before device implantation. Currently, it is known that about one-third of patients receiving CRT do not show a favorable response.[1-8] A number of methods have been used to characterize non-responders to CRT, including hemodynamic, clinical and echocardiographic variables. A commonly used definition of acute hemodynamic response is a gain in pulse pressure of 5% or more, while improvement in dP/dt_{max} has also been suggested. The definition of clinical response is highly variable, ranging from the use of single or multiple assessment measures (e.g., New York Heart Association (NYHA) functional class, 6-minute hall walk distance, and heart failure-related quality-of-life score) to hard clinical endpoints (e.g., heart failure hospitalization, mortality, and composite clinical score).[2-5,10] Lastly, echocardiographic response usually focuses on left ventricular (LV) reverse remodeling (e.g., reduction of LV end-systolic volume (LVESV)) or improvement of systolic function (e.g., increase in LV ejection fraction (LVEF), cardiac output, or stroke volume).[6,8,11,12] It is important to realize that clinical and echocardiographic responses, although they seem to be related, do not always occur simultaneously in the same patient.[13] This chapter will discuss the role of myocardial tissue imaging by echocardiography in predicting CRT response.

IMPORTANCE OF EARLY ECHOCARDIOGRAPHIC RESPONSE AFTER CRT

Early echocardiographic response signifies a favorable cardiac structural and functional response to CRT. When resynchronization of systolic contraction of the LV is achieved by pacing, systolic intraventricular asynchrony is decreased. As a result, systolic contractile efficacy is enhanced; i.e., there is improvement of forward pump function with a volume-unloading effect.[14] Together with reduction of mitral regurgitation, this explains why systolic parameters and LV volume measured by echocardiography are improved.[15,16] Our recent study in 50 patients illustrated that, immediately after CRT, although there was a significant gain in LVEF (2%) and a reduction in LVESV (8%), there was no change in LV mass in the acute assessment.[17] On the other hand, reassessment after CRT for 3 months showed a cumulative increase in LVEF by 7.7% and a decrease in LV volume by 22%. This was accompanied by a significant decrease in LV mass by 8% and a decrease in LV regional wall thickness. In fact, responders to LV reverse remodeling had a gain in LVEF of 11.8% and a reduction of LV mass by 15.5%.[17] Therefore, LV reverse remodeling after CRT not only signifies

LV functional improvement, but also favorable structural alteration in response to the functional and hemodynamic improvement.

The beneficial change in LV reverse remodeling after CRT for 3–6 months is also a predictor of favorable long-term clinical outcome. A recent study examined 141 patients receiving CRT from two centers and followed up for a mean duration of 1.9 years. It was reported that patients receiving CRT and with ≥10% LV reverse remodeling (as measured by LVESV) had lower all-cause mortality rate (6.9% vs 30.6%; log-rank $\chi^2=13.26$, $p=0.0003$), cardiovascular mortality rate (2.3% vs 24.1%; log-rank $\chi^2=17.1$, $p<0.0001$), heart failure event rate (11.5% vs 33.3%; log-rank $\chi^2=8.71$, $p=0.0032$) and composite endpoint of all-cause mortality or cardiovascular hospitalization.[18] This is in contrast to improvements in heart failure symptoms and exercise capacity, which were unable to predict clinical outcome. Therefore, prediction of echocardiographic reverse remodeling and improvement in cardiac function is clinically relevant in the context of CRT. Furthermore, prediction of CRT responders will also allow the therapy to be more cost-effective, and possibly avoid subjecting heart failure patients to the risky procedure of device implantation without significant potential benefit.

ROLE OF MYOCARDIAL IMAGING IN IDENTIFYING RESPONDERS TO CRT

Tissue Doppler velocity

Tissue Doppler velocity is the fundamental data obtained from tissue Doppler imaging (TDI). The latter is the most common imaging modality employed to predict CRT response. The aim of TDI is to detect low-frequency, high-amplitude myocardial movement. Different imaging modes of TDI are available, including spectral pulse TDI for online measurement, color TDI for offline analysis, and color M-mode TDI. Of these, color TDI is the imaging mode most frequently employed in CRT studies.

As LV free-wall delay is suggested to be a common mechanical consequence of QRS prolongation, basal septal-to-lateral delay has been assessed by two-dimensional (2D) color TDI. CRT abolished septal-to-lateral delay acutely,

resulting in a gain in LVEF and a decrease in LV volume.[19] In a study of 25 patients receiving CRT, a septal-to-lateral delay at baseline ≥60 ms had a sensitivity of 76% and a specificity of 87.5% in predicting an increase in LVEF by ≥5%.[20] Improvement in clinical status was also mainly observed in these responders. Subsequently, the same investigators examined 85 patients, who were followed up for 1 year. The clinical response rate was 73%, with response being defined as an improvement in NYHA functional class by ≥1 score and a gain in 6-minute hall walk distance by ≥25%.[21] A septal-to-lateral delay ≥65 ms had a sensitivity and specificity of 80% to predict clinical response, and a sensitivity and specificity of 92% to predict LV reverse remodeling (defined as a reduction in LVESV ≥15%).[21]

The two-segment approach can be oversimplified and may miss some other complex patterns of systolic dyssynchrony. Therefore, a multiple segment approach has been adopted by many researchers to create various models of intraventricular dyssynchrony in order to predict a favorable response to CRT. Examples of these models include the use of six basal LV segments, of six basal and six mid-LV segments, and the use of septal versus LV free-wall segments.

Penicka et al[21] measured the time to onset of systolic contraction in the ejection phase of the myocardial velocity curve using spectral pulse TDI in 49 patients. They defined intraventricular dyssynchrony as the maximum electromechanical delay among the three basal LV segments (septal, lateral, and posterior wall), and interventricular dyssynchrony as the maximum delay between the basal right ventricular (RV) segment and the three LV sites. They suggested that summing intra- and interventricular dyssynchrony with a cut-off value of 102 ms has an accuracy of 88% in predicting a relative increase in LVEF by 25%.

Most of the published studies to date have been based on offline analysis of color TDI images. Notobartolo et al[11] measured the time to highest peak velocity in either the ejection phase or post-systolic shortening from the three apical views, and calculated the maximum time difference among the six basal LV segments as the 'peak velocity difference'. In 49 patients receiving CRT, a peak velocity difference of >110 ms at baseline predicted LV reverse remodeling at 3-month follow up with a sensitivity of 97%, although the specificity was only 55%.

Examination of the myocardial velocity curve, focusing on the ejection phase velocity, is another common way of assessing CRT response. Yu et al[10] measured the standard deviation of the time to peak systolic velocity in the ejection phase in the six-basal, six-midsegmental model and calculated the asynchrony index (Ts-SD) (Figure 17.1). With a population-derived cut-off value of 32.6 ms, this index was able to divide responders from non-responders with LV reverse remodeling from a preliminary study of 30 patients. Since the degree of QRS prolongation might have impacted on the response rate to CRT, a further study was conducted to examine whether such a difference exists between patients with narrower (>120–150 ms) and wider (>150 ms) QRS complex.[22] It was found that the response rate of LV reverse remodeling was lower in the narrower-QRS group (46%) than in those with QRS >150 ms (68%), as the former group had a lower prevalence of pre-pacing systolic dyssynchrony. The sensitivity and specificity of predictive LV reverse remodeling for the runover-QRS group were 83% and 86%, respectively, and were 100% and 78%, respectively, in those with QRS >150 ms.

Two studies have examined the role of echocardiography in predicting a favorable response after CRT by comparing multiple echocardiographic indices of systolic asynchrony at the same time. Bordacher et al[23] compared septal-to-posterior wall motion delay using M-mode, interventricular delay using Doppler echocardiography, percentage segment with delayed longitudinal contraction using TDI, asynchrony index, and pulse TDI measures of intraventricular delay using the maximum difference in the time to onset or peak systolic velocity of 12 LV segments in 41 patients. The endpoint measures were gain in cardiac output and reduction of mitral regurgitation after CRT for 3 months. It was concluded that the asynchrony index of 12 LV segments correlated mostly strongly with changes in cardiac output ($r=-0.67$, all $p<0.001$) and mitral regurgitation ($r=0.68$, all $p<0.001$). The correlation was much weaker for delayed longitudinal contraction, and not significant for interventricular dyssynchrony.

Another study examined 18 echocardiographic parameters derived from TDI or strain rate imaging, and compared the predictive value for LV reverse remodeling after CRT for 3 months.[8] The parameters consisted of interventricular delay, septal-to-lateral wall delay, septal-to-posterior wall delay, medial-to-free-wall delay, 6 LV basal segments and 12 LV segments. Of these, the asynchrony index has the greatest predictive value (correlation coefficient -0.74, $p<0.001$; receiver operating characteristics (ROC) curve area 0.94, $p<0.001$).[8] A cut-off value of the asynchrony index of 31.4 ms was derived, which gives a sensitivity of 96% and a specificity of 78%. The predictive value dropped when a smaller number of LV segments were measured, while interventricular dyssynchrony failed to predict LV reverse remodeling.

Tissue synchronization imaging

Tissue synchronization imaging (TSI) works in principle highly similar to tissue Doppler velocity measurement, and is derived from TDI itself. The measured positive values of time to peak systolic velocity are transformed into color maps. Therefore, in addition to quantitative analysis by TDI, it allows rapid qualitative estimation of regional delay. As the user needs to define the beginning and end of time measurement by TSI, a thorough understanding of myocardial velocity curves is important for interpretation of TSI data. In the study by Gorcsan et al,[9] the TSI detection window was set to begin with the pre-ejection period and end with early diastole, which included post-systolic shortening, if present. This acute study defined a positive response as an increase in stroke volume of ≥15% within 48 hours after CRT. In 29 patients receiving CRT, a delay between anterior septum and posterior wall of >65 ms predicted the gain in stroke volume with a sensitivity of 87% and a specificity of 100%.[9] However, a late response was observed in 5 of the 7 acute non-responders with decrease in LV end-systolic volume ≥15%, which suggests that acute response underestimates long-term response.

Another larger study by Yu et al[24] compared the predictive value of TSI when set to ejection phase only (between aortic valve opening and closure) and to include both ejection phase and

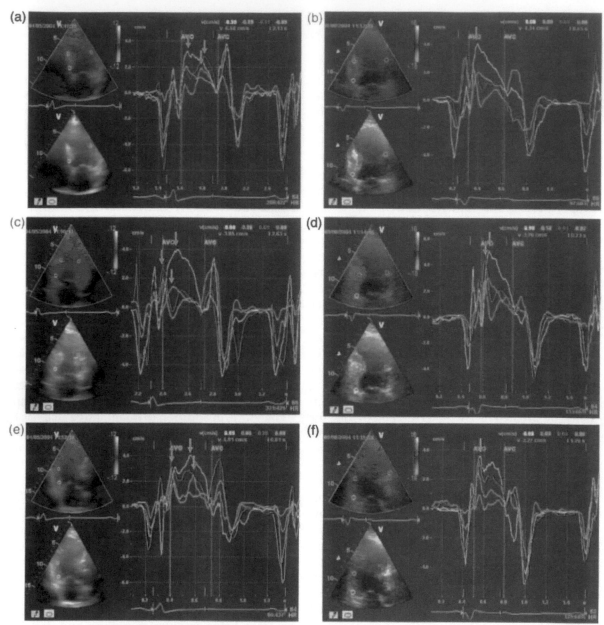

Figure 17.1 Color tissue Doppler imaging with myocardial velocity curves reconstructed in the apical four-chamber (a, b) apical two-chamber (c, d), and long-axis (e, f) views before (a, c, e) and after (b, d, f) CRT. The use of three apical views can establish the six-basal, six-midsegmental model to examine for systolic dyssynchrony. Aortic valve opening (AVO) and closure (AVC) markers are tagged relative to the electrocardiogram signal to provide a temporal guidance on 'ejection' period. Before CRT, delay in the time to peak systolic velocity is evident in the lateral wall in the four-chamber view, the anterior wall in the two-chamber view, and the mid-anterior septum in the long-axis view (arrows). After CRT, there is realignment of the contractile profile and the peak systolic velocities occur at about the same time.

post-systolic shortening in 56 patients treated for 3 months. This study also included multiple parameters of systolic dyssynchrony, ranging from 2 to 12 LV segments. Among the various methods, calculation of the asynchrony index from 12 LV segments yielded a sensitivity and specificity of 87% and 81%, respectively (Figure 17.2). However, the predictive value decreased precipitously when post-systolic shortening was included in the measurement. Qualitative analysis illustrated that the most severe delay region occurring at the lateral wall is a specific predictor of a LV reverse remodeling response, although the sensitivity is low.[25] Therefore, TSI appears to be a useful screening tool for systolic dyssynchrony, before contemplating quantitative assessment.

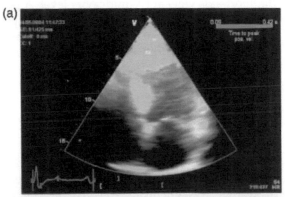

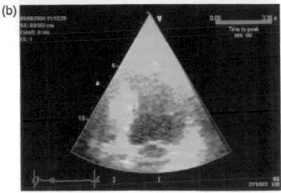

Figure 17.2 Tissue synchronization imaging (TSI) of the same patient as in Figure 17.1. The apical four-chamber view at baseline (a) shows evidence of systolic dyssynchrony with moderate delay in the lateral wall (yellow color coding) when compared with the septal wall (green color coding). The lateral wall delay was abolished after CRT (b).

Strain rate imaging

Strain rate imaging is a post-processing imaging procedure derived from fundamental tissue velocity data. It is a deformation mapping that examines the rate of deformation between two points a predefined distance apart. Although thought to have the theoretical advantage of avoiding translational motion being measured as active contraction, parameters derived from strain rate have not been shown to predict a CRT response in a study that examined a large number of parameters derived from 2–12 LV segments.[8] Currently, no further study has ascertained the role of strain rate in predicting CRT response. Technical improvements in strain rate imaging will be necessary before it can be used in clinical practice, including a high signal-to-noise ratio and good reproducibility.

Strain imaging

Strain imaging is another post-processing imaging procedure derived from fundamental tissue velocity data. It is another deformation mapping that examines the cumulative amount of linear deformation between two points a predefined distance apart. In a normal heart, systolic strain reaches its maximum value during end-systole. In patients with LV dyssynchrony, variations of the timing to peak negative strain may occur. An acute study by Dohi et al[25] examined radial strain in the short-axis view in 38 patients receiving CRT. Responders were defined as those with an acute increase in stroke volume ≥15%, which was present in 55% of patients. It was observed that a septal-to-posterior delay of ≥130 ms predicted responders with a sensitivity of 95% and a specificity of 88%.

Another study examined 37 patients for CRT response.[26] Responders were defined as those with an increase in LVEF by ≥20% and/or a decrease in LVESV ≥15% at 6 months. Criteria for systolic dyssynchrony included septal-to-posterior motion delay by M-mode (SPWMD), septal-to-posterior thickening delay by M-mode plus strain imaging (SPWTD), and the standard deviation of the time to peak strain of 12 LV segments in apical views (TPS-SD). The study observed that SPWMD was unable to predict echocardiographic response. On the other hand, the two parameters from strain imaging predicted a favorable response, although TPS-SD gave a tighter correlation coefficient than SPWTD for both change in LVEF ($r=0.86$, $p<0.001$) and LVESV ($r=-0.73$, $p<0.001$). A median cut-off value of TPS-SD ≥ 60 ms has been suggested, although its sensitivity and specificity have yet to be determined.

Another recent study by Yu et al[27] compared tissue velocity, tissue strain, and displacement mapping in predicting LV reverse remodeling (reduction of LVESV) and gain in LVEF in 55 patients. Both the correlation coefficient and ROC curve area were compared for different models of systolic dyssynchrony, including the standard deviation and maximum time-difference methods for 12 and 6 basal LV segments, and septal-to-lateral as well as septal-to-posterior wall delay. Ts-SD from 12 segments (i.e., the asynchrony index) had the best performance in predicting LV reverse remodeling ($r=-0.76$, $p<0.001$) and gain in LVEF ($r=0.65$, $p<0.001$) than all the other parameters derived from tissue velocity. Interestingly, a similar parameter derived from displacement mapping has a much weaker predictive power for both LV reverse remodeling ($r=-0.36$, $p<0.05$) and LVEF ($r=0.28$, $p<0.05$). On the other hand, none of the strain-imaging-derived parameters predicts such improvement (Figure 17.3).[28] Therefore, further studies are needed to ascertain the role of strain imaging in identifying dyssynchrony and predicting a favorable response to CRT.

Post-systolic shortening (delayed longitudinal contraction)

Post-systolic shortening (PSS) denotes a state of delayed contraction that occurs after aortic valve closure. It is also called delayed longitudinal contraction. Counting the number of LV segments with PSS has been suggested as a marker of dyssynchrony. A study by Sogaard et al[28] observed that delayed longitudinal contraction was present in the basal LV segments in heart failure patients, and was reduced after CRT. A cut-off value to predict a favorable response has not been identified. Furthermore, in two other studies, TDI assessment of time to peak systolic contraction has been shown to be superior to

PSS in predicting favorable LV reverse remodeling or improvement in cardiac function/mitral regurgitation.[8,24] A negative role in ischemic patients has also been suggested, as PSS could be a marker of myocardial ischemia and hibernation rather than dyssynchrony in this group.[8]

Speckle tracing

Another new technology of detecting regional function is speckle tracking. From high-resolution 2D imaging, software detects frame-to-frame migration of 2D speckle signals from the myocardium. This tool has the advantage of being angle-independent. Integration of the data obtained allows calculation of regional strain.[30] A recent study by Suffoletto et al[29] examined 48 patients using 2D speckle tracking and measured the time to peak radial strain in the short-axis view at LV midcavity level. A peak septal-to-posterior wall strain ≥ 130 ms predicted $\geq 15\%$ increase in stroke volume with 91% sensitivity and 75% specificity. In 50 patients, at a mean follow-up of 8 ± 5 months after CRT, the same cut-off value predicted $\geq 15\%$ increase in LVEF with 89% sensitivity and 83% specificity.[29]

SUMMARY

There have been a large number of parameters of systolic dyssynchrony derived by TDI and related post-processing techniques (Table 17.1). The main application of these parameters relies on their capacity to predict a favorable response, in particular an echocardiographic response. As early LV reverse remodeling is also a powerful predictor of favorable long-term outcome measures, any parameter that predicts early LV reverse remodeling is potentially useful in clinical practice. In TDI, for example, the presence of septal-to-lateral wall delay ≥ 65 ms has been shown to predict a favorable 1-year clinical outcome.[20] Currently, the PROSPECT study is the largest of those examining the role of echocardiographic parameters of systolic dyssynchrony in predicting LV reverse remodeling and clinical outcome assessed by a composite clinical score. The study has enrolled about 450 patients.

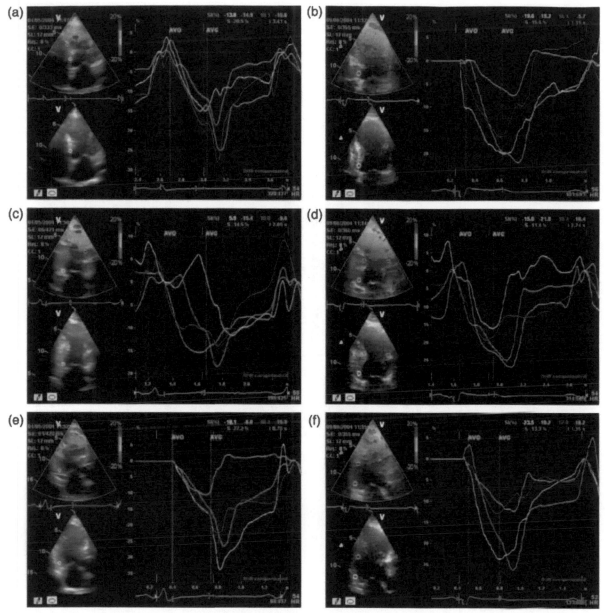

Figure 17.3 Strain imaging derived by tissue Doppler imaging of the same patient as in Figure 17.1, showing apical four-chamber (a, b), two-chamber (c, d), and long-axis (e, f) views before (a, c, e) and after (b, d, f) CRT. The normal systolic strain in apical views is negative, with the largest cumulative values occurring during end-systole, i.e., at the time of aortic valve closure (AVC). In the apical four-chamber view (a), this patient exhibited post-systolic shortening in most of the segments at baseline, and therefore peak negative strain in most segments occurred after AVC. After CRT (b), although peak systolic velocities are aligned at the same time, peak negative strain in the midseptal and midlateral segments remains delayed. In the apical two-chamber view, delay of peak strain also occurs in most of the segments, except the midanterior segment (c), although it remains delayed in the midanterior and inferior segments after CRT (d). In the apical long-axis view, the delay in strain occurs mainly in the midanteroseptal segment (e). However, it becomes delayed in the midanteroseptal and midposterior segments after CRT (f). Therefore, this case illustrates that tissue velocity demonstrates an obvious improvement in systolic dyssynchrony after CRT – but not tissue strain. However, this patient is a responder with LV reverse remodeling and shows an improvement in systolic function.

Table 17.1 Echocardiographic parameters for assessing systolic dyssynchrony with cut-off values predicting a favorable response to cardiac resynchronization therapy

Ref.	N	Follow-up period (months)	Echocardiographic technique	Methodology for dyssynchrony	Main findings	Sensitivity (%)	Specificity (%)
19	25	Acute	Tissue Doppler velocity	Septal-to-lateral delay of Ts in ejection phase	Septal-to-lateral delay of Ts ≥60 ms predicts ↑LVEF ≥5%	76	87.5
8	54	3	Tissue Doppler velocity, strain rate	Ts-SD of 12 LV segments in ejection phase (and 17 other parameters)	Ts-SD of 12 LV segments >31.4 ms predicts ↓LVESV >15%	96	78
21	49	6	Tissue Doppler velocity	Ts (onset) of 3 basal LV and 1 basal RV segments	Summation of inter- and intraventricular delay >102 ms predicts relative ↑LVEF ≥25%	96	71
20	85	12	Tissue Doppler velocity	Septal-to-lateral delay of Ts in ejection phase	Septal-to-lateral delay >65 ms predicts improvement of ≥1 NYHA class, >25% ↑6-min hall walk distance; and is associated with lower event rate	80	80
11	49	3	Tissue Doppler velocity	Maximum difference in Ts in 6 basal segments (both ejection phase and post-systolic shortening)	Maximum difference in Ts in 6 basal segments >110 ms predicts ↓LVESV >15%	97	55
9	29	Acute	Tissue Doppler velocity	Septal-to-posterior delay (both ejection phase and post-systolic shortening)	Septal-to-posterior delay ≥65 ms predicts ↑stroke volume ≥15%	87	100
30	56	3	TSI	Ts-SD of 12 LV segments in ejection phase	Ts-SD of 12 LV segment in ejection phase >34.4 ms predicts ↓LVESV >15%	87	81
25	38	Acute	Tissue strain	Septal-to-posterior radial strain	Septal-to-posterior delay ≥130 ms predicts ↑stroke volume ≥15%	95	88
29	50	8±5	2D speckle tracking	Septal-to-posterior radial strain	Septal-to-posterior delay ≥130 ms predicts ≥15% ↑LVEF with 89% sensitivity and 83% specificity	89	83

LV, left ventricular; LVEF, LV ejection fraction; LVESV, LV end-systolic volume; NYHA, New York Heart Association; RV, right ventricular; Ts, time to peak myocardial systolic velocity; Ts(onset), time to onset of myocardial systolic velocity; Ts-SD, standard deviation of time to peak myocardial systolic velocity (asynchrony index).

REFERENCES

1. Nelson GS, Curry CW, Wyman BT, et al. Predictors of systolic augmentation from left ventricular preexcitation in patients with dilated cardiomyopathy and intraventricular conduction delay. Circulation 2000; 101:2703–9.

2. Alonso C, Leclercq C, Victor F, et al. Electrocardiographic predictive factors of long-term clinical improvement with multisite biventricular pacing in advanced heart failure. Am J Cardiol 1999;84:1417–21.

3. Reuter S, Garrigue S, Barold SS, et al. Comparison of characteristics in responders versus nonresponders with biventricular pacing for drug-resistant congestive heart failure. Am J Cardiol 2002;89:346–50.

4. Abraham WT, Fisher WG, Smith AL, et al. Cardiac resynchronization in chronic heart failure. N Engl J Med 2002;346:1845–53.

5. Young JB, Abraham WT, Smith AL, et al. Combined cardiac resynchronization and implantable cardioversion defibrillation in advanced chronic heart failure: the MIRACLE ICD Trial. JAMA 2003;289:2685–94.

6. Stellbrink C, Breithardt OA, Franke A, et al. Impact of cardiac resynchronization therapy using hemodynamically optimized pacing on left ventricular remodeling in patients with congestive heart failure and ventricular conduction disturbances. J Am Coll Cardiol 2001;38: 1957–65.

7. Yu CM, Fung JWH, Zhang Q, Sanderson JE. Understanding nonresponders of cardiac resynchronization therapy – current and future perspectives. J Cardiovasc Electrophysiol 2005;16:1117–24.

8. Yu CM, Fung JW, Zhang Q, et al. Tissue Doppler imaging is superior to strain rate imaging and postsystolic shortening on the prediction of reverse remodeling in both ischemic and nonischemic heart failure after cardiac resynchronization therapy. Circulation 2004; 110:66–73.

9. Auricchio A, Stellbank C, Block M, Sach S, Vogt J, Bakker P, Klein H, Kramer A, Ding J, Salo R, Tockman B, Pocnet T, Spinelli J. Effect of pacing chamber and atrioventricular delay on acute systolic function of paced patients with congestive heart failure. The Pacing Therapies for Congestive Heart Failure Study Group. The Guidant Congestive Heart Failure Research Group. Circulation 1999;99: 2993–3001.

10. Gorcsan J, III, Kanzaki H, Bazaz R, Dohi K, Schwartzman D. Usefulness of echocardiographic tissue synchronization imaging to predict acute response to cardiac resynchronization therapy. Am J Cardiol 2004;93:1178–81.

11. Yu CM, Fung JWH, Lin H, et al. Predictors of left ventricular reverse remodeling after cardiac resynchronization therapy for heart failure secondary to idiopathic dilated or ischemic cardiomyopathy. Am J Cardiol 2003;91:684–8.

12. Notabartolo D, Merlino JD, Smith AL, et al. Usefulness of the peak velocity difference by tissue Doppler imaging technique as an effective predictor of response to cardiac resynchronization therapy. Am J Cardiol 2004;94:817–20.

13. Bleeker GB, Bax JJ, Fung JW, et al. Clinical versus echocardiographic parameters to assess response to cardiac resynchronization therapy. Am J Cardiol 2006;97:260–3.

14. Yu CM, Chau E, Sanderson JE, et al. Tissue Doppler echocardiographic evidence of reverse remodeling and improved synchronicity by simultaneously delaying regional contraction after biventricular pacing therapy in heart failure. Circulation 2002;105:438–45.

15. Breithardt OA, Sinha AM, Schwammenthal E, et al. Acute effects of cardiac resynchronization therapy on functional mitral regurgitation in advanced systolic heart failure. J Am Coll Cardiol 2003;41:765–70.

16. Kanzaki H, Bazaz R, Schwartzman D, et al. A mechanism for immediate reduction in mitral regurgitation after cardiac resynchronization therapy: insights from mechanical activation strain mapping. J Am Coll Cardiol 2004;44:1619–25.

17. Zhang Q, Fung JW, Auricchio A, et al. Differential change in left ventricular mass and regional wall thickness after cardiac resynchronization therapy for heart failure. Eur Heart J 2006;27:1423–30.

18. Yu CM, Bleeker GB, Fung JW, et al. Left ventricular reverse remodeling but not clinical improvement predicts long-term survival after cardiac resynchronization therapy. Circulation 2005;112:1580–6.

19. Yu CM, Lin H, Fung WH, et al. Comparison of acute changes in left ventricular volume, systolic and diastolic functions, and intraventricular synchronicity after biventricular and right ventricular pacing for heart failure. Am Heart J 2003;145:E18.

20. Bax JJ, Marwick TH, Molhoek SG, et al. Left ventricular dyssynchrony predicts benefit of cardiac resynchronization therapy in patients with end-stage heart failure before pacemaker implantation. Am J Cardiol 2003;92: 1238–40.

21. Bax JJ, Bleeker GB, Marwick TH, et al. Left ventricular dyssynchrony predicts response and prognosis after cardiac resynchronization therapy. J Am Coll Cardiol 2004;44:1834–40.

22. Penicka M, Bartunek J, de Bruyne B, et al. Improvement of left ventricular function after cardiac resynchronization therapy is predicted by tissue Doppler imaging echocardiography. Circulation 2004;109:978–83.

23. Yu CM, Fung JW, Chan CK, et al. Comparison of efficacy of reverse remodeling and clinical improvement

for relatively narrow and wide QRS complexes after cardiac resynchronization therapy for heart failure. J Cardiovasc Electrophysiol 2004;15:1058–65.

24. Bordachar P, Lafitte S, Reuter S, et al. Echocardiographic parameters of ventricular dyssynchrony validation in patients with heart failure using sequential biventricular pacing. J Am Coll Cardiol 2004;44:2157–65.

25. Yu CM, Zhang Q, Fung JW, et al. A novel tool to assess systolic asynchrony and identify responders of cardiac resynchronization therapy by tissue synchronization imaging. J Am Coll Cardiol 2005;45:677–84.

26. Dohi K, Suffoletto MS, Schwartzman D, et al. Utility of echocardiographic radial strain imaging to quantify left ventricular dyssynchrony and predict acute response to cardiac resynchronization therapy. Am J Cardiol 2005; 96:112–16.

27. Mele D, Pasanisi G, Capasso F, et al. Left intraventricular myocardial deformation dyssynchrony identifies responders to cardiac resynchronization therapy in patients with heart failure. Eur Heart J 2006;27:1070–8.

28. Yu C-M, Zhang Q, Chan Y-S, et al. Tissue Doppler velocity is superior to displacement and strain mapping in predicting left ventricular reverse remodelling response after cardiac resynchronisation therapy. Heart 2006;92:1452–6.

29. Sogaard P, Egeblad H, Kim WY, et al. Tissue Doppler imaging predicts improved systolic performance and reversed left ventricular remodeling during long-term cardiac resynchronization therapy. J Am Coll Cardiol 2002;40:723–30.

30. Suffoletto MS, Dohi K, Cannesson M, Saba S, Goresan J, III. Novel speckle-tracking radial strain from routine black-and-white echocardiographic images to quantify dyssynchrony and predict response to cardiac resynchronization therapy. Circulation 2006;113: 960–8.

31. Yu C-M, Abraham WT, Bax J, et al. Predictors of response to cardiac resynchronization therapy (PROSPECT) – Study design. Am Heart J 2005; 149:600–609.

18

Echocardiographic determination of response to cardiac resynchronization therapy

John Gorcsan

Introduction • Acute response to CRT • Chronic response to CRT

INTRODUCTION

Echocardiography not only plays a major role in quantifying cardiac mechanical dyssynchrony before cardiac resynchronization therapy (CRT), but also contributes to determining response to this important therapy. There has been increasing interest in refining patient selection for CRT, because the rate of non-responders may be 25–35%.[1,2] The definition of response to CRT has varied from study to study, including clinical response measures, such as New York Heart Association (NYHA) functional class, 6-minute walk distance, or a quality-of-life score questionnaire. These indices have been useful in several previous heart failure clinical trials. More objective measures of left ventricular (LV) structure and function have been promising following CRT in several investigations. Accordingly, this chapter will focus on the use of echocardiographic measures to quantify response to CRT.

ACUTE RESPONSE TO CRT

Determining response to CRT may be considered in two broad areas: acute and chronic. An acute hemodynamic response may result immediately from coordination of septal free-wall dyssynchrony with multisite pacing, which improves ejection efficiency.[3] These results have been observed in acute hemodynamic studies in the cardiac catheterization laboratory with recordings of LV pressure, dP/dt, pressure–volume loops, and aortic pulse pressure. Since acute responders appear to manifest an increase in LV stroke volume, Doppler echocardiographic measures of ejection velocity have been useful as a surrogate of stroke volume.[4] This is done by measuring the diameter of the aortic annulus, usually from the parasternal long-axis view, and converting this to a circular cross-sectional area: area = $P \times d^2$. Either pulsed or continuous-wave Doppler can be used to measure LV ejection velocity. The integral of the spectral Doppler velocity over time, known as the flow velocity integral, is multiplied by the cross-sectional area to determine the stroke volume (Figure 18.1). Stroke volume can also then be multiplied by the heart rate to determine the cardiac output.

The sample volume of pulsed Doppler must be carefully placed in the LV outflow close to the aortic valve, but before flow acceleration occurs. The disadvantage of this measure is that the velocity may vary if placement is not carefully attended to. This measurement is reproducible in most laboratories, but others prefer the use of continuous-wave Doppler to assess stroke volume. A disadvantage of continuous wave Doppler is that the maximum velocity along the entire beam is represented. Continuous-wave Doppler may not accurately represent volumetric

(a)

(b)

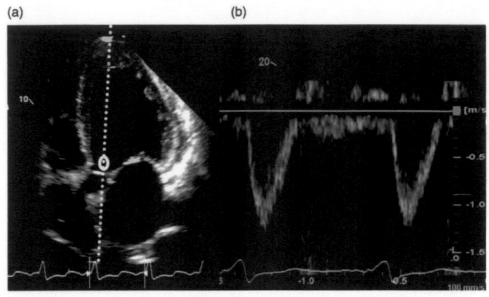

Figure 18.1 Apical view with imaging of left ventricular outflow tract and placement of pulsed Doppler sample volume (a) and the corresponding spectral Doppler velocity tracing over time (b) for estimation of stroke volume.

stroke volume in situations where the cross-sectional area through the aortic valve is not represented by the cross-sectional area of the measured aortic annulus in low-flow states where the valve leaflets do not separate fully. Accordingly, the pulsed Doppler method may be advantageous in the assessment of heart failure patients with diminished stroke volume. The relative advantages and disadvantages of pulsed versus continuous-wave Doppler become less important when patients are assessed before and acutely after CRT, where one assesses changes from baseline and individual patients serve as their own controls. Another important factor is the presence of heart rate changes that may affect results. Acute increases in Doppler measures of stroke volume following CRT have been predicted by the presence of longitudinal dyssynchrony by tissue Doppler velocities and also radial dyssynchrony by either tissue Doppler or speckle tracking measures of radial strain.[5-7] In a group of 29 patients studied by longitudinal color-coded tissue Doppler – known as tissue synchronization imaging – CRT was associated with acute favorable effects on LV function for the entire study group: stroke volume by pulsed Doppler increased from 56 ± 12 ml to 63 ± 12 ml ($p < 0.001$).[5]

The presence of an opposing wall delay in the time to peak velocity ≥ 65 ms was predictive of favorable response. In a separate study, small but significant increases in stroke volume from 31 ± 16 ml to 35 ± 16 ml ($p < 0.001$) occurred following CRT, and radial dyssynchrony ≥ 130 ms by speckle tracking of radial strain predicted an acute response with 91% sensitivity (95% confidence interval (CI) 76–97%) and 75% specificity (95% CI 51–90%).[7] Increases in LV ejection fraction (LVEF) can be detected in these same patients with an acute response to CRT. However, these changes are usually subtle in individual patients – perhaps due to variability in tracing LV volumes by the biplane Simpson's rule. For example, small but significant acute increases in LVEF were observed from 24% ± 6% to 26% ± 6% ($p < 0.005$) in the tissue Doppler study mentioned above[5] and from 26% ± 7% to 29% ± 7% ($p < 0.0005$) in the speckle tracking radial strain study in patients studied the day after CRT.[7]

Acute improvements in stroke volume, as assessed by Doppler echocardiography, have been correlated with acute improvements in dyssynchrony following CRT. In a study of 33 patients with measures of stroke volume and radial dyssynchrony by tissue Doppler strain before and the day after CRT, changes in radial dyssynchrony correlated with acute changes in stroke volume ($r = 0.83$, $p < 0.0001$).[6] Changes in stroke volume correlated with the degree of baseline dyssynchrony until 200 ms ($r = 0.93$, $p < 0.0001$); thereafter, a plateau was observed, similar to the pattern observed by Bax et al[8] with longitudinal velocities. It appears that reductions in LV end-systolic volume (LVESV) and improvements in LVEF associated with reverse remodeling are preferred for determining long-term or chronic response to CRT. Although Doppler estimates of stroke volume are very useful in determining acute responses, they are difficult to obtain in the electrophysiology laboratory at the time of implantation because of logistical difficulties with the sterile field and fluoroscopy equipment, which may limit access to the patient's echocardiographic windows. Accordingly, these acute non-invasive hemodynamic studies can be done more easily in the echocardiography laboratory or at the patient's bedside following CRT implantation. An alternative method to assess acute changes in LV function following CRT is to estimate dP/dt using continuous-wave Doppler assessment of the mitral regurgitant jet.[9]

CHRONIC RESPONSE TO CRT

Echocardiography is an important means to follow the clinical progress of patients with heart failure. Accordingly, it is an important means to quantify response to CRT. Clinical trials have used clinical endpoints to determine clinical response, but several trials have included measures of LV volumes and LVEF as part of their protocol. CRT appears to exert favorable effects on LV structure and function that are known as reverse remodeling. This was demonstrated in the MIRACLE trial, where 453 patients who had a device successfully implanted were randomized either to the control group of 225 with biventricular pacing turned off or to the CRT group of 228 with biventricular pacing turned on.[10] Quantitative echocardiography preformed by an expert core laboratory revealed a significant decrease in LV end-diastolic volume (LVEDV) and LVESV ($p < 0.001$) and an increase in group

mean LVEF by 3.6% in the CRT group versus 0.4% in the control group 6 months after CRT ($p < 0.001$). These results have been a consistent finding in several randomized trials of CRT where improvements in LVESV and LVEF were observed in the CRT treatment groups.[1,2] The echocardiographic quantitative standard for determining these chronic changes is application of the biplane Simpson's rule, or method of disks, to the apical four- and two-chamber views[11] (Figure 18.2). Yu et al[12] demonstrated a dramatic dynamic relationship between CRT and reverse remodeling in a series of 25 patients in whom CRT was instituted, resulting in decreases in LVESV and increases in LVEF followed by a period of time where CRT was turned off. These beneficial changes in LVESV and LVEF were lost with cessation of CRT after 4 weeks, followed by return of the favorable effects on LV function following reinstitution of CRT. Bleeker et al[13] examined the agreement between clinical and echocardiographic parameters of reverse remodeling following CRT. In 144 patients following CRT, they observed an agreement between clinical response (a reduction in $\geqslant 1$ NYHA class) after 3–6 months of CRT and echocardiographic response (defined as a decrease of >15% in LVESV in 76%: 74 patients (51%) had reductions in NYHA class and LVESV and 36 patients (25%) had no reductions in either NYHA class or LVESV. However, clinical improvement without a >15% reduction in LVESV was observed in 27 patients (19%), and 7 patients (5%) with no clinical response had reductions in LVESV. Thus, in 34 patients (24%), a disagreement between clinical and echocardiographic responses was noted; this disagreement was mainly due to patients with clinical responses without echocardiographic responses. This was hypothesized to be related to factors other than LV function or to a placebo effect, which is a common feature of clinical therapeutic trials. Yu et al[14] also reported results in 141 patients with advanced heart failure who had echocardiographic measures of reverse remodeling, as defined by a decreases in LVESV. Specifically, they observed a decrease in LVESV of $\geqslant 9.5\%$ to have a sensitivity of 70% and a specificity of 70% in predicting all-cause mortality, and of 87% and 69%, respectively, in predicting

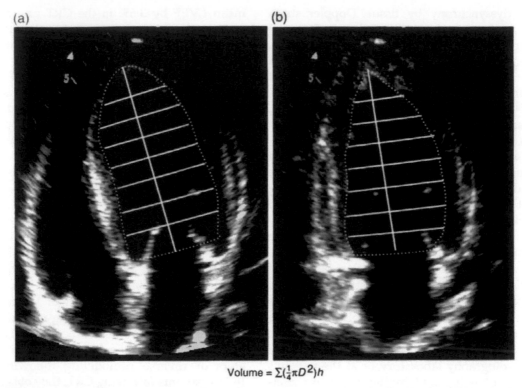

$$\text{Volume} = \Sigma(\tfrac{1}{4}\pi D^2)h$$

Figure 18.2 Apical four-chamber (a) and two-chamber (b) views with computer-assisted tracing of endocardial borders from digital images for calculation of volumes and ejection fraction using the biplane Simpson's rule (method of disks). *D*, diameter of disk; *h*, height of disk.

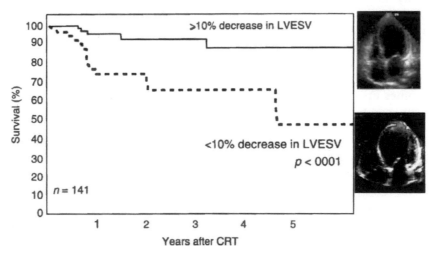

Figure 18.3 Kaplan–Meier survival curve of patients with reductions in left ventricular end-systolic volume (LVESV) of ⩾10% following cardiac resynchronization therapy (CRT), compared with the curve for those who did not demonstrate evidence of reverse remodeling.

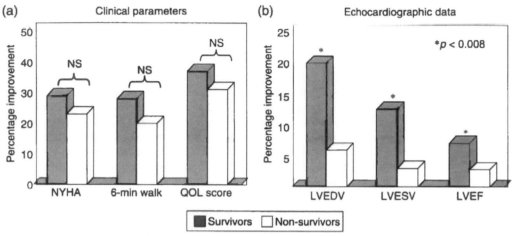

Figure 18.4 Comparison of clinical predictors of response to cardiac resynchronization therapy with echocardiographic measures of left ventricular end-diastolic and end-systolic volumes (LVEDF and LVESV) and ejection fraction (LVEF), demonstrating greater predictive valve of echocardiographic data (b) versus clinical markers of response (a). NYHA, New York Heart Association functional class; QOL, quality-of-life questionnaire; NS, not significant.

cardiovascular mortality. Accordingly, a decrease in LVESV of at least 10% was found to be a clinically relevant marker of reverse remodeling, and to actually predict survival better than routine clinical markers (Figure 18.3). They found LVESV to be a better predictor of survival and heart failure events after CRT than NYHA functional class, 6-minute walk distance or quality-of-life score by questionnaire (Figure 18.4). This supports the important and objective nature of echocardiographic determination of LVEDV, LVESV, and LVEF in predicting outcome in heart failure patients following CRT.

Suffoletto et al[15] reported a preliminary experience with examining the relationship of acute hemodynamic response to chronic reverse remodeling in 33 patients who were studied the day after CRT and 7 ± 5 months (all > 3 months) following CRT. An acute hemodynamic response, defined as ≥15% increase in stroke volume by Doppler echocardiography, occurred in 22 of 33 patients (67%), 19 of whom (86%) went on to reverse remodeling 7±5 months after CRT and whose LVEF increased from 25%±7% to 34%±11% ($p<0.001$). A subset of patients who did not have an acute hemodynamic response still went on to demonstrate decreases in LVESV and increases in LVEF. Baseline dyssynchony by tissue Doppler was found to be statistically

predictive of both acute hemodynamic response and later reverse remodeling. A relationship of acute to chronic response was observed, but there were patients in whom chronic reverse remodeling could occur, despite the lack of an acute response.

REFERENCES

1. Abraham WT, Fisher WG, Smith AL, et al. MIRACLE Study Group. Cardiac resynchronization in chronic heart failure. N Engl J Med 2002;346:1845–53.
2. Cleland JG, Daubert JC, Erdmann E, et al. Cardiac Resynchronization–Heart Failure (CARE-HF) Study Investigators. The effect of cardiac resynchronization on morbidity and mortality in heart failure. N Engl J Med 2005; 352:1539–49.
3. Kass DA, Chen CH, Curry C, et al. Improved left ventricular mechanics from acute VDD pacing in patients with dilated cardiomyopathy and ventricular conduction delay. Circulation 1999;99:1567–73.
4. Lewis JF, Kuo LC, Nelson JG, Limacher MC, Quinones MA. Pulsed Doppler echocardiographic determination of stroke volume and cardiac output: clinical validation of two new methods using the apical window. Circulation 1984;70:425–31.
5. Gorcsan J III, Kanzaki H, Bazaz R, Dohi K, Schwartzman D. Usefulness of echocardiographic tissue synchronization imaging to predict acute response to cardiac resynchronization therapy. Am J Cardiol 2004;93:1178–81.

6. Dohi K, Suffoletto MS, Schwartzman D, et al. Utility of echocardiographic radial strain imaging to quantify left ventricular dyssynchrony and predict acute response to cardiac resynchronization therapy. Am J Cardiol 2005;96:112–16.

7. Suffoletto M, Dohi K, Cannesson M, Saba S, Gorcsan J. Novel speckle-tracking radial strain from routine black and white echocardiographic images to quantify dyssynchrony and predict response to cardiac resynchronization therapy. Circulation 2006;113:960–8.

8. Bax JJ, Bleeker GB, Marwick TH, et al. Left ventricular dyssynchrony predicts response and prognosis after cardiac resynchronization therapy. J Am Coll Cardiol 2004;44:1834–40.

9. Heist E, Taub C, Fan D, et al. Usefulness of a novel 'response score' to predict hemodynamic and clinical outcome from cardiac resynchronization therapy. Am J Cardiol 2006;97:1732–6.

10. St John Sutton MG, Plappert T, Abraham WT, et al. Multicenter InSync Randomized Clinical Evaluation (MIRACLE) Study Group. Effect of cardiac resynchronization therapy on left ventricular size and function in chronic heart failure. Circulation 2003;107:1985–90.

11. Lang RM, Bierig M, Devereux RB, et al. Recommendations for chamber quantification: a report from the American Society of Echocardiography's Guidelines and Standards Committee and the Chamber Quantification Writing Group. J Am Soc Echocardiogr 2005;18:1440–63.

12. Yu CM, Chau E, Sanderson JE, et al. Tissue Doppler cardiographic evidence of reverse remodeling and improved synchronicity by simultaneously delaying regional contraction after biventricular pacing therapy in heart failure. Circulation 2002;105:438–45.

13. Bleeker GB, Bax JJ, Fung JW, et al. Clinical versus echocardiographic parameters to assess response to cardiac resynchronization therapy. Am J Cardiol 2006;97:260–3.

14. Yu CM, Bleeker GB, Fung JW, et al. Left ventricular reverse remodeling but not clinical improvement predicts long-term survival after cardiac resynchronization therapy. Circulation 2005;112:1580–6.

15. Suffoletto MS, Cannesson M, Tanabe M, Saba S, Gorcsan J. Relationship of tissue doppler dyssynchrony and acute hemodynamic response to later reverse remodeling after resynchronization therapy. J Am Coll Cardiol 2006;47:11A (abst).

19

Impact of cardiac resynchronization therapy on mitral regurgitation

Ole-A Breithardt

Introduction • **Pathophysiology of functional mitral regurgitation in heart failure** • **Effects of CRT on functional mitral regurgitation** • **Summary**

INTRODUCTION

Functional mitral regurgitation (MR) contributes significantly to the poor hemodynamic status of patients with advanced systolic heart failure. Its presence is an unfavorable prognostic marker in patients with systolic heart failure and is associated with worsening clinical symptoms, a decrease in exercise capacity, and decreased survival. In a prospective trial including 128 consecutive patients with left ventricular (LV) dysfunction (LV ejection fraction (LVEF) <50%, average 31% ± 9%), more than 80% of all patients presented with more than trace functional MR.[1] Another study reported a 30% incidence of severe MR in patients with severely depressed LV function.[2] The severity of functional MR has been associated with an adverse outcome in terms of mortality and hospitalization,[2-5] particularly in patients after myocardial infarction.[6] This motivated the development of numerous different therapeutic strategies to reduce the severity of functional MR, ranging from pharmacologic treatment[7] to corrective surgical measures[8] and more recently percutaneous approaches for mitral annuloplasty.[9] Conservative medical treatment with vasodilator agents such as angiotensin-converting enzyme (ACE) inhibitors is of limited success, with a 2-year survival rate of less than 60% in patients with

severe MR,[4] and mainly effective in patients with arterial hypertension.[10] Surgical approaches to reduce severe functional MR in dilated cardiomyopathies have focused on downsizing the mitral annulus, and have been comparatively successful, with 2-year survival rates ranging between 71% and 85%.[11,12] Despite these promising results, many physicians and patients refrain from open-heart surgery because of the significant perioperative morbidity and the early mortality rate of 5–9%.[13] Less-invasive percutaneous approaches are currently under investigation, but long-term results are still missing.

LV-based pacing might be an alternative strategy to reduce the severity of functional MR in selected patients with advanced systolic heart failure and mechanical LV dyssynchrony. Already in the very first patients who underwent 'multisite pacing for end-stage heart failure' – nowadays referred to as cardiac resynchronization therapy (CRT) – it was noted that CRT not only improved the systolic function of the LV, but, almost as a side-effect, also reduced the severity of functional MR, as measured by the mean pulmonary capillary v-wave.[14,15] These early observations obtained by right-heart catheterization were confirmed in many subsequent studies using more direct measures for quantification of MR severity. All investigators consistently reported that CRT is associated with a significant decrease in functional MR, both acutely[16–18] and in long-term follow-up.[19–28] To understand the mechanisms responsible for this CRT-related improvement in the severity of functional MR, it is necessary to take a closer look at the complex pathophysiology of this phenomenon.

PATHOPHYSIOLOGY OF FUNCTIONAL MITRAL REGURGITATION IN HEART FAILURE

The term 'functional MR' implies the presence of MR in the absence of structural damage to the mitral valve leaflets. In the presence of systolic heart failure, the incomplete systolic closure of the mitral leaflets is provoked by several contributing factors:

- LV remodeling (i.e., spherical dilatation)
- regional wall motion abnormalities
- depressed LV systolic function

The most frequently cited (and probably somewhat overemphasized) responsible condition for the occurrence of functional MR is progressive dilatation of the mitral annulus in the failing heart. It has been postulated that the mitral leaflet area is insufficient to compensate for the dilatation of the mitral annulus in heart failure patients,[29] but anatomic studies have demonstrated that the actual available mitral leaflet area is theoretically large enough to

compensate for an amount of annular dilatation that is usually beyond the degree observed in heart failure patients.[30] Thus, mitral annular dilatation alone cannot sufficiently explain the occurrence of functional MR. Simultaneous with the dilatation of the mitral annulus, the LV undergoes spherical LV remodeling with a progressively increasing distance between the mitral leaflets and the papillary muscles. Since the chordal apparatus is inelastic, the increased distance will in turn lead to an increased tethering force that drags on the leaflet edges during systole and delays or even completely prevents complete leaflet coaptation during systole (Figure 19.1).[31,32] The amount of tethering can be quantified by measuring the outward displacement of the mitral leaflets, the so-called 'tenting' area.[31,33] These observations led to the experimental concept of selective chordal cutting to reduce the tethering forces and thereby the severity of functional MR.[34] Furthermore, it has been well documented not only that regional dysfunction in the area of papillary muscle insertion after myocardial infarction may cause or aggravate functional MR,[1] but also that an additional isolated loss of papillary muscle contraction may paradoxically reduce the amount of MR. While any regional dysfunction of the myocardium around the papillary muscle insertion may augment the tethering forces, the additional loss of contractile function within the papillary muscle itself will counterbalance the increased tethering

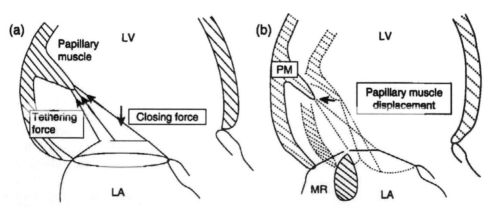

Figure 19.1 (a) Balance of forces acting on the mitral valve. (b) Left ventricular (LV) dilatation displaces the papillary muscle (PM) and increases the mitral tethering forces. This restricts complete mitral valve closure and causes functional mitral regurgitation (MR). LA, left atrium. (Reproduced from Otsuji Y, Handschumacher MD, Schwammenthal E, et al. Insights from three-dimensional echocardiography into the mechanism of functional mitral regurgitation: in vivo demonstration of altered leaflet tethering geometry. Circulation. 1997; 96(6):1999–2008.[31])

forces and cause less apical tenting and a decrease in the effective orifice area.[35]

The increased tethering force is counterbalanced by the LV 'closing force', which is determined by the effective transmitral pressure gradient. LV dilatation will not cause significant functional MR as long as myocardial contractility is still preserved and as long as the LV is able to generate enough force to overcome the increased tethering force. An example is the patient with severe aortic regurgitation and preserved LV function who develops LV dilatation (eccentric remodeling) but no significant functional MR. However, if LV myocardial contractility is also depressed – as it is by definition in patients with systolic heart failure – then the pressure rise in the LV will be delayed and diminished. Thus, the closing force that is required to overcome the increased tethering forces cannot be generated, and functional MR will be further aggravated.[36] This concept is supported by the observations that inotropic stimulation (e.g., by dobutamine stress) in a patient with heart failure will decrease the severity of functional MR, while dynamic physical exercise, with an increase in afterload but only a modest increase in inotropy, will aggravate functional MR.[37,38] The dependence of the effective

MR orifice area on the LV pressure rise also explains the dynamic changes of the effective regurgitant orifice area (EROA) during systole.[39] Delayed, asynchronous electrical activation of the LV as is typically seen in patients with left bundle branch block (LBBB) is another independent cause of functional MR mediated by the delayed LV pressure rise.[40] A prolonged atrioventricular interval further delays the onset of LV contraction and pressure rise. In the presence of an abnormally tethered mitral valve, this situation predisposes to incomplete mitral valve closure with the occurrence of pre-systolic (diastolic) MR (Figure 19.2a).[41] The end-diastolic pressure reversal may not exert enough force to close the restricted mitral leaflets (Figure 19.3).[42] The critical value for the PR interval for the appearance of diastolic MR has been determined to be around 0.23 s.[43]

In summary, the progressive spherical remodeling of the LV during the evolutionary process of systolic heart failure increases the mitral annulus diameter and the distance between the mitral leaflets and the papillary muscles. Both effects will decrease the mitral leaflet coaptation area and increase the tethering forces on the leaflets, thereby increasing the EROA. Severe regional wall motion abnormalities around the

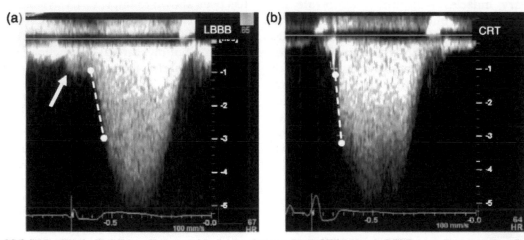

Figure 19.2 (a) A patient with left bundle branch block, showing a prolonged PR interval of 280 ms and pre-systolic mitral regurgitation (MR) on continuous-wave (CW) Doppler (arrow). (b) Cardiac resynchronization therapy (CRT) with atrioventricular delay optimization eliminates pre-systolic MR, and LV dP/dt_{max} increases from 530 mmHg/s to approximately 1000 mmHg/s, as indicated by the steeper slope of the regurgitant signal during CRT (dashed lines in (a) and (b)). Note that CW Doppler tends to overestimate the improvement in LV dP/dt_{max}. Reprinted from The American Journal of Cardiology: Vol 97: Nof E, Glikson M, Bar-Lev D, et al. Mechanism of Diastolic Mitral Regurgitation in candidates for Cardiac Resynchronization therapy. Issue II, pages 1611–1614. (2006). With permission from Elsevier.

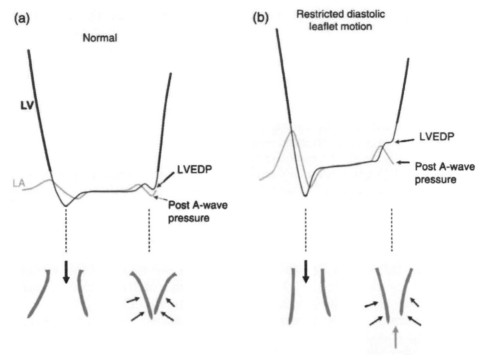

Figure 19.3 The effect of the left ventricular end-diastolic pressure (LVEDP) gradient on a normally (a) and abnormally (b) tethered mitral valve. If diastolic leaflet motion is restricted due to increased tethering forces, the end-diastolic reversal of the left ventricular (LV) – left atrial (LA) pressure gradient may not exert enough force to close the leaflets sufficiently. (Reproduced from Am J Cardiol. Vol 97. Nof E, et al. Mechanism of diastolic mitral regurgitation in candidates for cardiac resynchronization therapy. Pages 1611–14 (2006). With permission from Elsevier.[42])

papillary muscles will further aggravate the severity of MR, but papillary dysfunction in itself will not further contribute to functional MR. Electrical conduction delays as in first-degree atrioventricular (AV) block and bundle branch block contribute independently to the problem. The volume overload of the LV contributes further to LV dilatation and the progressive deterioration in LV function, which in turn again increases MR severity. Thus, it is often quoted that 'MR begets MR'.[44]

EFFECTS OF CRT ON FUNCTIONAL MITRAL REGURGITATION

On the basis of the pathophysiology described above, it becomes evident that any therapy that improves global LV systolic function and that simultaneously reduces wall motion abnormalities will also help to decrease the severity of functional MR. CRT is such a therapy, and

has been shown to improve LV systolic function as measured by an acute increase in LV dP/dt_{max} and pulse pressure[45,46] mediated by an improved synchrony of myocardial contraction.[22,47–49]

The diastolic (pre-systolic) component of functional MR is mainly dependent on delayed AV coupling, which can be identified by a prolonged PR interval. It is eliminated by pacing with a short (optimized) AV delay, independent of the ventricular pacing site (Figure 19.2b). Thus, diastolic MR can theoretically also be effectively treated by conventional right ventricular (RV) pacing; however, this approach might aggravate mechanical LV dyssynchrony and thereby the systolic MR component.

As explained above, the systolic MR component is mainly determined by the imbalance between the tethering and closing forces on the leaflets. This led to the assumption that the CRT-related acute improvement in LV systolic function will augment the closing force on the mitral leaflet and thereby immediately produce a more rapid and more effective closure of the valves. This was tested in an acute experiment with reprogramming of the CRT device at rest to on-and-off pacing in 24 patients with an implanted CRT device.[17] The severity of MR was quantified with echocardiography by the proximal isovelocity surface area (PISA) method and compared with the non-invasively determined changes in LV systolic function (LV dP/dt_{max} by continuous-wave Doppler). As postulated, a linear correlation between the EROA and LV dP/dt_{max} was observed in this small study, demonstrating the close relationship between the accelerated rise in the systolic closing force and the severity of functional MR (Figure 19.4 and 19.5). This is in good agreement with the observations by Fukuda et al,[28] who showed in a detailed color flow Doppler analysis

of the dynamic behavior of functional MR that CRT reduced only the amount of early-systolic MR, but not the late-systolic MR fraction (Figure 19.6).

Kanzaki et al[26] were able to confirm the relationship between the increase in LV dP/dt_{max} and severity of MR. In addition, they analyzed the deformation sequence of the papillary muscles by strain rate imaging and found a relationship between the interpapillary muscle activation time delay and the improvement in the degree of MR by CRT (Figures 19.7 and 19.8). Similar observations were made by Porciani et al,[50] who demonstrated that the improvement in MR was mainly related to the improved ventricular synchrony in the midventricular level. Thus, the immediate reduction in severity of MR can be attributed to an improved coordination of ventricular contraction, including resynchronized

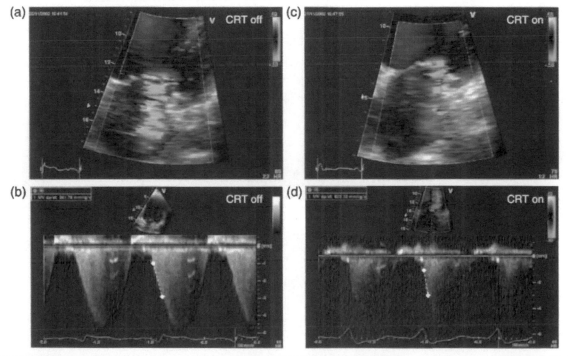

Figure 19.4 Effect of CRT on functional mitral regurgitation. Color Doppler shows moderate mitral regurgitation during no pacing (LBBB) (a), and the estimated LV dP/dt_{max} <400 mmHg/s (b). During CRT, the mitral regurgitant velocity is smaller, corresponding to mild mitral regurgitation (c). The simultaneously acquired LV dP/dt_{max} by continuous-wave Doppler has improved significantly, as indicated by the faster rise of the regurgitant velocity (d). (Reprinted from J Am Coll Cardiol. Vol 46. Bax JJ et al. Part 2–Issues During And After Device Implantation and Unresolved Questions. Pages 2168–82 (2005). With permission from American College of Cardiology Foundation.)

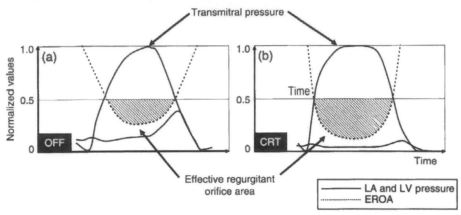

Figure 19.5 Schematic representation of the relationship between the increase in transmitral pressure (TMP, the instantaneous difference between left ventricular (LV) and left atrial (LA) pressure) and the decrease in effective regurgitant orifice area (EROA). During no pacing (a), LV contractility is low and results in a slow rise in the LV pressure curve and TMP, with a relatively late systolic maximum. Due to the slow LV pressure rise with delayed development of an effective transmitral closing force (~TMP), EROA remains large for a relatively long period until it finally reaches its minimum value. In contrast, during CRT (b) LV contractility improves, TMP rises faster and to a higher maximum value, which is also reached earlier. Consequently, the reduction in EROA occurs earlier, and EROA reaches lower values and for a prolonged period of time. The shaded area represents the time in systole during which EROA is <50% of its initial value. Note that in the example chosen here, the reduction in the height of the V-wave following a decrease in the initial mitral regurgitation will contribute to a preserved TMP during the latter half of systole. (Reprinted from J Am Coll Cardiol. Vol 41. Breithart OA, et al. Acute effects of cardiac resynchronization therapy on functional mitral regurgitation in advanced systolic heart failure. Pages 765–70 (2003). With permission from American College of Cardiology Foundation.[17])

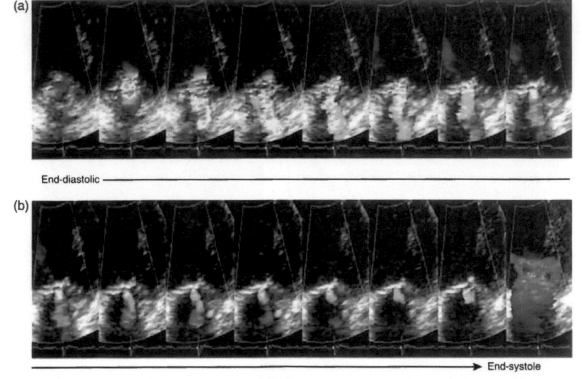

Figure 19.6 Dynamic behavior of the mitral regurgitant (MR) jet throughout systole. (a) Before CRT, the mitral jet area and the proximal flow convergence zone are much larger during early systole compared with late systole. (b) CRT reduces the total amount of MR and reverses this pattern, with a late systolic peak of the MR jet. (Reproduced from Fukuda S et al. J Am Coll Cardiol 2005;46:2270–6.[28])

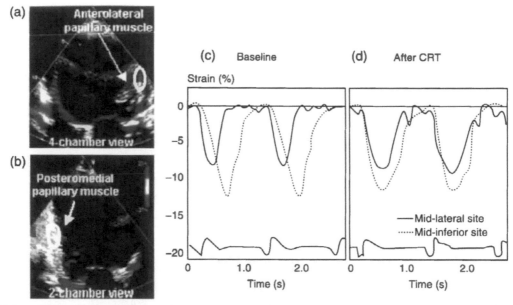

Figure 19.7 (a, b) Parametric strain images from the apical four-chamber and two-chamber views. (c, d) Time–strain plots from the LV myocardial segments adjacent to the papillary muscles, showing the extent of segmental shortening before and during CRT. At baseline (c), clear dyssynchrony is observed, with delayed peak shortening of the mid-inferior segment. After CRT (d), both segments shorten simultaneously. (Reprinted from American College of Cardiology Foundation. Vol 44. Kanzaki H, et al. A mechanism for immediate reduction in mitral regurgitation after cardiac resynchronization therapy: insights from mechanical activation. Pages 1619–25 (2004). With permission from American College of Cardiology Foundation.[26])

papillary muscle activation, which results in improved systolic function and reduced mitral leaflet tethering forces.

The effect of CRT on MR is largely independent of the underlying disease, and is found both in ischemic and non-ischemic cardiomyopathy patients.[25] The immediate reduction of the MR volume approaches about 30–40% on average at rest.[17,22,26] A further 10–20% improvement can be observed in the long term after some months of CRT, and is probably partly related to LV reverse remodeling,[22] although a direct relationship between reverse remodeling and MR reduction has not yet been demonstrated.[51] However, even a modest decrease in the MR volume will improve the volume load to the LV and contribute to long-term LV reverse remodeling.

Recent studies have also demonstrated that the improvement in functional MR is not limited to resting conditions, but can also be observed during exercise. Lafitte et al[52] found that about 30–40% of heart failure patients with a normal QRS width (<120 ms) and 60–70% of patients with a prolonged QRS width (>120 ms) demonstrate significant echocardiographic dyssynchrony at rest. Of those patients, about 30–40% show a deterioration of the degree of dyssynchrony during exercise, which is accompanied by a worsening of the severity of their MR. The exercise-related increase in MR can be reduced by appropriate biventricular pacing, as demonstrated by Lancellotti et al[18] (Figure 19.9). It was concluded that the inadequate rise in the mitral closing force (i.e., LV dP/dt_{max}) during bicycle exercise was the main determinant for the increase in MR in non-synchronized patients (CRT off at rest and during exercise). In already-resynchronized patients (CRT on at rest and during exercise), the residual increase in MR was mainly determined by geometrical factors (namely the residual tenting area) and independent of the increase in LV dP/dt_{max}.

The acute beneficial effects of CRT on MR are sustained during mid- and long-term follow-up and contribute significantly to the observed long-term benefit of CRT. Yu et al[22] demonstrated that

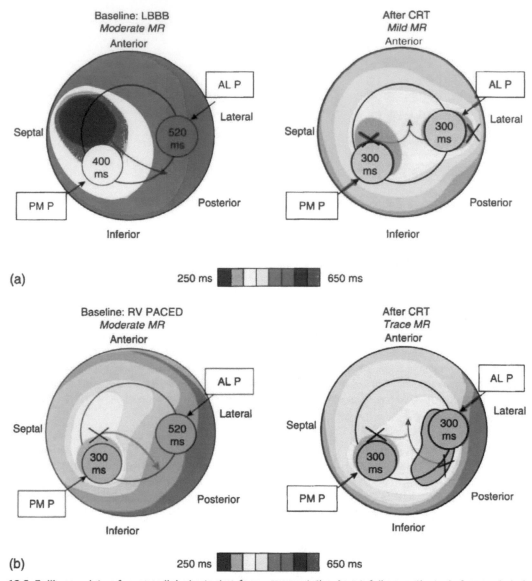

Figure 19.8 Bull's-eye plots of myocardial shortening from representative heart failure patients before and during CRT: (a) a patient with LBBB; (b) a patient with RV pacing. The time to peak systolic strain is color-coded with lines representing isochrones of mechanical shortening (activation) times at 50 ms intervals. The 'X' indicates the site of lead placement and the arrow indicates the direction of the propagating mechanical shortening. The time to peak strain is shown for sites adjacent to the anterolateral (AL P) and posteromedial (PM P) papillary muscles. (Reprinted from J Am Coll Cardiol. Vol 44. Kanzaki H, et al. A mechanism for immediate reduction in mitral regurgitation after cardiac resynchronization therapy: insights from mechanical activation strain mapping. Pages 1619–25 (2004). With permission from American College of Cardiology Foundation.[26])

brief cessation of CRT after 3 months of active pacing led to a return of MR to baseline levels (Figure 19.10). Even after more than 1 year, abrupt cessation of active CRT will worsen the severity of MR, indicating that the clinical and hemodynamic benefit of CRT persists over time.[27]

In general, the reduction in MR seems to be independent of the etiology of heart failure (ischemic vs non-ischemic).[25] However, in another series of 169 patients, the magnitude of the CRT response, defined as an increase in LVEF, was larger in non-ischemic patients with a lesser extent of scar

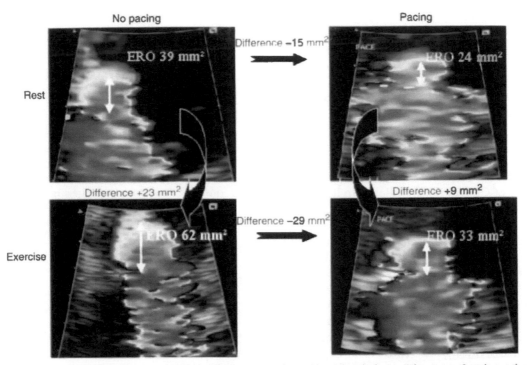

Figure 19.9 Proximal flow convergence zone in a representative patient with pacing during rest (upper row) and exercise (lower row) without CRT (left) and with active CRT (right). CRT reduced MR at rest (calculated effective regurgitant orifice area (ERO) from 39–24 mm²) and diminished the relative increase during exercise. (Reprinted from Am J Cardiol. Vol 94. Lancellotti P, et al. Effect of cardiac resynchronization therapy on functional mitral regurgitation in heart failure. Pages 1462–5 (2004). With permission from Elsevier.[18])

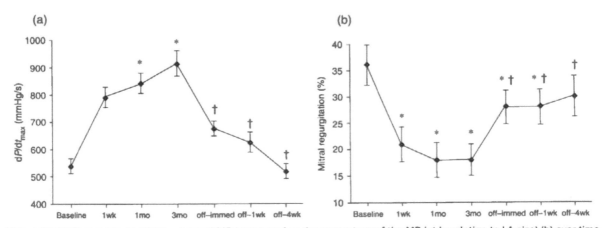

Figure 19.10 Changes in LV dP/dt$_{max}$ (a) and MR (expressed as the percentage of the MR jet in relation to LA size) (b) over time during CRT. Both parameters improve with CRT and return towards baseline levels after cessation of CRT after 3 months of active pacing. *Significant difference versus baseline. †Significant difference versus 3 months. (Reproduced from Yu CM et al. Tissue Doppler echocardiographic evidence of reverse remodeling and improved synchrony by simultaneously delaying regional contraction after biventricular pacing therapy in heart failure. Circulation 2002;40:111–18.[22])

segments and a lower wall motion score index.[53] Patients with a marked response (LVEF increase >10%) showed a greater improvement in severity of MR than moderate responders (LVEF increase 4–10%), while LVEF non-responders (LVEF increase ≤4%) experienced no change in MR.

SUMMARY

It has become evident that the clinical long-term benefit of CRT is closely related to its acute and long-term effects on mitral valve competence. The most impressive improvement is observed in patients with non-ischemic cardiomyopathies and with mild to moderate functional MR. Preliminary evidence suggests that the response to CRT might be more dubious in patients with very severe MR. These patients usually respond less to pacing, and should probably also be evaluated for reconstructive mitral valve surgery. Among the multiple clinical and procedural factors that determine the success of CRT, the effects on the mitral valve are of utmost clinical and prognostic importance. A patient with a CRT-related improvement in functional MR is also likely to experience a significant clinical and prognostic long-term benefit.

REFERENCES

1. Yiu SF, Enriquez-Sarano M, Tribouilloy C, Seward JB, Tajik AJ. Determinants of the degree of functional mitral regurgitation in patients with systolic left ventricular dysfunction: a quantitative clinical study. Circulation 2000;102:1400–6.
2. Trichon BH, Felker GM, Shaw LK, Cabell CH, O'Connor CM. Relation of frequency and severity of mitral regurgitation to survival among patients with left ventricular systolic dysfunction and heart failure. Am J Cardiol 2003;91:538–43.
3. Robbins JD, Maniar PB, Cotts W, et al. Prevalence and severity of mitral regurgitation in chronic systolic heart failure. Am J Cardiol 2003;91:360–2.
4. Grigioni F, Enriquez-Sarano M, Zehr KJ, Bailey KR, Tajik AJ. Ischemic mitral regurgitation: long-term outcome and prognostic implications with quantitative doppler assessment. Circulation 2001;103:1759–64.
5. Grigioni F, Detaint D, Avierinos JF, et al. Contribution of ischemic mitral regurgitation to congestive heart failure after myocardial infarction. J Am Coll Cardiol 2005;45:260–7.
6. Lamas GA, Mitchell GF, Flaker GC, et al. Clinical significance of mitral regurgitation after acute myocardial infarction. Survival and Ventricular Enlargement Investigators. Circulation 1997;96:827–33.
7. Seneviratne B, Moore GA, West PD. Effect of captopril on functional mitral regurgitation in dilated heart failure: a randomised double blind placebo controlled trial. Br Heart J 1994;72:63–8.
8. Bolling SF. Mitral reconstruction in cardiomyopathy. J Heart Valve Dis 2002;11(Suppl 1):S26–31.
9. Rogers JH, Macoviak JA, Rahdert DA, et al. Percutaneous septal sinus shortening: a novel procedure for the treatment of functional mitral regurgitation. Circulation 2006;113:2329–34.
10. Harris KM, Aeppli DM, Carey CF. Effects of angiotensin-converting enzyme inhibition on mitral regurgitation severity, left ventricular size, and functional capacity. Am Heart J 2005;150:1106.
11. Bolling SF, Pagani FD, Deeb GM, Bach DS. Intermediate-term outcome of mitral reconstruction in cardiomyopathy. J Thorac Cardiovasc Surg 1998;115:381–6.
12. Szalay ZA, Civelek A, Hohe S, et al. Mitral annuloplasty in patients with ischemic versus dilated cardiomyopathy. Eur J Cardiothorac Surg 2003;23:567–72.
13. Braun J, Bax JJ, Versteegh MI, et al. Preoperative left ventricular dimensions predict reverse remodeling following restrictive mitral annuloplasty in ischemic mitral regurgitation. Eur J Cardiothorac Surg 2005;27:847–53.
14. Cazeau S, Ritter P, Lazarus A, et al. Multisite pacing for end-stage heart failure: early experience. Pacing Clin Electrophysiol 1996;19:1748–57.
15. Blanc JJ, Etienne Y, Gilard M, et al. Evaluation of different ventricular pacing sites in patients with severe heart failure: results of an acute hemodynamic study. Circulation 1997;96:3273–7.
16. Breithardt OA, Kuhl HP, Stellbrink C. Acute effects of resynchronisation treatment on functional mitral regurgitation in dilated cardiomyopathy. Heart 2002;88:440.
17. Breithardt OA, Sinha AM, Schwammenthal E, et al. Acute effects of cardiac resynchronization therapy on functional mitral regurgitation in advanced systolic heart failure. J Am Coll Cardiol 2003;41:765–70.
18. Lancellotti P, Melon P, Sakalihasan N, et al. Effect of cardiac resynchronization therapy on functional mitral regurgitation in heart failure. Am J Cardiol 2004;94:1462–5.
19. Lau CP, Yu CM, Chau E, et al. Reversal of left ventricular remodeling by synchronous biventricular pacing in heart failure. Pacing Clin Electrophysiol 2000;23:1722–5.
20. Etienne Y, Mansourati J, Touiza A, et al. Evaluation of left ventricular function and mitral regurgitation during left ventricular-based pacing in patients with heart failure. Eur J Heart Fail 2001;3:441–7.

21. Kim WY, Sogaard P, Mortensen PT, et al. Three dimensional echocardiography documents haemodynamic improvement by biventricular pacing in patients with severe heart failure. Heart 2001;85:514–20.

22. Yu CM, Chau E, Sanderson JE, et al. Tissue Doppler echocardiographic evidence of reverse remodeling and improved synchronicity by simultaneously delaying regional contraction after biventricular pacing therapy in heart failure. Circulation 2002;105:438–45.

23. Linde C, Leclercq C, Rex S, et al. Long-term benefits of biventricular pacing in congestive heart failure: results from the MUltisite STimulation in Cardiomyopathy (MUSTIC) study. J Am Coll Cardiol 2002;40:111–18.

24. Chan KL, Tang AS, Achilli A, et al. Functional and echocardiographic improvement following multisite biventricular pacing for congestive heart failure. Can J Cardiol 2003;19:387–90.

25. St John Sutton MG, Plappert T, Abraham WT, et al. Effect of cardiac resynchronization therapy on left ventricular size and function in chronic heart failure. Circulation 2003;107:1985–90.

26. Kanzaki H, Bazaz R, Schwartzman D, et al. A mechanism for immediate reduction in mitral regurgitation after cardiac resynchronization therapy: insights from mechanical activation strain mapping. J Am Coll Cardiol 2004;44:1619–25.

27. Brandt RR, Reiner C, Arnold R, et al. Contractile response and mitral regurgitation after temporary interruption of long-term cardiac resynchronization therapy. Eur Heart J 2006;27:187–92.

28. Fukuda S, Grimm R, Song JM, et al. Electrical conduction disturbance effects on dynamic changes of functional mitral regurgitation. J Am Coll Cardiol 2005;46:2270–6.

29. Boltwood CM, Tei C, Wong M, Shah PM. Quantitative echocardiography of the mitral complex in dilated cardiomyopathy: the mechanism of functional mitral regurgitation. Circulation 1983;68:498–508.

30. Otsuji Y, Kumanohoso T, Yoshifuku S, et al. Isolated annular dilation does not usually cause important functional mitral regurgitation: comparison between patients with lone atrial fibrillation and those with idiopathic or ischemic cardiomyopathy. J Am Coll Cardiol 2002;39:1651–6.

31. Otsuji Y, Handschumacher MD, Schwammenthal E, et al. Insights from three-dimensional echocardiography into the mechanism of functional mitral regurgitation: direct in vivo demonstration of altered leaflet tethering geometry. Circulation 1997;96:1999–2008.

32. Nielsen SL, Nygaard H, Fontaine AA, et al. Chordal force distribution determines systolic mitral leaflet configuration and severity of functional mitral regurgitation. J Am Coll Cardiol 1999;33:843–53.

33. Godley RW, Wann LS, Rogers EW, Feigenbaum H, Weyman AE. Incomplete mitral leaflet closure in patients with papillary muscle dysfunction. Circulation 1981;63:565–71.

34. Messas E, Guerrero JL, Handschumacher MD, et al. Chordal cutting: a new therapeutic approach for ischemic mitral regurgitation. Circulation 2001;104:1958–63.

35. Messas E, Guerrero JL, Handschumacher MD, et al. Paradoxic decrease in ischemic mitral regurgitation with papillary muscle dysfunction: insights from three-dimensional and contrast echocardiography with strain rate measurement. Circulation 2001;104:1952–7.

36. Hung J, Otsuji Y, Handschumacher MD, Schwammenthal E, Levine RA. Mechanism of dynamic regurgitant orifice area variation in functional mitral regurgitation: physiologic insights from the proximal flow convergence technique. J Am Coll Cardiol 1999;33:538–45.

37. Keren G, Laniado S, Sonnenblick EH, Lejemtel TH. Dynamics of functional mitral regurgitation during dobutamine therapy in patients with severe congestive heart failure: a Doppler echocardiographic study. Am Heart J 1989;118:748–54.

38. Lebrun F, Lancellotti P, Pierard LA. Quantitation of functional mitral regurgitation during bicycle exercise in patients with heart failure. J Am Coll Cardiol 2001;38:1685–92.

39. Schwammenthal E, Chen C, Benning F, et al. Dynamics of mitral regurgitant flow and orifice area. Physiologic application of the proximal flow convergence method: clinical data and experimental testing. Circulation 1994;90:307–22.

40. Erlebacher JA, Barbarash S. Intraventricular conduction delay and functional mitral regurgitation. Am J Cardiol 2001;88:83–6.

41. Brecker SJ, Xiao HB, Sparrow J, Gibson DG. Effects of dual-chamber pacing with short atrioventricular delay in dilated cardiomyopathy. Lancet 1992;340:1308–12.

42. Nof E, Glikson M, Bar-Lev D, et al. Mechanism of diastolic mitral regurgitation in candidates for cardiac resynchronization therapy. Am J Cardiol 2006;97:1611–14.

43. Ishikawa T, Kimura K, Miyazaki N, et al. Diastolic mitral regurgitation in patients with first-degree atrioventricular block. Pacing Clin Electrophysiol 1992;15:1927–31.

44. Carabello BA. Ischemic mitral regurgitation and ventricular remodeling. J Am Coll Cardiol 2004;43:384–5.

45. Auricchio A, Stellbrink C, Block M, et al. Effect of pacing chamber and atrioventricular delay on acute systolic function of paced patients with congestive heart failure. Circulation 1999;99:2993–3001.

46. Kass DA, Chen CH, Curry C, et al. Improved left ventricular mechanics from acute VDD pacing in patients with dilated cardiomyopathy and ventricular conduction delay. Circulation 1999;99:1567–73.

47. Leclercq C, Faris O, Tunin R, et al. Systolic improvement and mechanical resynchronization does not require electrical synchrony in the dilated failing heart with left bundle-branch block. Circulation 2002;106:1760–3.

48. Breithardt OA, Stellbrink C, Kramer AP, et al. Echocardiographic quantification of left ventricular asynchrony predicts an acute hemodynamic benefit of cardiac resynchronization therapy. J Am Coll Cardiol 2002;40:536–45.

49. Breithardt OA, Stellbrink C, Herbots L, et al. Cardiac resynchronization therapy can reverse abnormal myocardial strain distribution in patients with heart failure and left bundle-branch block. J Am Coll Cardiol 2003;42:486–94.

50. Porciani MC, Macioce R, Demarchi G, et al. Effects of cardiac resynchronization therapy on the mechanisms underlying functional mitral regurgitation in congestive heart failure. Eur J Echocardiogr 2006;7:31–9.

51. Stellbrink C, Breithardt OA, Franke A, et al. Impact of cardiac resynchronization therapy using hemodynamically optimized pacing on left ventricular remodeling in patients with congestive heart failure and ventricular conduction disturbances. J Am Coll Cardiol 2001;38:1957–65.

52. Lafitte S, Bordachar P, Lafitte M, et al. Dynamic ventricular dyssynchrony: an exercise–echocardiography study. J Am Coll Cardiol 2006;47:2253–9.

53. Mangiavacchi M, Gasparini M, Faletra F, et al. Clinical predictors of marked improvement in left ventricular performance after cardiac resynchronization therapy in patients with chronic heart failure. Am Heart J 2006;151:477.

20

Non-responders and patient selection from an echocardiographic perspective

Richard A Grimm

Introduction • Clinical approach to the non-responder once non-responder status has been established • Symptoms and/or LVEF worsened • AV optimization • V–V timing • Re-evaluation of intraventricular dyssynchrony • Symptomatic improvement, LVEF unchanged • Symptoms and LVEF unchanged • Conclusions

INTRODUCTION

It has been reported that 10–30% of patients undergoing CRT either do not experience an improvement or in fact may worsen following implantation of a biventricular (BiV) pacing system and therefore have been termed 'non-responders'.[1-3] Managing and troubleshooting these patients can be challenging, yet a rational systematic approach utilizing echocardiographic imaging to diagnose problems and optimize pacing settings can be useful in maximizing the potential of the therapy. Moreover, echocardiographic data may play a key role in determining when pacing therapy is poorly deployed or even detrimental.[4] Significant controversy persists, however, regarding the definition of non-response, as some experts would argue that evidence of reverse remodeling (defined as a decrease in end-systolic volume of >15%) is necessary in order to categorize a patient as a responder,[1,3,5,6] whereas others maintain that parameters such as functional class (New York Heart Association (NYHA) classification), global quality-of life-scores, and hospitalizations should be included in defining success or failure of the therapy. This controversy is dealt with elsewhere in this book. This chapter will focus on the clinical and echocardiographic evaluation of the patient once a *no-response* status has been determined, regardless of whether that means failure to demonstrate an improved left ventricular (LV) ejection fraction (LVEF) or lack of an improved functional status. Yet another important consideration should be the time interval following implantation that should be allowed before re-evaluating function. Although some patients may experience an immediate response (either positive or negative), most studies would suggest that of the two-thirds of patients who experience a benefit, most will experience evidence of reverse remodeling 3–6 months following the procedure.[7] Unless clear clinical or ventricular function deterioration is apparent, allowing a minimum of 1 and at least 3 months for evidence of response would seem most representative of the true impact of the therapy.

CLINICAL APPROACH TO THE NON-RESPONDER ONCE NON-RESPONDER STATUS HAS BEEN ESTABLISHED

The standard approach to problem-solving in these patients involves a clinical as well as an echocardiographic examination, as this allows for a comprehensive evaluation of cardiac structure, function, and hemodynamics that is readily available to all cardiologists. Utilizing this method, one can evaluate the impact of pacing on chamber size and ventricular function, as well as electromechanical events including interventricular, intraventricular and atrioventricular (AV) synchrony.

When first encountering a non-responder, the first consideration should be to review the patient's criteria for implant. Re-evaluation of selection criteria must include a search for reversible causes of heart failure and LV dysfunction (i.e., valve disease, coronary artery disease, pulmonary disease, and congenital heart disease), as well as the degree of baseline LV dysfunction, the presence and degree of intraventricular mechanical delay, and QRS duration pre-implant. Patients with borderline LVEF or borderline QRS durations as well as a QRS morphology other than left bundle branch block (LBBB) (i.e., right bundle branch block (RBBB) or intraventricular conduction delay (IVCD)) may be less likely to demonstrate a positive response as compared with those with non-ischemic cardiomyopathies, LVEF <35% and a QRS >150 ms, and LBBB. Precise knowledge of this information may be able to provide insights into why a patient may have realized a suboptimal response. Non-responders often present with either symptoms or persistent or worsening LV dysfunction, or both. Classifying these cases as they present may be helpful in determining an etiology and generating a management strategy.

SYMPTOMS AND/OR LVEF WORSENED

It is typically very clear that these patients have not experienced the desired effect of CRT, and therefore investigation must proceed to determine whether a specific reason for this lack of response can be uncovered and if so whether it can be corrected. A systematic approach may be useful in managing these cases – specifically, one that addresses issues related to intraventricular, interventricular, and AV synchrony.

AV OPTIMIZATION

Once appropriate patient selection has been assured, and assuming that the optimal lead position has been achieved, evaluation of AV and interventricular (V–V) timing intervals is recommended. In comparison with the importance and impact of correction of intraventricular dyssynchrony, AV and V–V timing are minor contributors to the overall impact of CRT.[8] However, data clearly demonstrate that, in selected patients, optimizing the AV delay does improve hemodynamics.[8-10] The optimal AV

delay has been defined as that which enables completion of atrial filling prior to ventricular contraction, thereby allowing for an optimal diastolic filling time.[11] Evidence demonstrating a clinical benefit or positive impact of AV delay optimization on outcome, however, is lacking. Despite this lack of definitive data supporting its utility, several centers have advocated various methods for evaluating AV delay and optimizing AV intervals in patients undergoing CRT. These protocols range from routinely evaluating hemodynamics with Doppler echocardiography in all patients undergoing CRT and optimizing as indicated, to only evaluating AV synchrony and ultimately optimizing AV delay if the patient is considered a non-responder. In our center, we have found it both useful and practical to evaluate diastolic filling parameters (mitral inflow) by Doppler echocardiography in all patients undergoing CRT and to proceed with an AV optimization procedure only if the hemodynamics are suboptimal[9] (Figure 20.1). If E–A wave reversal is present, there is adequate separation of the E and A waves, the A wave terminates at least 40 ms after the onset of the QRS

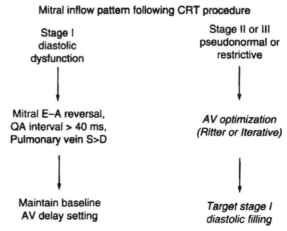

Mitral inflow pattern following CRT procedure

Stage I diastolic dysfunction → Mitral E–A reversal, QA interval > 40 ms, Pulmonary vein S>D → Maintain baseline AV delay setting

Stage II or III pseudonormal or restrictive → *AV optimization (Ritter or Iterative)* → *Target stage I diastolic filling*

Figure 20.1 Recommended algorithm utilizing pulsed Doppler of mitral inflow to assess diastolic function for approaching CRT patients being considered for AV optimization. If the patient presents with stage I diastolic dysfunction or delayed relaxation abnormality, the QA interval is >40 ms, and the pulmonary vein flow pattern is systolic > diastolic (S>D), then the baseline AV delay settings are maintained. If, on the other hand, pseudonormal (stage II) or restrictive (stage III) physiology is present, then AV optimization is performed.

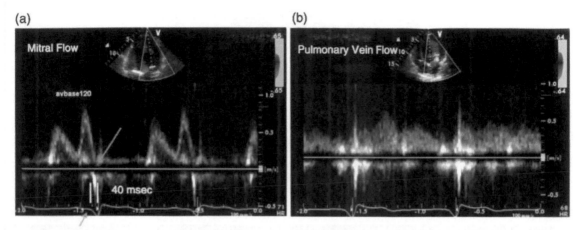

Figure 20.2 Because the mitral inflow pattern (a) demonstrates E–A reversal, adequate E–A wave separation, and a QA interval >40 ms, and the pulmonary vein flow (b) reveals S>D, no further optimization is necessary, as further modifications are unlikely to improve hemodynamics.

complex, and the systolic flow velocity is greater than the diastolic flow velocity on pulmonary vein flow assessment, then the baseline 'out-of-the-box' setting is maintained (Figure 20.2).

Regardless of a given institution's preference in routinely evaluating AV delay settings, it is clear that AV delay is worth interrogating in the non-responder population. Several Doppler methods for optimization have been described in the literature, all of which utilize a Doppler parameter of either systolic or diastolic function to determine functional response to various AV delay settings. The two most commonly reported Doppler parameters are pulsed-wave Doppler assessment of mitral inflow and continuous-wave Doppler assessment of aortic outflow (stroke volume estimate).[12] Also reported to be useful in this setting is the Tei index,[10] which evaluates both systolic and diastolic function. The utility of mitral inflow assessment is based upon the ability to time the termination of the atrial contribution to filling with the onset of ventricular contraction, in addition to its ability to assess diastolic function. This was initially proposed to be useful in this context by Ritter et al.[13] The Doppler assessment of aortic flow is a systolic parameter and is an estimation of stroke volume. In our experience, mitral inflow assessment has been more robust in regard to ease of acquisition, interpretation, and prognostic value relative to the aortic flow parameter.

Utilizing the Doppler mitral inflow method as a parameter to assess myocardial function and the relationship between the termination of the atrial contribution to filling and the onset of ventricular systole, the optimal AV delay can be determined using either an iterative or a Ritter method. The iterative method simply attempts to target stage 1 diastolic filling or early relaxation, which is an optimal diastolic function status in a heart failure population. The AV delay is set to an abnormally prolonged setting while maintaining BiV capture if conduction is presumed to be relatively normal at baseline, and the mitral inflow is sampled. The AV delay intervals are decreased in 20 ms increments, with the mitral inflow being sampled at each stage. Optimal AV delay is achieved when E–A reversal is present, adequate separation of an A wave is appreciated, and the A wave terminates at least 40 ms after the onset of the QRS complex, representing minimum electrical–mechanical delay. If there is evidence of intraatrial or AV conduction delay at baseline, the AV delay can be adjusted in increasing increments, again targeting delayed relaxation abnormality, stage I diastolic dysfunction (Figure 20.3). The Ritter method achieves this same endpoint by initially setting the AV delay to an inappropriately short setting, sampling mitral inflow, measuring the QA interval (QRS onset to A-wave termination) and comparing this measure with the QA interval at an

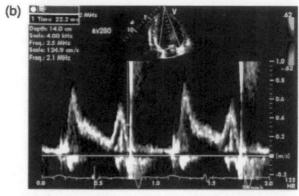

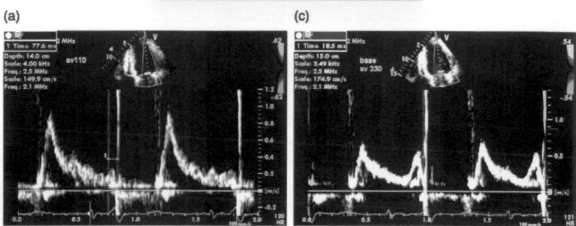

Figure 20.3 This patient was a 69-year-old male with ischemic cardiomyopathy and s/p aortic valve replacement, atrial fibrillation, ventricular tachycardia, and heart failure who had recently undergone implantation of a biventricular (BiV) pacemaker. At a baseline setting of 110 ms, there was no discernible A wave (a). The AV delay was then extended to 280 ms while maintaining BiV capture (c). At an AV delay of 280 ms, the termination of the A wave fell before QRS onset, resulting in suboptimal diastolic filling and the potential for diastolic mitral regurgitation. The AV delay was then empirically decreased to 230 ms, where a more physiologic relationship between the end of the A wave and QRS onset could be realized. The AV delay setting was therefore maintained at 230 ms.

inappropriately long AV delay setting. The optimal AV delay is then calculated from the difference of the QA intervals at each setting plus the short AV delay setting.

Data from our institution suggests that most patients (60%) exhibit optimal diastolic filling or delayed relaxation (stage I) at an out-of-the-box setting of approximately 100–140 ms. Furthermore, approximately 10% of patients with suboptimal diastolic filling hemodynamics (stage II or III) will exhibit improved diastolic filling with optimization of the AV delay (Figure 20.4). The predictors of a longer than normal (optimal) AV delay include a paced

rhythm, AV block, and an enlarged left atrium (LA) (Figure 20.5), suggesting that intraatrial conduction delay necessitates an abnormally prolonged AV delay in order to optimize diastolic filling.[9] Although there are no known data supporting the utility or impact of AV optimization on outcome, data from several centers experienced in performing these procedures suggest that this intervention may positively impact a segment (albeit small) of the non-responder group.[9,14] Because conduction times may vary over time – likely related to reverse remodeling – regular interrogation at 6- to 12-month intervals seems prudent.[15]

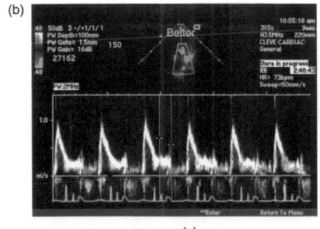

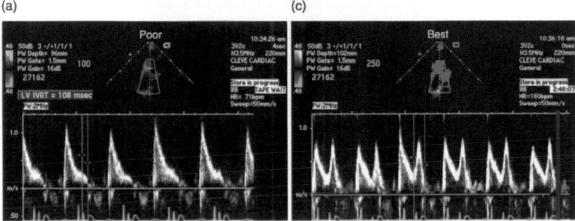

Figure 20.4 Using an iterative method for AV delay optimization, the AV delay was extended in this 69-year-old male with known underlying conduction disease. There is no effective late diastolic filling (no A wave) at the baseline AV delay setting of 100 ms (a), which was set in the laboratory during the CRT procedure. At an AV delay of 150 ms (b), the Doppler mitral inflow pattern has improved, as an A wave is unmasked, whereas optimal diastolic filling is realized only when the AV delay is prolonged to 250 ms. Notably, at this prolonged AV delay setting of 250 ms (c), the A-wave termination falls clearly after the QRS onset – hence, a relatively physiologic electrical–mechanical delay can be assumed.

V–V TIMING

V–V timing is another parameter that can be modified in patients undergoing BiV pacing, especially in the non-responder group. As with AV optimization, optimization of V–V timing has little data to support its utility and impact on outcome measures. Additionally, similar to AV timing, V–V timing likely contributes relatively little to the overall impact of CRT. However, in selected cases, V–V timing may have a significant impact. Preliminary studies have demonstrated improvement in hemodynamics.[16–18]

It has been speculated that this may in part be the result of compensation for suboptimal lead position.[19] Sogaard et al,[20] for example, suggested that patients with ischemic cardiomyopathies benefit from a right ventricular (RV) pre-offset, whereas patients with dilated cardiomyopathies benefit from an LV pre-offset. Furthermore, Porciani et al[10] demonstrated that tailored BiV pacing was advantageous. Bordacher et al[17] demonstrated that V–V optimization resulted in a significant reduction in mitral regurgitation, whereas Van Gelder et al[18] reported that

(a)   (b)   (c)

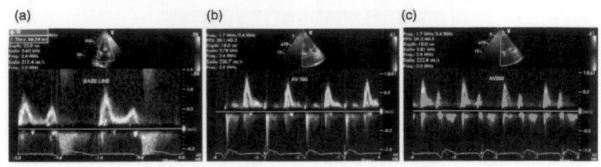

Figure 20.5 This patient is a 76-year-old female with ischemic cardiomyopathy, ischemic mitral regurgitation, hypertension, and paroxysmal atrial fibrillation who was s/p Carpentier–Edwards mitral valve replacement. She had recently undergone CRT and now presented for an AV optimization procedure. The AV delay was set at 320 ms at the time of the BiV implant. Further investigation revealed that the interatrial conduction times had been measured at time of BiV implant in the endocardial prosthesis laboratory and found to be very abnormally prolonged (350 ms) as the patient had biatrial enlargement with an LA diameter of 6 cm and an area of 34 cm². It was decided to modify the AV delay to investigate whether changes in diastolic filling could be elicited. Mitral inflow is shown at AV delays of 320 ms (a), 150 ms (b), and 250 ms (c). The optimal diastolic filling was confirmed to be at an AV delay of 320 ms.

most patients (83%) benefited from LV-first pre-activation in a series of 53 patients. One of the major challenges, however, is to agree or settle on the best non-invasive parameter available in our armamentarium that can be practically employed to assist in detecting whether simultaneous versus LV pre-offset versus RV pre-offset is best in a given patient.

Clearly, further investigation is needed to guide appropriate adjustment of this capability. However, in the absence of definitive guidelines, and particularly in patients with a suboptimal response to CRT, it is certainly reasonable to optimize hemodynamics utilizing one or more parameters of cardiac function. The protocol utilized in our laboratory is to measure aortic outflow (stroke volume estimate) and the Tei index (aortic outflow and mitral inflow by pulsed Doppler) with simultaneous pacing, and four LV and four RV pre-offsets at 20 ms intervals. Simultaneous pacing is maintained in most cases, and only if both parameters exhibit a consistent positive improvement in function at a given setting will we recommend modification of the V–V timing. The evaluation will then be repeated in 6 months to reassess the patients' clinical status, as well as the associated hemodynamic parameters.

RE-EVALUATION OF INTRAVENTRICULAR DYSSYNCHRONY

Once AV and V–V timing has been optimized, and if no improvement in symptoms or ventricular function has been realized, then a reassessment of intraventricular dyssynchrony using Doppler tissue imaging could be informative. Importantly, comparison with baseline or pre-implant dyssynchrony information, as well as precise knowledge of the coronary sinus lead location, are necessary in order to provide the greatest possible insight into the impact of BiV stimulation on ventricular mechanical function. Evaluating intraventricular dyssynchrony post implant without pre-implant baseline dyssynchrony data and without precise information on lead location can be problematic, as residual dyssynchrony will likely be present (Figure 20.6) – and, without baseline data, much less meaningful. Improvement in intraventricular dyssynchrony may be useful to document but is not necessary for success of therapy (Figure 6 and 7).

If LV function is poor (≤ 35%), unchanged from baseline, or worse as compared with baseline, and significant intraventricular dyssynchrony persists, particularly if the segment of most significant delay does not correspond to

(a)   (b)

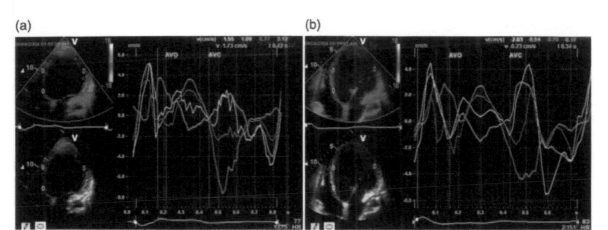

Figure 20.6 Basal and mid myocardial velocity data pre and post CRT obtained using Doppler Tissue Imaging from a 49 y/o female with a dilated cardiomyopathy and LBBB who responded favorably with improvement in symptoms and EF from 20% to 30%. The left panel is pre implant and demonstrates significant intraventricular dyssynchrony (opposing wall time to peak velocity difference of 112ms from the apical 4 chamber view). The right panel is post implant and reveals persistent residual intraventricular dyssynchrony (opposing wall time to peak velocity difference of 120ms) despite satisfactory lead placement and a favorable clinical response to CRT.

the site of the coronary sinus lead placement, then it would seem reasonable to consider revising lead placement either transvenously or surgically with an epicardial lead. The recognition of an anterior lead location combined with a non-responder status would also favor proceeding with lead repositioning (Figure 20.8). When a clear discordance between lead position and dyssynchrony data cannot be determined with a high degree of confidence, attempting an empiric lead revision should be avoided.

Finally, if no clear explanation of the patient's failure to respond can be confidently diagnosed, a trial of allowing intrinsic conduction by discontinuing pacing therapy should be attempted. Global ventricular function as well as re-acquisition of dyssynchrony parameters can be re-evaluated during intrinsic conduction, along with a clinical

(a)   (b)

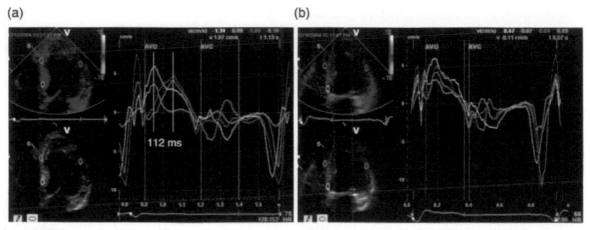

Figure 20.7 Base and mid myocardial velocity data pre and post CRT within 3 days of implant of a CRT device obtained using Doppler Tissue Imaging. The left panel is pre implant and demonstrates significant intraventricular dyssynchrony (opposing wall time to peak velocity difference of 100 ms from the apical 4 chamber view at the base) with improvement in dyssynchrony (right panel) as the systolic peaks align nearly perfectly. The patient responded favorably with an improvement in symptoms and LV function.

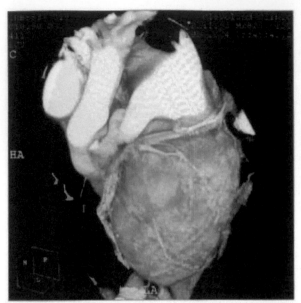

Figure 20.8 Multislice computed tomographic (MSCT) scan of the heart, and more specifically of the coronary veins. This is a 65-year-old male who underwent CRT and was designated a non-responder, as after 3 months and then 6 months, his LVEF was unchanged and his symptomatology was not improved. Further diagnostics were performed, including a MSCT scan to assess precise lead placement. The coronary sinus lead here is seen traversing the great cardiac vein on the anterior aspect of the heart, and could well explain the suboptimal response described clinically.

evaluation for a trial period. Clearly, pacing can be detrimental to LV function – even BiV pacing with the RV lead positioned in the RV apex.[21]

SYMPTOMATIC IMPROVEMENT, LVEF UNCHANGED

This group of patients may or may not be categorized as non-responders, depending on whether or not reverse remodeling is considered necessary to define success. The placebo effect may be implicated as an explanation for improvement in this subgroup, and therefore a neutral effect on ventricular function could be consistent with this outcome. Yet another possibility, however, is that functional status is in fact truly improved yet traditional methods of evaluating ventricular function are suboptimal for measuring a real increase in ventricular contractility. In these cases, demonstrating improved

intraventricular synchrony as described above by comparing pre- and post-implant dyssynchrony measures may be clinically useful.[22]

Even though no objective improvement in ventricular function may be realized when using standard measures of function such as LVEF, an assessment of intraventricular dyssynchrony may be worth documenting. This scenario would contrast with that of a patient whose ventricular function has clearly improved by two-dimensional echocardiographic assessment of LVEF by volumes and in whom an assessment of intraventricular dyssynchrony could therefore be considered irrelevant and potentially even misleading to the uninformed.

The time to peak velocity measurements as determined by color Doppler tissue imaging utilizing the opposing-wall method (a standard measure of intraventricular mechanical dyssynchrony) is recommended as a parameter that could be collected pre and post implant for comparison.[5,23] It is important to note that opposing-wall time to peak velocity measurements made in isolation post-implant will have little meaning unless pre-implant data are readily available for comparison.[22,24] As reported by Yu et al,[23] segmental opposing-wall times to peak velocity (Ts) post BiV implant remain abnormally prolonged (anteroseptum 191 ± 32 ms and lateral wall 213 ± 44 ms); however, the coefficient of regional variation relative to pre-implant is improved as a result of a more synchronized segmental delay among regions of the LV.

SYMPTOMS AND LVEF UNCHANGED

If at 1–3 months post-implant a patient exhibits no objective improvement in either symptoms or ventricular function, most clinicians would consider this to be in the non-responder category. In these cases, a systematic investigation of possible explanations for the lack of response should be initiated. After reviewing the baseline data, including the patient selection criteria to assure appropriate candidacy and to rule out other potential reversible causes of ventricular dysfunction, procedural issues (operative notes) should be reviewed and pacing setting optimization should be considered.

Lead position should be reviewed and confirmed with a postero-anterior and lateral chest X-ray. If the lead position is in a location typically considered suboptimal (i.e., anterior), if the RV/cardiac sinus lead distance is not maximized, or if intraventricular dyssynchrony can be confidently determined to be increased or even unchanged as compared with the pre-implant evaluation, then serious consideration should be given to repositioning the LV lead. Finally, useful information may be obtained by re-examining intraventricular mechanical dys-synchrony by color TDI with the pacemaker in both the off and the on mode and comparing more acutely the real-time impact of the BiV pacing therapy on ventricular synchrony and function. On occasion, it can be determined that ventricular function and/or intraventricular dyssynchrony are worsened with BiV pacing.

CONCLUSIONS

Improving our understanding of the mechanisms underlying CRT, (which will lead to improved selection criteria and implantation technique), will be the basis for minimizing the non-responder population. However, until this progress can be realized, evaluation and management of the non-responder population must be thoughtful, careful, and thorough.

Because of the many limitations and uncertainties clinicians have before them in trying to identify and problem-solve this population of patients, it is imperative that they accurately define the problem with objective data, review expectations with their patients, and pursue a redirection of therapy only once definitive diagnosis can be delineated. Additionally, appreciating the utility as well as the limitations of echocardiography can be extremely valuable in arriving at a correct diagnosis and ultimately applying the appropriate corrective therapy – which may well include no therapy.

REFERENCES

1. Cazeau S, Leclercq C, Lavergne T, et al. ftMSiCS Investigators. Effects of multisite bi-ventricular pacing in patients with heart failure and intra-ventricular conduction delay. N Engl J Med 2001;344:873–80.
2. Bristow M, Saxon L, Boehmer J, et al. Cardiac-resynchronization therapy with or without an implantable defibrillator in advanced chronic heart failure. COMPANION Investigators. N Engl J Med 2004;350:2140–50.
3. Cleland J, Daubert J, Erdmann E, et al. CARE-HF Study Investigators. The effect of cardiac resynchronization on morbidity and mortality in heart failure. N Engl J Med 2005;352:1539–49.
4. Bax JJ, Abraham T, Barold SS, et al. Cardiac resynchronization therapy: Part I: Issues before device implantation. J Am Coll Cardiol 2005;46:2153–67.
5. Yu CM, Bleeker GB, Fung JW, et al. Left ventricular reverse remodeling but not clinical improvement predicts long-term survival after cardiac resynchronization therapy. Circulation 2005;112:1580–6.
6. Young JB, Abraham WT, Smith AL. Multicenter Insync ICD Randomized Clinical Evaluation (MIRACLE ICD) Trial Investigators. Combined cardiac resynchronization and Implantable cardioversion defibrillation in advanced chronic heart failure: the MIRACLE ICD trial. JAMA 2003;289:2685–94.
7. St John Sutton MG, Plappert T, Abraham WT, et al. Effect of cardiac resynchronization therapy on left ventricular size and function in chronic heart failure. Circulation 2003;107:1985–90.
8. Auricchio A, Stellbrink C, Block M, et al. Effect of pacing chamber and atrioventricular delay on acute systolic function of paced patients with congestive heart failure: the Pacing Therapies for Congestive Heart Failure Study Group: the Guidant Congestive Heart Failure Research Group. Circulation 1999;99:2993–3001.
9. Kedia N, Ng K, Apperson-Hansen C, et al. Usefulness of atrioventricular delay optimization using Doppler assessment of mitral inflow in patients undergoing cardiac resynchronization therapy. Am J Cardiol 2006; 98:780–5.
10. Porciani MC, Dondina C, Macioce R, et al. Echocardiographic examination of atrioventricular and interventricular delay optimization in cardiac resynchronization therapy. Am J Cardiol 2005;95:1108–10.
11. Ronaszeki A. Hemodynamic consequences of the timing of atrial contraction during complete AV block. Acta Biomed Lovaniensia 1989;15.
12. Faddis MN, Waggoner AD, Sawhney N. AV delay optimization by aortic VTI is superior to the pulsed Doppler mitral inflow method for cardiac resynchronization therapy. Pacing Clin Electrophysiol 2003; 26:1042.
13. Ritter P, Padeletti L, Gillio-Meina L, et al. Determination of the optimal atrioventricular delay in DDD pacing: comparison between echo and peak endocardial acceleration measurements. Europace 1999; 1:126–30.
14. Sawhney NS, Waggoner AD, Garhwal S, et al. Randomized prospective trial of AV delay programming for cardiac resynchronization therapy. Heart Rhythm 2004;1:562–7.

15. O'Donnell D, Nadurata V, Hamer A, Kertes S, Mohammed W. Long term variations in optimal programming of CRT devices. Pacing Clin Electrophysiol 2005;(Suppl 1):S27–30.

16. Mortensen PT, Sogaard P, Mansour H, et al. Sequential biventricular pacing: evaluation of safety and efficacy. Pacing Clin Electrophysiol 2004;27:339–45.

17. Bordachar P, Lafitte S, Reuter S, et al. Echocardiographic parameters of ventricular dyssynchrony validation in patients with heart failure using sequential biventricular pacing. J Am Coll Cardiol 2004;44:2154–65.

18. Van Gelder BM, Bracke FA, Meijer A, Lakerveld LJ, Pijls NH. Effect of optimizing the VV interval on left ventricular contractility in cardiac resynchronization therapy. Am J Cardiol 2004;93:1500–3.

19. Greenberg J, Delurgio DBM, Mera F. Left ventricular lead location in biventricular pacing with variable RV–LV timing does not affect optimal stroke volume. In: North American Society for Pacing and Electrophysiology (NASPE), 2002:151.

20. Sogaard P, Egeblad H, Pedersen AK, et al. Sequential versus simultaneous biventricular resynchronization for severe heart failure: evaluation by tissue Doppler imaging. Circulation 2002;106:2078–84.

21. Willkoff BL, Cook JR, Epstein AE, et al. Dual-chamber pacing or ventricular back-up pacing in patients with an implantable defibrillator; the Dual chamber And VVI Implantable Defibrillator (DAVID) trial. JAMA 2002;288:3115–23.

22. Gorcsan J, Kanzaki H, Bazaz R, Dohi K, Schwartzman D. Usefulness of echocardiographic tissue synchronization imaging to predict acute response to cardiac resynchronization therapy. Am J Cardiol 2004;93: 1178–81.

23. Yu CM, Chau E, Sanderson JE, et al. Tissue Doppler echocardiographic evidence of reverse remodeling and improved synchronicity by simultaneously delaying regional contraction after biventricular pacing therapy in heart failure. Circulation 2002;105:438–45.

24. Yu CM, Lin H, Fung WH, et al. Comparison of acute changes in left ventricular volume, systolic and diastolic functions, and intraventricular synchronicity after biventircular and right ventricular pacing for heart failure. Am Heart J 2003;145:E18.

21

Use of devices with both cardiac resynchronization and cardioverter–defibrillator capabilities

Arthur M Feldman, Reginald T Ho, and Behzad Pavri

Introduction • Clinical studies • Cost of CRT-D devices • Caveats regarding CRT-D therapy • Summary

INTRODUCTION

As detailed in other chapters of this textbook, two unique and distinct devices have been evaluated for the treatment of patients with congestive heart failure: implantable cardioverter–defibrillators (ICD) and cardiac resynchronization devices (CRT). The development of each of these devices was based on a unique hypothesis. In the case of the ICD, investigators hypothesized that because a large number of heart failure patients died suddenly,[1] presumably secondary to a lethal tachy- or bradyarrhythmia, the ability of an implanted device to sense and defibrillate a tachyarrhythmia or to sense and pace a bradyarrhythmia would be beneficial. Alternatively, the observation that nearly 30% of patients with heart failure had dyssynchronous left ventricular (LV) contraction and that cardiac dyssynchrony was associated with worsened ventricular function, increased myocardial oxygen demand, maladaptive ventricular remodeling, and increased mortality[2-5] led investigators to assume that resynchronizing the pattern of ventricular contraction would have salutary benefits. Indeed, these assumptions proved true, as both individual trials[6,7] and meta-analysis have demonstrated salutary benefits of both ICD therapy[8] and CRT[9] in patients with heart failure.

Interestingly, the development of both the ICD and CRT devices was facilitated by similar advances in engineering that provided miniaturization of the required electronics as well as the capacity to both detect and transmit electrical signals across wires that could readily be placed in contact with the ventricular myocardium. Furthermore, the utility of the CRT device was enhanced by the development of techniques and equipment for reaching the LV myocardium via a percutaneous approach through the coronary sinus. Engineers were also able to combine both the technology for biventricular pacing and requisite technology for defibrillation into the same relatively small device, thereby overcoming the problems associated with the device–device interactions that had plagued separately implanted pacemakers and defibrillators. Intuitively, the combination of an ICD and a CRT device seemed logical because each would be expected to interact with different physiologic pathways in the ventricular myocardium and thus provide salutary benefits through different mechanisms. However, the combined use of an ICD and a CRT device has not been without controversy. Indeed, the recent American College of Cardiology/American Heart Association (ACC/AHA) Guidelines note that the balance of risks and benefits of ICD implantation in an individual patient is complex, particularly in patients with advanced heart failure or other comorbidities, in whom the survival benefit obtained with an ICD implantation might not be evident for several years[10-12] or may be overshadowed by competing causes of mortality. Therefore, in this chapter, we will review the available data on the combined use of an ICD and a resynchronization device (CRT-D), address some of the ongoing controversies, including the combined cost of both devices versus the cost of either device alone, and provide some pragmatic recommendations for the use of CRT-D.

CLINICAL STUDIES

InSync

The first prospective multicenter study to evaluate an implantable CRT device was reported in 2002.[13] The InSync study enrolled patients who met indications for implantation of an ICD because of symptomatic sustained ventricular tachycardia (VT) and/or survival of a cardiac arrest. Patients were required to have an LV ejection fraction (LVEF) <35%, an LV end-diastolic diameter >55 mm, and a QRS duration >130 ms. In comparison with baseline measures, the 81 patients in whom the LV lead was successfully implanted demonstrated an improvement in 6-minute walk time, classification of New York Heart Association (NYHA) symptoms, and LV fractional shortening, as well as decreases in both end-systolic and end-diastolic dimensions. Of 81 patients, 26 experienced a total of 472 episodes of spontaneous sustained VT, with all episodes being successfully terminated (with the exception of 16 episodes in a single patient who had incessant VT). Although interpretation of the study was limited because of the lack of a control arm, it was the first to demonstrate in a modest-sized population of heart failure patients that an ICD and a CRT could be used together with favorable clinical outcomes.

CONTAK-CD

The CONTAK-CD study was a double-blind, randomized, controlled study in patients with symptomatic heart failure who also had indications for placement of an ICD.[14] All patients had typical enrollment criteria, including NYHA class II–IV symptoms, an LVEF ≤35%, and a

QRS interval ≥120 ms. Because the patients enrolled in the study had an immediate need for an ICD, the total system was implanted but the patient was not randomized to CRT or no CRT until after a period of at least 30 days. The study began as a crossover study after a period of 3 months, but was then changed to a parallel design because of regulatory concerns. A total of 501 patients were implanted with the device system, although 11% of patients received the device via a transthoracic intervention. Patients were then randomized to either CRT or control for up to 6 months, with the primary endpoint being heart failure progression as defined by the combination of all-cause mortality, hospitalization for heart failure, and VT/ventricular fibrillation (VF) requiring device intervention. Randomization to the active treatment group was associated with a trend towards an improvement in heart failure progression, but, this trend was not statistically significant. However, patients randomized to CRT demonstrated an improvement in functional capacity, a reduction in ventricular size, and an improvement in LV function – but not a change in NYHA symptoms. Patients with NYHA class III and IV symptoms appeared to have the most robust response to CRT. Importantly, there were no differences in the incidence or frequency of ventricular tachyarrhythmias in the two treatment groups, and patients who experienced spontaneous monomorphic VT were successfully treated in 88% of the episodes. Because of the relatively short follow-up period of the trial, investigators could not assess the effect of long-term therapy with CRT-D in this patient population. Nonetheless, it confirmed early studies demonstrating improvements in functional capacity in patients with heart failure, as well as further documenting the safety of combining an ICD with a CRT.

MIRACLE ICD

Similar to CONTAK-CD, the MIRACLE (Multicenter Insync Randomized Clinical Evaluation) ICD trial enrolled patients with LVEF ≤35%, QRS duration ≥130 ms, and a high risk of life-threatening ventricular arrhythmias but who had NYHA class III or IV symptoms.[15]

Patients received a CRT-D device but were randomized to having the CRT turned on or turned off. After 6 months of therapy, patients in whom the CRT was activated demonstrated an improvement in quality-of-life score and in functional class, but showed no difference in the distance walked in six minutes. However, both peak oxygen consumption (VO_{2max}) and exercise duration increased in the CRT group when compared with controls. As was noted in earlier trials, use of the CRT option in the device was not associated with an increase in arrhythmias, nor did it interfere with the ability of the ICD to terminate arrythmias. However, this relatively small study did not demonstrate a change in LV size or function, survival, or rates of hospitalization with CRT.

COMPANION

Because earlier studies had assessed outcomes with CRT or CRT-D over relatively short periods of time and were not powered to assess the effects of either CRT or CRT-D on survival, the COMPANION (Comparison of Medical Therapy, Pacing, and Defibrillation in Chronic Heart Failure) trial was undertaken to assess whether the long-term use of CRT alone or of CRT-D could influence morbidity and mortality in patients with heart failure who remained symptomatic despite optimal medical therapy.[16] COMPANION was an open-label, prospective, multicenter, randomized clinical trial. Patients were randomized to receive optimal pharmacologic therapy, optimal pharmacologic therapy plus CRT, or optimal pharmacologic therapy plus CRT-D. Because of ethical concerns, the randomization ratio was 1:2:2 (i.e., one patient was assigned to the control arm for every four patients assigned to active therapy). The primary endpoint of the trial was the combination of all-cause mortality and all-cause hospitalizations. Patients who received an intravenous inotrope or vasoactive drug in either an emergency room or unscheduled office visit setting were considered to have reached an event endpoint. By definition, the study was designed to compare each of the active treatment arms with optimal pharmacologic therapy – but not to compare CRT with CRT-D.

A total of 1520 patients with NYHA class III or IV heart failure symptoms were enrolled into the COMPANION trial.[16] As with earlier CRT trials, patients had a QRS interval $\geq$120 ms, were predominantly males, and had a mean LVEF of 22%; however, in contrast with earlier studies, nearly 90% of patients were receiving either an angiotensin-converting enzyme (ACE) inhibitor or an angiotensin-receptor blocker, 66% were receiving a beta-blocker, and 55% were being treated with spironolactone. Both CRT alone and CRT-D effected a marked decrease in the risk of patients reaching the primary endpoint (hazard ratio 0.81 for CRT and 0.80 for CRT-D). Furthermore, the risk of the combined endpoint of death from or hospitalization for heart failure was reduced by 34% in the CRT group and by 40% in the CRT-D group (Figure 21.1). There was a trend towards a reduction in the risk of the secondary endpoint of all-cause mortality in the CRT group (24%; $p = 0.059$); however, the combination of a CRT device and an ICD significantly reduced the risk of death by 36% ($p = 0.003$). The salutary benefits of both CRT and CRT-D on the primary and secondary endpoints were not influenced by age, gender, NYHA classification, LVEF, or medical therapy (Figure 21.2). However, there was a suggestion that the benefit of resynchronization therapy was greater in those patients with a wider QRS interval – a finding that was difficult to rely upon because of the limitations of retrospective subgroup analysis. In addition to having a benefit on the primary endpoints of the trial, both CRT and CRT-D effected an improvement in 6-minute walk distance, an increase in quality of life, and an improvement in NYHA class symptoms. Interestingly, the institution of either CRT or CRT-D increased systolic blood pressure over a period of 3 months but had no effect on diastolic blood pressure, thereby supporting the contention that 'resynchronization' could improve cardiovascular inotropy.

The COMPANION trial was criticized because there was a disproportionately higher withdrawal rate in the group that received pharmacologic therapy when compared with the two groups who received devices. This was due in large part to the fact that each of the devices utilized in the study became available

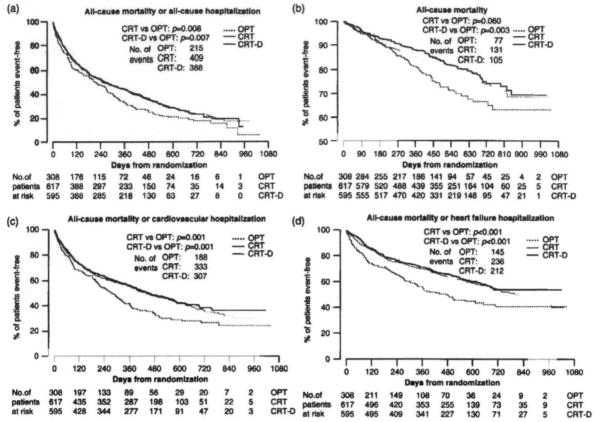

Figure 21.1 Kaplan–Meier curves for various endpoints. (a) Time to death or all-cause hospitalization (primary endpoint). The 12-month event rates for optimal pharmacologic therapy (OPT), OPT plus cardiac resynchronization therapy (CRT), and OPT plus CRT combined with an implantable cardioverter–defibrillator (CRT-D) were 67.8%, 55.4%, and 55.8%, respectively. The median follow-up for OPT, CRT, and CRT-D was 11.7, 16.0, and 15.5 months, respectively. (b) Time to all-cause death. The 12-month event rates for OPT, CRT, and CRT-D were 18.9%, 14.9%, and 12.1%, respectively. The median follow-up for OPT, CRT, and CRT-D was 14.6, 16.3, and 15.8 months, respectively. (c) Time to death or cardiovascular hospitalization. The 12-month event rates for OPT, CRT, and CRT-D were 59.9%, 44.6%, and 43.7%, respectively. (d) Time to death or heart failure hospitalization. The 12-month event rates for OPT, CRT, and CRT-D were 45.3%, 30.5%, and 28.7%, respectively.

commercially during the course of the trial and neither investigators nor patients were blinded to whether the patient did or did not receive a device. To address these concerns, we excluded patients receiving elective implantation of devices from analyses of the primary endpoint and other hospitalization endpoints and obtained 'reconsent' from patients who had withdrawn from the trial to 'cross-over' to a device implantation in order that these patients could be subsequently evaluated to ascertain whether or not they had met a mortality or hospitalization endpoint. By including these patients in the data analyses, we reduced the

potential effect of withdrawal rate on the end-point analyses as well as taking a very conservative approach to the data analyses.

It is notable that the addition of a defibrillator to CRT therapy did not influence the combined outcomes of death from or hospitalization for any cause. However, this endpoint was heavily influenced by the hospitalization endpoint, as approximately 78% of the events were hospitalizations. By contrast, the addition of a defibrillator to CRT incrementally increased the survival benefit over that seen with CRT alone. Although the study design did not allow for a statistical comparison between CRT alone and CRT-D, this

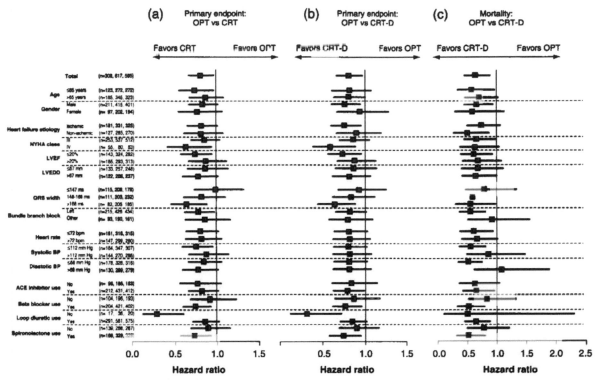

Figure 21.2 Hazard ratios and 95% confidence intervals for subgroup analyses: (a) for mortality or all-cause hospitalization, CRT versus OPT; (b) for mortality or all-cause hospitalization, CRT-D versus OPT; (c) for mortality, CRT-D versus OPT. CRT, cardiac resynchronization therapy; OPT, optimal pharmacologic therapy; CRT-D, CRT with an implantable cardioverter–defibrillator; NYHA, New York Heart Association; LVEF, left ventricular ejection fraction; LVEDD, LV end-diastolic diameter; BP, blood pressure; ACE, angiotensin-converting enzyme.

finding suggests that the addition of the ICD to the CRT device clearly offers beneficial effects in terms of survival. Additional information supporting the hypothesis that CRT-D improves mortality over and above the effects of CRT alone comes from an analysis of the mode of death in patients enrolled in the COMPANION trial.[17] In 78% of patients enrolled in COMPANION, the primary cause of death was cardiac: 44% were due to pump failure and; 26.5% were due to sudden cardiac death. While both CRT and CRT-D tended to reduce pump failure deaths, only CRT-D significantly reduced the number of cardiac deaths by 56%. Therefore, these data supported the concept that the addition of an ICD to a CRT device provided additional benefits – in particular, an improvement in survival. Anecdotal case reports notwithstanding, this large randomized trial provided substantive

evidence that CRT therapy does not increase the risk of ICD shocks.

It was interesting to note that the curves for sudden cardiac death in the COMPANION trial separated later than the pump failure curves. One might expect that the opposite would have occurred, i.e., that the CRT-D device in particular would have had an earlier benefit. Interestingly, this same phenomenon was seen in both the MADIT-II and SCD-HeFT trials.[11,12] Moss et al[18] suggested that this phenomenon was due at least in part to an early preponderance of non-sudden cardiac events in a large population of heart failure patients. This theory fits with the findings of COMPANION, as well as those of CARE-HF.[19] In the latter study, the use of a CRT alone resulted in a marked decrease in mortality, leading some investigators to suggest that patients could be adequately treated with a CRT alone. While this hypothesis is intriguing, a careful assessment of the CARE-HF data suggests otherwise. The primary difference between COMPANION and CARE-HF was that CARE-HF followed patients for over 4 years, in a population that was not as severely ill as that studied in COMPANION. Furthermore, the primary endpoint in COMPANION was assessed at 1 year, whereas the CARE-HF study followed patients for over 4 years. Therefore, when one looks at the survival curves in CARE-HF at 1 year, they closely mirror those seen in COMPANION. Thus, there is overwhelming data to suggest that the combination of a CRT and an ICD provides synergistic and additive benefits over and above the benefits of CRT alone.

COST OF CRT-D DEVICES

One concern regarding the combined use of a CRT and ICD device is the obvious increase in cost. However, we modeled the data from the COMPANION trial to estimate the cost-effectiveness of CRT-D and CRT combined with a pacemaker (CRT-P) relative to optimal pharmacologic therapy over a base-case 7-year treatment episode[20] (Table 21.1). For the first 2 years, follow-up hospitalization costs were based on trial data. However, the model assumed equalization of hospital rates beyond 2 years; i.e., it assumed that neither device provided benefit over and above the time line of the trial. Over 2 years, follow-up hospitalization costs were reduced by 29% for CRT-D and 37% for CRT-P. However, extending the cost-effectiveness analysis to a 7-year base-case time period, the incremental cost-effectiveness ratio for CRT-P was $19 600 per quality-adjusted life-year and the incremental cost-effectiveness ratio for CRT-D was $43 000 per quality-adjusted life-year relative to optimal pharmacologic therapy (Table 21.1). These values are consistent with data obtained from an analysis of eight randomized trials assessing the effectiveness of the prophylactic use of an ICD.[21] The cost per quality-adjusted life-year for CRT-D is quantitatively consistent with the cost of many therapeutic interventions used in patients with cardiovascular disease, including percutaneous coronary intervention with stenting, thrombolytic therapy, and long-term treatment for hypertension. While these cost analyses suggest that the benefits of CRT are economically viable, the societal costs for an innovative therapy must be based on comparisons with cost-effectiveness benchmarks for new technologies and an overall assessment of the impact of the disease on society.[22]

CAVEATS REGARDING CRT-D THERAPY

From a simplistic standpoint, the combination of a CRT device with an ICD is rational. The electrical resynchronization afforded by CRT improves the hemodynamic properties of the heart by synchronizing left and right ventricular contractility. This in turn leads to biological

---

Table 21.1 Summary results of cost-effectiveness analysis of the COMPANION trial

Outcome[a]	CRT-D	CRT-P	OPT
Total cost over 7 years (all-cause readmission)	$75 671	$59 870	$46 021
Years of survival	4.15	3.87	3.37
Quality-adjusted life-years of survival	3.69	3.40	2.83
Incremental cost (versus OPT)	$29 650	$13 849	–
Incremental survival (versus OPT)	0.78	0.49	–
Incremental quality-adjusted life-years gained (versus OPT)	0.84	0.71	–
Incremental cost per life-year gained (versus OPT)	$38 225	$28 061	–
Incremental cost per quality-adjusted life-years gained (versus OPT)	$35 195	$19 557	–

[a] Discounted at 3% per annum.

CRT-D, cardiac resynchronization therapy combined with an implantable cardioverter–defibrillator; CRT-P, CRT combined with a pacemaker; OPT, optimal pharmacologic therapy.

alterations in the myocardial cells and to 'reverse' remodeling. At the same time, the use of an ICD provides protection from lethal ventricular arrhythmias. However, while the COMPANION trial suggests that the combined devices have added effects in terms of decreasing hospitalizations and death, the risks associated with implantation and use of the combined device might also be additive over the long term. For example, the implantation of a CRT-D device carries the same attendant risks associated with implantation of a CRT device: a transvenous success rate of only approximately 90%, requiring that some patients undergo epicardial lead placement; the risk of a perforation or dissection of the coronary sinus; loss of resynchronization over time; inadequate lead placement resulting in a failure to resynchronize; a loss of effective biventricular pacing due to changes in intrinsic electrical conduction; and frequent premature ventricular contractions or rapid ventricular rates during paroxysmal atrial fibrillation that inhibit pacing output.[23] In addition, the implantation of a CRT-D device also carries the unique risks associated with an ICD: larger device size, with increased risk of erosion in cachectic patients; lead malfunctions; fractures in a lead or failure in the insulation, which can cause false signals and inappropriate shocks; changes in medical therapy or defibrillation threshold that result in unnecessary shocks; frequent but appropriate shocks that adversely after cardiac performance as well as causing patient discomfort; and psychological effects associated with shocks.[6]

In addition to the risks associated with both placement and use of a CRT-D device, the use of the combined device in patients with advanced heart failure raises other controversial issues. For example, while patients with advanced heart failure might be anxious to improve their quality of life – something that may be accomplished with a CRT device – they may not be willing to prolong their survival, particularly if this entails receiving a shock. It is probable that defibrillators alter the mode of death (by preventing sudden arrhythmic death, thereby making electromechanical dissociation or pump failure more likely to be the terminal events), which may be a potential concern for some patients.

Alternatively, if a patient feels better by virtue of receiving a CRT, they may decide that they also want to extend their life. As a result, it is virtually impossible to dogmatically identify those patients who are candidates for combined therapy of CRT and ICD, and advanced age, by itself, should not be the only criterion in guiding device selection. Rather, the decision to use a CRT-D device in a given patient should be made only after all of the issues and options have been carefully reviewed with both the patient and their family. Furthermore, the use of a CRT-D device should be carefully considered in patients with comorbidities that would limit their survival. Finally, it should be recognized that implantation does not preclude discontinuation of either the CRT or ICD component of the device and that patients should receive continued counseling and follow-up during the course of their disease and be able to discontinue therapy in the face of changes in their disease status or prognosis.

SUMMARY

In summary, the ability to combine an ICD and a CRT in a single device is a technological breakthrough that provides a new and important option for the treatment of patients with congestive heart failure and cardiac dyssynchrony. As detailed in other chapters of this book, ongoing studies of both the ICD and CRT components will help us to better understand how to best select patients for these two therapeutic interventions individually and how to best choose patients for the combined device. It is likely that, in the future, echocardiographic indices of dyssynchrony will replace QRS duration as selection criteria to decide candidacy for CRT. In addition, both ongoing and future studies will help us to optimize the use of CRT through more selective lead placement and timing.

REFERENCES

1. Uretsky BF, Sheahan RG. Primary prevention of sudden cardiac death in heart failure: will the solution be shocking? J Am Coll Cardiol 1997;30:1589–97.
2. Eriksson P, Hansson PO, Eriksson H, et al. Bundle-branch block in a general male population: the study of men born 1913. Circulation 1998;98:2494–500.

3. Grines CL, Bashore TM, Boudoulas H, et al. Functional abnormalities in isolated left bundle branch block. The effect of interventricular asynchrony. Circulation 1989;79:845–53.

4. Little WC, Reeves RC, Arciniegas J, et al. Mechanism of abnormal interventricular septal motion during delayed left ventricular activation. Circulation 1982;65:1486–91.

5. Baldasseroni S, Opasich C, Gorini M, et al. Left bundle-branch block is associated with increased 1-year sudden and total mortality rate in 5517 outpatients with congestive heart failure: a report from the Italian network on congestive heart failure. Am Heart J 2002;143:398–405.

6. DiMarco JP. Implantable cardioverter–defibrillators. N Engl J Med 2003;349:1836–47.

7. Saxon LA, Ellenbogen KA. Resynchronization therapy for the treatment of heart failure. Circulation 2003;108:1044–8.

8. Nanthakumar K, Epstein AE, Kay GN, et al. Prophylactic implantable cardioverter–defibrillator therapy in patients with left ventricular systolic dysfunction: a pooled analysis of 10 primary prevention trials. J Am Coll Cardiol 2004;44:2166–72.

9. Bradley DJ, Bradley EA, Baughman KL, et al. Cardiac resynchronization and death from progressive heart failure: a meta-analysis of randomized controlled trials. JAMA 2003;289:730–40.

10. Hunt SA. ACC/AHA 2005 Guideline Update for the Diagnosis and Management of Chronic Heart Failure in the Adult: a report of the American College of Cardiology/American Heart Association Task Force on Practice Guidelines (Writing Committee to Update the 2001 Guidelines for the Evaluation and Management of Heart Failure). J Am Coll Cardiol 2005;46:e1–82.

11. Bardy GH, Lee KL, Mark DB, et al. Amiodarone or an implantable cardioverter–defibrillator for congestive heart failure. N Engl J Med 2005;352:225–37.

12. Moss AJ, Zareba W, Hall WJ, et al. Multicenter Automatic Defibrillator Implantation Trial II Investigators. Prophylactic implantation of a defibrillator in patients with myocardial infarction and reduced ejection fraction. N Engl J Med 2002;346:877–83.

13. Kuhlkamp V. Initial experience with an implantable cardioverter–defibrillator incorporating cardiac resynchronization therapy. J Am Coll Cardiol 2002; 39:790–7.

14. Higgins SL, Hummel JD, Niazi IK, et al. Cardiac resynchronization therapy for the treatment of heart failure in patients with intraventricular conduction delay and malignant ventricular tachyarrhythmias. J Am Coll Cardiol 2003;42:1454–9.

15. Young JB, Abraham WT, Smith AL, et al. Combined cardiac resynchronization and implantable cardioversion defibrillation in advanced chronic heart failure: the MIRACLE ICD trial. JAMA 2003;289:2685–94.

16. Bristow MR, Saxon LA, Boehmer J, et al. Cardiac-resynchronization therapy with or without an implantable defibrillator in advanced chronic heart failure. N Engl J Med 2004;350:2140–50.

17. Carson P, Anand I, O'Connor C, et al. Mode of death in advanced heart failure: the Comparison of Medical, Pacing, and Defibrillation Therapies in Heart Failure (COMPANION) trial. J Am Coll Cardiol 2005;46:2329–34.

18. Moss AJ, Vyas A, Greenberg H, et al. MADIT-II Research Group. Temporal aspects of improved survival with the implanted defibrillator (MADIT-II). Am J Cardiol 2004;94:312–15.

19. Cleland JG, Daubert JC, Erdmann E, et al. The effect of cardiac resynchronization on morbidity and mortality in heart failure. N Engl J Med 2005;352:1539–49.

20. Feldman AM, de Lissovoy G, Bristow MR, et al. Cost effectiveness of cardiac resynchronization therapy in the Comparison of Medical Therapy, Pacing, and Defibrillation in Heart Failure (COMPANION) trial. J Am Coll Cardiol 2005;46:2311–21.

21. Sanders GD, Hlatky MA, Owens DK. Cost-effectiveness of implantable cardioverter–defibrillators. N Engl J Med 2005;353:1471–80.

22. Mark DB, Hlatky MA. Medical economics and the assessment of value in cardiovascular medicine: Part II. Circulation 2002;106:626–30.

23. Abraham WT, Hayes DL. Cardiac resynchronization therapy for heart failure. Circulation 2003;108:2596–603.

Efficacy of cardiac resynchronization therapy in atrial fibrillation

Cecilia Linde

Introduction • Acute studies • Long-term studies • Studies with patient inclusion mainly due to atrial fibrillation • CRT impact on reverse remodeling, morbidity and mortality, and the importance of AV junction ablation • Conclusions

INTRODUCTION

In the last few years, controlled crossover trials and parallel comparisons of cardiac resynchronization therapy (CRT) with control treatment have convincingly demonstrated symptomatic improvement in patients with severe heart failure and intraventricular conduction disturbances.[1-5] Importantly, two trials[6,7] showed a reduced need for hospitalization and one[7] a reduced total mortality with CRT compared with control treatment. All trials almost exclusively included patients in sinus rhythm.

The prevalence of atrial fibrillation in severe heart failure is substantial (16–21%), as indicated by the CIBIS II[8] and MERIT HF[9] studies. Atrial fibrillation in heart failure becomes more prevalent with time, reflecting remodelling of both the left ventricle (LV) and left atrium (LA) and thus the severity of the underlying heart disease. There is a broad consensus about the negative effect of atrial fibrillation on hemodynamics, whereas its impact on prognosis remains controversial.[10] A clear survival disadvantage in combination with left bundle branch block (LBBB) was demonstrated by Baldasseroni et al.[11] Therefore, atrial fibrillation patients are probably worse off in terms of both prognosis and hemodynamics. These circumstances indicate

that this patient group could be in even greater need of supplementary device therapy such as CRT than patients in sinus rhythm. Although the evidence for the efficacy of CRT is in patients in sinus rhythm, there is also some evidence from acute hemodynamic and long-term studies that atrial fibrillation patients may also benefit from CRT.

ACUTE STUDIES

Blanc et al[12] demonstrated an acute hemodynamic benefit of LV-based pacing in 23 patients, 6 of whom were in atrial fibrillation. These observations were confirmed in a similar study by Etienne et al[13] comprising 10 atrial fibrillation and 17 sinus rhythm patients. In this study, LV pacing and biventricular pacing provided the same benefit concerning pulmonary capillary wedge pressure, systolic blood pressure, and mitral incompetence, irrespective of whether patients were in sinus rhythm or atrial fibrillation. These observations indicate that ventricular resynchronization, rather than atrioventricular (AV)-synchrony, explained the acute hemodynamic benefits. However, it is not self-evident that acute hemodynamic improvements imply a long-term benefit.

The first early non-randomized study of CRT included atrial fibrillation patients.[14] In this

French pilot study, a beneficial effect by biventricular pacing was observed in 14 atrial fibrillation patients followed for a mean of 15 months.

LONG-TERM STUDIES

The MUSTIC study is the only controlled study that has included heart failure patients with atrial fibrillation.[1-3] Patients were included if they had severe New York Heart Association (NYHA) class III heart failure in stable condition for at least 1 month and if they were on optimal medical treatment including angiotensin-converting enzyme (ACE) inhibitors and diuretics. The LV ejection fraction (LVEF) had to be below 35% and the LV end-diastolic diameter (LVEDD) > 60 mm. All patients had to have persistent (> 3 months) atrial fibrillation requiring a permanent pacemaker due to slow ventricular rhythm, either spontaneously or induced by bundle of His ablation. The paced QRS duration had to be > 20 ms. A 6-week (non-ablated patients) to 12-week (ablated patients) observation period in right ventricular (RV) ventricular inhibited rate-adaptive (VVIR) pacing was performed to verify stability of the heart failure condition and to allow for reversal of any tachycardia-induced cardiomyopathy. The study began with a single-blind crossover comparison of 3 months each of biventricular pacing and RV-VVIR pacing, both at a basic rate of 70 bpm. Following the end of the crossover phases, patients were programmed according to their preferred study period and followed every 3 months for another 6 months. Patient characteristics are presented in Table 22.1.

Sixty-three percent of patients had undergone AV junction ablation. After the crossover phase, four of the patients preferred to be programmed to RV VVIR pacing, while the rest preferred biventricular pacing. Forty-one patients completed the crossover period and 33 patients the 12-month follow up. The clinical results were not as good as for the sinus rhythm patients in the MUSTIC study. Results from patients in sinus rhythm and in atrial fibrillation are presented in Tables 22.2 and 22.3. At 1 year significant symptomatic improvements were seen in both groups of patients. In a long-term follow up, Leclercq et al[15] demonstrated that the benefits observed at 1 year were maintained in the 26 patients completing a 2-year follow-up. In the MUSTIC study, hospitalizations for heart failure were three times less during biventricular pacing than during RV-VVIR pacing for the atrial fibrillation group.

Over the duration of the MUSTIC study, the magnitudes of improvements in the sinus rhythm group were overall more impressive than for the atrial fibrillation group. There are a multitude of possible explanations for this finding. Among these are the high dropout rate in the MUSTIC study (attributed to events in the long run-in period) and the heterogeneity of the atrial fibrillation group. Moreover, the potentially harmful effect of RV pacing during the run-in could have contributed. Finally, to treat atrial fibrillation patients with biventricular pacing requires complete rate control in order to prevent intrinsic rhythm obviating biventricular stimulation. In fact, two patients in the MUSTIC study were not paced due to insufficient rate control. Moreover, the paced QRS duration during biventricular stimulation was in fact longer in the atrial fibrillation group (170 ms) compared with the sinus rhythm group (156 ms). This could indicate that a lesser degree of ventricular synchronization was obtained in the atrial fibrillation group.

Leon et al[16] studied 20 consecutive patients with chronic atrial fibrillation and NYHA class III–IV, with LVEF < 35%. They all had prior AV junction ablation and RV pacing for a mean of 26.4 months (Table 22.4). Patients were upgraded from RV pacing to CRT and followed for 6 months. In this non-randomized trial,

---

Table 22.1 Baseline characteristics in the MUSTIC atrial fibrillation group (64 patients)[2,3]

Mean age	65 ± 9 years
Sex: M/F	52/12 (81%/19%)
NYHA class III	64 (100%)
Ischemic/non-ischemic	17/47 (27%/73%)
LVEF	26% ± 10%
LVEDD	68 ± 7 mm
QRS duration	206 ± 19 ms

NYHA, New York Heart Association; LVEF, left ventricular ejection fraction; LVEDD, LV end-diastolic diameter.

Table 22.2 Evolution of the 6-minute walk distance, peak oxygen consumption (VO$_{2max}$), quality of life (QoL), and NYHA class at 6, 9 and 12 months in the MUSTIC study sinus rhythm and atrial fibrillation groups[3]

	Randomization	6 months	9 months	12 months
Sinus rhythm group				
6-min walk distance (m)	354 ± 82 (*n*=43)	396 ± 104 (*n*=43)	411 ± 113 (*n*=38)	418 ± 112 (*n*=38)
	346 ± 96 (*n*=38)			*p*=0.0001
	348 ± 98 (*n*=38)			
VO$_{2max}$ (ml/kg/min)	14.2 ± 4.6 (*n*=41)	15.5 ± 4.6 (*n*=41)	NA	16.6 ± 3.6 (*n*=32)
	14.9 ± 4.7 (*n*=32)			*p*=NS
Minnesota QoL score	47 ± 22 (*n*=46)	31 ± 22 (*n*=46)	30 ± 20 (*n*=41)	30 ± 22 (*n*=41)
(0–105)	45 ± 21 (*n*=41)			*p*=0.0001
	47 ± 23 (*n*=41)			
NYHA class (I–IV)	2.8 ± 0.4 (*n*=46)	2.1 ± 0.5 (*n*=46)	2.1 ± 0.4 (*n*=40)	2.1 ± 0.5 (*n*=41)
	2.8 ± 0.4 (*n*=40)			*p*=0.0001
	2.8 ± 0.4 (n=41)			
Atrial fibrillation group				
6-min walk distance (m)	338 ± 87 (*n*=37)	363 ± 101 (*n*=37)	368 ± 97 (*n*=27)	370 ± 87 (*n*=27)
	320 ± 82 (*n*=27)			*p*=0.004
	315 ± 80 (*n*=27)			
VO$_{2max}$ (ml/kg/min)	12.8 ± 4.7 (*n*=37)	14.3 ± 4.1 (*n*=37)	NA	13.9 ± 3.5 (*n*=24)
	12.8 ± 3.6 (*n*=24)			*p*=NS
Minnesota QoL score	44 ± 22 (*n*=40)	34 ± 20 (*n*=40)	34 ± 22 (*n*=31)	31 ± 17 (*n*=28)
(0–105)	45 ± 22 (*n*=31)			*p*=0.0002
	45 ± 23 (*n*=28)			
NYHA class (I–IV)	3.0 ± 0 (*n*=38)	2.3 ± 0.5 (*n*=38)	2.1 ± 0.4 (*n*=29)	2.2 ± 0.5 (*n*=28)
	3.0 ± 0 (*n*=29)			*p*=0.0001
	3.0 ± 0 (*n*=28)			

NA, not applicable; NS, not significant (p > 0.0125 Bonferroni adjustment); NYHA, New York Heart Association.

significant 6-month improvements in NYHA class and quality of life were found by CRT (Figure 22.1). There was evidence of LV reverse remodeling, with a mean absolute improvement in LVEF of 9.4% and a decrease in LV dimensions by an absolute mean value of 4.5 mm for LVEDD and 4.8 mm for LV end-systolic diameter (LVESV) (Figure 22.2). Importantly, hospital admissions 1 year before upgrading compared with 1 year after were also significantly reduced (Figure 22.3).

In an observational study, Dorszewski et al[17] compared 1-year outcome between 69 patients with atrial fibrillation and 450 patients in sinus rhythm given CRT due to NYHA class II–III heart failure, LVEF < 30%, and QRS > 150 ms. The patients in atrial fibrillation were on medication for rate control to avoid intrinsic rate, but had not undergone AV junction ablation. At baseline, there were no significant differences in sex or age distribution or in underlying heart disease between patients in atrial fibrillation compared with those in sinus rhythm (Table 22.5). The results are reported in Figure 22.4. The NYHA class, 6-minute walk distance, and peak oxygen consumption (VO$_{2max}$) increased significantly in both the atrial fibrillation and sinus rhythm groups. In contrast, there was no evidence of reverse LV remodeling in the atrial fibrillation group compared with the sinus rhythm group. The incidence of severe cardiac events such as need for heart transplantation or death did not differ between groups.

Table 22.3 Echocardiographic data and ejection fraction at 6, 9 and 12 months in the MUSTIC sinus rhythm and atrial fibrillation groups

	Randomization	6 months	9 months	12 months
Sinus rhythm group				
LVEDD (mm)	74 ± 9 (*n*=46) 73 ± 9 (*n*=42) 74 ± 10 (*n*=40)	69 ± 11 (*n*=46)	68 ± 10 (*n*=42)	67 ± 12 (*n*=40)
LVESD (mm)	64 ± 10 (*n*=46) 64 ± 10 (*n*=42) 63 ± 10 (*n*=40)	58 ± 12 (*n*=46)	57 ± 11 (*n*=42)	58 ± 12 (*n*=40)
MR area (cm^2)	7.4 ± 6.8 (*n*=44) 8.0 ± 7.8 (*n*=39) 7.8 ± 7.8 (*n*=39)	5.6 ± 8.3 (*n*=44)	4.9 ± 4.6 (*n*=39)	4.3 ± 4.0 (*n*=39)
DFT (ms)	376 ± 134 (*n*=44) 372 ± 132 (*n*=42) 375 ± 136 (*n*=40)	430 ± 137 (*n*=44)	471 ± 154 (*n*=42)	425 ± 129 (*n*=40)
LVEF (%) radionuclides	24.5 ± 7.8 (*n*=26)	NA	NA	30.0 ± 12.1 (*n*=26)
Cardiothoracic ratio	0.60 ± 0.07 (*n*=41) 0.59 ± 0.07 (*n*=34) 0.60 ± 0.07 (*n*=36)	0.60 ± 0.07 (*n*=41)	0.56 ± 0.06 (*n*=34)	0.56 ± 0.06 (*n*=36)
Atrial fibrillation group				
LVEDD (mm)	69 ± 8 (*n*=28) 70 ± 9 (*n*=28)	NA	68 ± 10 (*n*=28)	68 ± 8 (*n*=28)
LVESD (mm)	59 ± 9 (*n*=28) 60 ± 10 (*n*=28)	NA	56 ± 11 (*n*=28)	58 ± 9 (*n*=28)
MR area (cm^2)	10.2 ± 13.7 (*n*=27) 10.8 ± 13.7 (*n*=26)	NA	6.4 ± 6.2 (*n*=27)	5.4 ± 3.4 (*n*=26)
DFT (ms)	349 ± 95 (*n*=27) 346 ± 99 (*n*=24)	NA	357 ± 133 (*n*=27)	405 ± 143 (*n*=24)
LVEF (%) radionuclides	26.7 ± 6.9 (*n*=19)	NA	NA	30.4 ± 7.8 (*n*=19)
Cardiothoracic ratio	0.61 ± 0.07 (*n*=36) 0.61 ± 0.07 (*n*=26) 0.61 ± 0.07 (*n*=27)	0.60 ± 0.07 (*n*=36)	0.60 ± 0.06 (*n*=26)	0.60 ± 0.07 (*n*=27)

DFT, diastolic filling time; LVEDD, left ventricular end-diastolic diameter; LVEF, LV ejection fraction; LVESD, LV end-systolic diameter; MR, mitral regurgitation; NA, not applicable.

STUDIES WITH PATIENT INCLUSION MAINLY DUE TO ATRIAL FIBRILLATION

Two small trials, OPSITE and PAVE, focused primarily on patients with atrial fibrillation[18,19] scheduled to undergo AV nodal ablation. Only a subset of patients in both trials had LV dysfunction and some were in NYHA class II–III heart failure. The results of both trials remain inconclusive regarding the primary endpoint. Therefore, the usefulness of CRT remains to be demonstrated in atrial fibrillation patients with or without heart failure in prospective randomized trials.

CRT IMPACT ON REVERSE REMODELING, MORBIDITY AND MORTALITY, AND THE IMPORTANCE OF AV JUNCTION ABLATION

The results of CRT treatment on reverse remodeling in patients with atrial fibrillation are controversial.[3,16,17] In a 1-year follow-up of the MUSTIC trial, Linde et al[3] reported significant reverse LV remodeling in the sinus rhythm patients. For patients in atrial fibrillation, reverse remodeling did not include LV dimensions and was restricted to improvements in LVEF, mitral regurgitation, and diastolic filling time (Table 22.3). These findings are in agreement with the German data[17] in

Table 22.4 Patient baseline characteristics in the study by Leon et al[17]

Age	69.9 ± 10.8 years
Gender: M/F	17/3
Duration of RV pacing	26.4 ± 12.2 months
Causes of CHF:	
Ischemic	11 (55%)
Idiopathic	5 (25%)
Hypertension	3 (15%)
Valvular	1 (5%)
Baseline medications:	
ACE inhibitor/receptor blocker	18 (90%)
Beta-blocker	5 (25%)
Diuretic	19 (95%)
Digoxin	12 (60%)
NYHA functional class:	
III	12 (60%)
IV	8 (40%)
Minnesota QoL score (0–105)	77.8 ± 23.6
Hospitalizations	1.9 ± 0.8
(1 year before BiVP)	
QRS width	213 ± 40 ms
LVEF	21.5% ± 6.9%
LVEDD	67.9 ± 8.3 mm
LVESD	56.3 ± 9.8 mm

ACE, angiotensin-converting enzyme; BiVP, biventricular pacing; CHF, congestive heart failure; LVEDD, left ventricular end-diastolic dimension; LVEF, LV ejection fraction; LVESD, LV end-systolic dimension; NYHA, New York Heart Association; RV, right ventricular.

which no signs of reverse LV remodeling were found, in spite of clinical improvement. In contrast, Leon et al[16] demonstrated significant reverse remodeling regarding both LV dimensions and LVEF (Figure 22.2). Gasparini et al[20] prospectively evaluated the long-term improvement due to CRT in 511 patients in sinus rhythm and 162 in permanent atrial fibrillation, 48 of whom had been subject to AV junction ablation. Reverse remodeling was as large in sinus rhythm and ablated atrial fibrillation patients, but was absent in non-ablated atrial fibrillation patients.

Early reports suggested that CRT could reduce the incidence of atrial fibrillation,[21] possibly by reversing left atrial (LA) remodelling.[22] However, in the larger CARE-HF trial, no such effect was shown. In CARE-HF, the development of atrial fibrillation was associated with a worse prognosis in both treatment groups.[23] In the CRT group, this was somewhat counterbalanced by the CRT treatment, meaning that control patients with atrial fibrillation had the worse outcome.

The impact of CRT on survival in heart failure patients with atrial fibrillation remains to be proven in randomized controlled trials. Neither the COMPANION nor the CARE-HF study included patients in atrial fibrillation. The 2-year

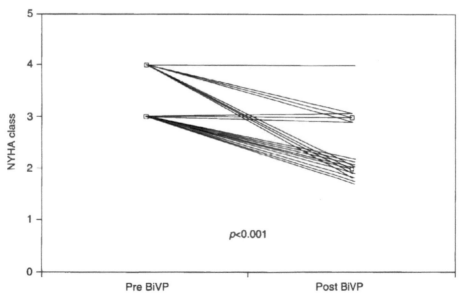

Figure 22.1 Results with regard to NYHA class from 1 year of CRT in patients upgraded from long-term right ventricular to biventricular pacing (BiVP). (Reproduced from Leon AR et al. J Am Coll Cardiol 2002;39:1258-63.[16])

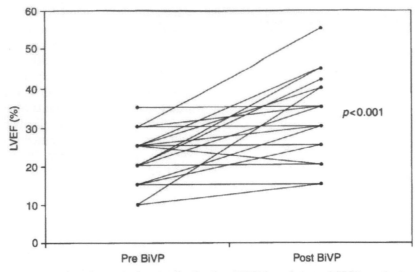

Figure 22.2 Results with regard to left ventricular ejection fraction (LVEF) from 1 year of CRT in patients upgraded from long-term right ventricular to biventricular pacing (BiVP). (Reproduced from Leon AR et al. J Am Coll Cardiol 2002;39:1258–63.[16])

survival curves from the MUSTIC study do not indicate any worse survival rate in the atrial fibrillation group compared with the sinus rhythm group, with a mean annual survival rate of 95.7% at 1 year and 82.6% at 2 years in the atrial fibrillation group and 87.9% at 1 year and 77.6% at 2 years in the sinus rhythm group.[24]

In contrast, Tolosana et al[25] reported a worse 12-month mortality during CRT in 31 patients with atrial fibrillation compared with 100 in sinus rhythm, despite otherwise favorable results of CRT, with 19% deaths due to heart failure in the atrial fibrillation group compared with 6% in the sinus rhythm group ($p = 0.019$). In the

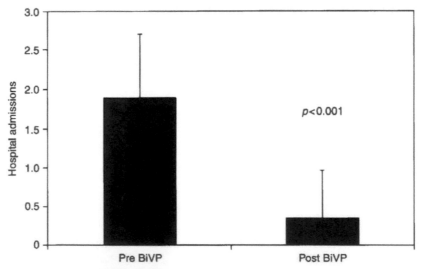

Figure 22.3 Results with regard to hospital admissions from 1 year of CRT in patients upgraded from long-term right ventricular to biventricular pacing (BiVP). (Reproduced from Leon AR et al. J Am Coll Cardiol 2002;39:1258–63.[16])

Table 22.5 Baseline characteristics in the study by Dorszewski et al[17]

Clinical characteristics	Atrial fibrillation (n = 69)	Sinus rhythm (n = 450)
Mean age (years)	62 ± 10	62 ± 11
Sex: M/F	54/15 (78%/22%)	343/107 (76%/24%)
NYHA class	3.1 ± 0.4	3.0 ± 0.4 (p < 0.05)
Non-ischemic etiology (%)	43	56
LVEF (%)	25 ± 8	24 ± 7
LVEDD (mm)	76 ± 9	78 ± 11
QRS duration (ms)	181 ± 37	183 ± 29

NYHA, New York Heart Association; LVEF, left ventricular ejection fraction; LVEDD, LV end-diastolic diameter.

MUSTIC atrial fibrillation group[31] and the study by Leon et al[16], CRT led to a clear reduction in hospital admissions.

In a recent open-label study, Gasparini et al[26] compared 4-year survival in 243 heart failure patients in atrial fibrillation with regard to whether or not they had been subject to AV nodal ablation. The yearly mortality rate was significantly better in the 118 ablated patients (4.3% per year) compared with the 125 non-ablated patients (15.2% per year) (p < 0.001). The existing evidence thus strongly suggests that CRT be combined with AV junction ablation in patients with atrial fibrillation.

CONCLUSIONS

Randomized studies of CRT to date have been almost exclusively restricted to patients in sinus rhythm. The prevalence of atrial fibrillation in patients with moderate to severe congestive heart failure is high, varying between 25% and 50%. This high prevalence contrasts with the low percentage (2%) of patients with atrial fibrillation, enrolled in randomized trials of CRT. Therefore, we have little knowledge of the clinical value of CRT in this population. The reasons for this lack of information are various. Patients suffering from heart failure, atrial fibrillation, and ventricular dyssynchrony are typically older and have a higher prevalence of associated illnesses, and a worse prognosis than patients in sinus rhythm. Outcomes are more difficult to measure, since both heart rate control and CRT may contribute to the observed changes in clinical status. Although the number of patients with atrial fibrillation participating

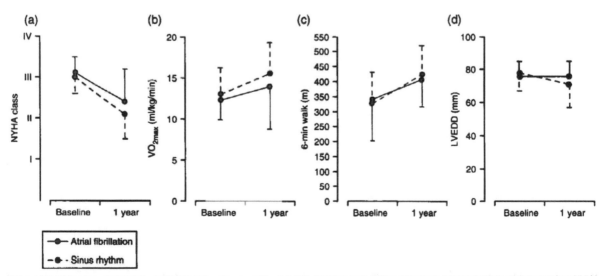

Figure 22.4 The 1-year results of CRT in 69 patients with atrial fibrillation and 450 patients in sinus rhythm with regard to NYHA class (a), peak oxygen consumption (VO_{2max}), (b), 6-minute walk distance (c), and left ventricular end-diastolic diameter (LVEDD) (d), in an open study by Dorszewksi et al.[17])

in studies of CRT so far has been small, the available evidence suggests that this treatment could be beneficial in these patients. AV junction ablation appears to be of crucial importance to ensure therapy delivery and clinical improvements.

Additional larger and better-designed studies are urgently needed in this area. In order to avoid confounding factors such as tachycardia-induced cardiomyopathy related to atrial fibrillation, studies need to focus on patients selected primarily on the basis of congestive heart failure and not for treatment of atrial fibrillation.

ACKNOWLEDGMENTS

This work was supported by the Swedish Heart and Lung Association.

REFERENCES

1. Cazeau S, Leclercq C, Lavergne T, et al, for the Multisite Stimulation in Cardiomyopathy. Effects of multisite biventricular pacing in patients with heart failure and intraventricular conduction delay. N Engl J Med 2001;12:873–80.

2. Leclercq C, Walker S, Linde C, et al. Comparative effects of permanent biventricular and right univentricular pacing in heart failure patients with chronic atrial fibrillation. Eur Heart J 2001;23:1780–7.

3. Linde C, Leclercq C, Rex S, et al. Long-term benefits of biventricular pacing in congestive heart failure. Results from the MUSTIC (Multisite Stimulation in Cardiomyopathy) study. J Am Coll Cardiol 2002;40: 111–18.

4. Auricchio A, Stellbrink C, Sack S, et al. Chronic effects of hemodynamically optimised cardiac resynchronisation therapy on patients with heart failure and ventricular conduction delay. J Am Coll Cardiol 2002;39:2026–33.

5. Abraham WT, Fisher WG, Smith AL, et al, for the Miracle Investigators and Coordinators. Multicentre InSync Randomized Clinical Evaluation (MIRACLE). Results of a randomized, double blind, controlled trial to assess cardiac resynchronisation therapy in heart failure patients. J Am Coll Cardiol 2001;38:595–6.

6. Bristow MR, Saxon KA, Boehmer J, et al, for the Comparison of Medical Therapy Pacing and Defibrillation in Heart Failure (COMPANION) Investigators. Cardiac resynchronization therapy with and without an implantable defibrillator in advanced chronic heart failure. N Engl J Med 2004;350:2140–50.

7. Cleland JGF, Daubert JC, Erdmann E, et al, for the Cardiac Resynchronization – Heart Failure (CARE-HF) Study Investigators. The effect of cardiac resynchronisation on morbidity and mortality in heart failure. N Engl J Med 2005;352:1539–49.

8. The CIBIS II Investigators and Committees. The Cardiac Insufficiency Bisoprolol Study II (CIBIS II): a randomised trial. Lancet 1999;353:9–13.

9. MERIT-HF Study Group. Effects of metoprolol CR/XL in chronic heart failure: Metoprolol CR/XL Randomised Intervention Trial in Congestive Heart Failure (MERIT.HF). Lancet 1999;353:2001–7.

10. Middlekauff HR, Stevenson WG, Stevenson LW. Prognostic significance of atrial fibrillation in advanced heart failure. Circulation 1991;84:40–8.

11. Baldasseroni S, de Biase L, Fresco C, et al, on behalf of the Italian Network on Congestive Heart Failure (IN-CHF) Investigators. Cumulative effect of complete left bundle branch block and chronical atrial fibrillation on 1-year mortality and hospitalisation in patients with congestive heart failure. Eur Heart J 2002;23: 1692–8.

12. Blanc JJ, Etienne Y, Gilard M, et al. Evaluation of different ventricular pacing sites in patients with severe heart failure. Circulation 1997;96:3273–7.

13. Etienne Y, Mansourati J, Gilard M. Evaluation of left ventricular based pacing in patients with congestive heart failure and atrial fibrillation. Am J Cardiol 1999; 83:1138–40.

14. Leclercq C, Cazeau S, Ritter P, et al. A pilot experience with permanent biventricular pacing to treat advanced heart failure. Am Heart J 2000;140:862–70.

15. Leclercq C, Linde C, Cazeau S, et al. Long term (2 years) clinical results of permanent biventricular pacing in patients with advanced heart failure and chronic atrial fibrillation: results from the MUSTIC trial. Pacing Clin Electrophysiol 2002;24:716 (abst).

16. Leon AR, Greenberg JM, Kanuro N, et al. Cardiac resynchronisation in patients with congestive heart failure and chronic atrial fibrillation. J Am Coll Cardiol 2002;39:1258–63.

17. Dorszewski A, Lamp B, Heintze J, et al. Long term outcome of cardiac resynchronisation therapy in patients with atrial fibrillation without AV-nodal ablation compared to sinus rhythm. Heart Rhythm 2006;3(Suppl):S292(abst).

18. Brignole F, Gammage M, Puggioni E, et al. Comparative assessment of right, left, and biventricular pacing in patients with permanent atrial fibrillation. Eur Heart J 2005;7:712–22.

19. Doshi RN, Daoud EG, Fellows C, et al; PAVE Study Group. Left ventricular-based cardiac stimulation post AV nodal ablation evaluation (the PAVE study). J Cardiovasc Electrophysiol 2005;16:1160–5.

20. Gasparini M, Auricchio A, Regoli F, et al. Four-year efficacy of cardiac resynchronization therapy on exercise tolerance and disease progression the importance of performing atrioventricular junction ablation in patients with atrial fibrillation. J Am Coll Cardiol 2006;48:734–43.

21. Fung JW, Yu CM, Chan JY, et al. Effect of cardiac resynchronization therapy on incidence of atrial fibrillation in patients with poor left ventricular systolic function. Am J Cardiol 2005;96:728–31.

22. Saxon LA, DeMarco T, Schafer J, et al. VIGOR Congestive Heart Failure Investigators. Effect of long term biventricular stimulation for resynchronization on echocardiographic measures of remodelling. Circulation 2002;105:1304–10.

23. Hoppe UC, Casares J, Eiskjer H, et al. Effect of cardiac resynchronization on the incidence of atrial fibrillation in patients with severe heart failure. J Am Coll Cardiol 2006;47:77A.

24. Daubert C, Linde C, Cazeau S, et al. Mortality in patients included in the MUSTIC study: long term (> 2 years) follow up. Pacing Clin Electrophysiol 2002; 24:558 (abst).

25. Tolosana JM, Macias A, Diaz Infante E, et al. High mortality in patients with permanent atrial fibrillation in spite of benefits of resynchronisation therapy. Heart Rhythm 2006;3(Suppl):s290(abst).

26. Gasparini M, Auricchio A, Lamp B, et al. Four year survival in 1285 patients undergoing cardiac resynchronisation therapy (CRT. The importance of atrioventricular junction ablation in patients with atrial fibrillation. Eur Heart J 2006;27(Suppl):25 (abst).

Cardiac resynchronization therapy in patients with an indication for permanent pacing for atrioventricular block or symptomatic bradycardia

Gustavo Lopera and Anne B Curtis

Introduction • Effects of chronic RV pacing: lessons from clinical trials • Selection of pacing mode in specific patient groups: To pace or not to pace? • Future perspectives in device therapy

INTRODUCTION

Cardiac pacing remains the only effective treatment for patients with symptomatic bradycardia due to sinus node dysfunction (SND) or atrioventricular block (AVB). However, the optimal pacing mode for these patients is still debated.

Right ventricular (RV) pacing, which is a form of iatrogenic left bundle branch block (LBBB), causes an altered electrical activation sequence with a significant delay between the onset of left ventricular (LV) and RV activation, contraction, and relaxation, resulting in ventricular dyssynchrony (Figure 23.1).[1,2] While most patients with permanent pacemakers appear to tolerate RV pacing well, induction of ventricular dyssynchrony by RV pacing may have adverse consequences that have only recently been appreciated. The result has been that clinicians have begun to rethink the way we approach permanent pacing in patients who have symptomatic bradycardia or atrioventricular (AV) block.

EFFECTS OF CHRONIC RV PACING: LESSONS FROM CLINICAL TRIALS

Chronic RV pacing has been associated with a higher incidence of heart failure and atrial fibrillation (AF) than atrial-based pacing modalities.[3-5]

In the MOST trial, 2010 patients with SND were randomized to single-chamber ventricular (VVI) pacing versus dual-chamber (DDD) pacing. The primary endpoint was overall mortality and non-fatal stroke. The mean follow-up was 33.1 months. The cumulative percentage of ventricular pacing (Cum% VP), rather than the specific pacing mode, was a strong predictor of heart failure hospitalization and AF. A Cum% VP >40% conferred a 2.6-fold increased risk of heart failure hospitalization in the DDD group compared with a lower percentage of pacing in similar patients. Similarly, the risk of AF was increased by about 1% for each 1% increase in Cum% VP in both pacing modalities (Figure 23.2).[3,4]

Andersen et al[5] randomized 225 patients with SND to single-chamber atrial (AAI) pacing or VVI pacing. During an 8-year follow-up period, atrial pacing was associated with significantly higher survival, less AF, less heart failure, and fewer thromboembolic complications. VVI pacing was associated with a significant increase in LV end-systolic diameter (LVESD) and dilatation of the left atrium (LA).[6] These findings also appeared to be time-dependent, since during the initial 3 years of follow-up, no significant changes in mortality or heart failure were observed.[7]

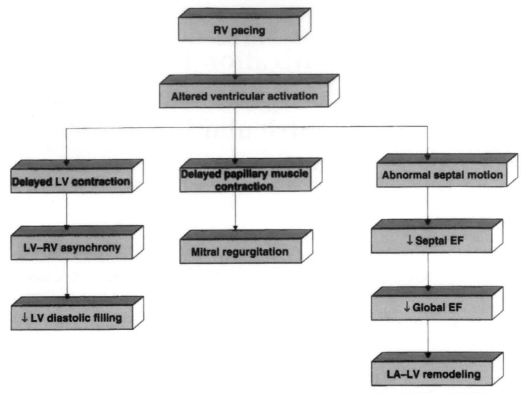

Figure 23.1 Detrimental effects of chronic right ventricular (RV) pacing. EF, ejection fraction; LA, left atrial; LV, left ventricular.

These findings could be explained by the asynchronous ventricular contraction caused by chronic RV pacing, suggesting that such pacing should be minimized in patients with SND and preserved intrinsic AV conduction.

Other prospective randomized clinical trials comparing DDD pacing and VVI pacing in patients with SND and AVB have only shown modest or negligible benefits on survival, heart failure, and AF.[8-10] These differences could be explained by a lack of detailed analysis of Cum% VP in the DDD group as compared with the VVI group. The lack of significant clinical benefit was observed despite the fact that AV synchrony was restored in the DDD group, suggesting that ventricular dyssynchrony induced by RV pacing may offset the benefits of preservation of AV synchrony with DDD pacing.

The effects of ventricular dyssynchrony induced by RV pacing may be more dramatic in patients with LV dysfunction or a previous history of HF. In the DAVID trial, 506 patients with an indication for an implantable cardioverter–defibrillator (ICD), LV ejection fraction (LVEF) <40%, and no indication for pacemaker therapy were randomized to the VVI mode with a lower rate of 40 bpm (VVI-40) versus the DDD mode with a lower rate of 70 bpm (DDDR-70). The mean follow-up was 8.4 months. The primary combined endpoint of death or hospitalization for heart failure was significantly increased at 1 year in the DDDR-70 group (22.6%) compared with the VVI-40 group (13.3%).[11,12] The worse outcome in the DDDR-70 group correlated with Cum% VP >40%. Patients in the DDDR-70 group who had <40% ventricular pacing had similar or better outcomes compared with the VVI-40 group (Figure 23.3).[13]

In the MADIT II trial, Cum% VP was available in 567 (76%) patients in the ICD arm. Patients with Cum% VP >50% had a significantly higher risk of heart failure and ventricular tachycardia (VT) or ventricular fibrillation (VF) requiring ICD therapy,[14] suggesting that

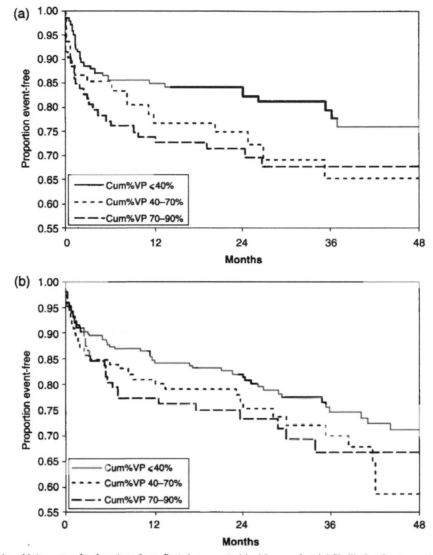

Figure 23.2 Kaplan–Meier rates for freedom from first documented incidence of atrial fibrillation by percent ventricular paced in the MOST trial: (a) DDDR pacing; (b) VVIR pacing.

ventricular dyssynchrony induced by RV pacing not only worsens heart failure, but also could be pro-arrhythmic.

In summary, data from randomized clinical trials have shown that Cum% VP >40% is associated with a higher incidence of heart failure and AF (Table 23.1). The adverse outcomes of ventricular dyssynchrony induced by RV pacing appear to be time-dependent and modulated by baseline LV systolic function, with an earlier

onset in follow-up (months as compared with several years) in patients with depressed LV systolic function. Moreover, these adverse clinical outcomes have been associated with concomitant atrial and ventricular remodeling.[2,6,13–16]

Results from observational studies and randomized clinical trials of cardiac resynchronization therapy (CRT) have consistently demonstrated significant improvement in quality of life, functional status, and exercise capacity in

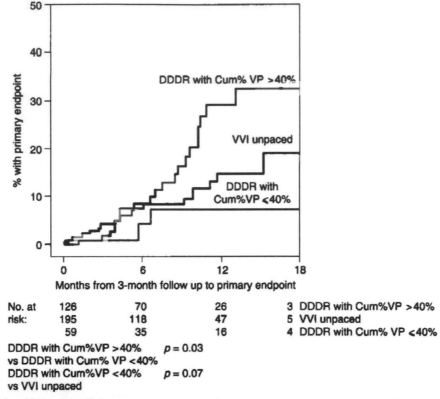

Figure 23.3 Kaplan–Meier plots of the composite outcome of death or hospitalization for heart failure based on cumulative percentage of ventricular pacing (Cum %VP) in the DAVID trial.

patients with New York Heart Association (NYHA) class III and IV heart failure symptoms, LVEF ≤35% and LBBB-induced ventricular dyssynchrony who received CRT without (CRT-P) and with (CRT-D) an ICD.[17,18] A survival benefit was also reported in the COMPANION and CARE-HF trials.[19–21]

The COMPANION trial randomized 1520 patients with NYHA functional class III–IV heart failure to optimal medical therapy versus CRT-P versus CRT-D. The trial showed a 20% reduction in the combined endpoint of all-cause hospitalization and mortality for both CRT-P and CRT-D, compared with optimal medical therapy

Table 23.1 Summary of detrimental effects of chronic right ventricular pacing in clinical trials

Study	Pacing modality	Mean follow-up	Findings/comments
MOST[3] (N = 2010)	VVI vs DDD	33.1 months	Cum% VP >40% increased risk of heart failure and AF
Andersen et al[5] (N = 225)	AAI vs VVI	8 years	VVI pacing was associated with significantly higher mortality, AF, and heart failure
DAVID trial[13] (N = 506)	VVI-40 vs DDDR-70	8 months	Cum% VP >40% was a strong predictor of death and heart failure
MADIT II[14] (N = 567)	46% DDD ICD vs 54% VVI ICD	20 months	Cum% VP >50% had a significantly higher risk of heart failure and VT/VF requiring ICD therapy

AF, atrial fibrillation; Cum% VP, cumulative percentage of ventricular pacing; ICD, implantable cardioverter–defibrillator; VF, ventricular fibrillation; VT, ventricular tachycardia.

($p = 0.01$), and showed that CRT-D reduced all-cause mortality by 36% ($p = 0.003$) as compared with medical therapy.[19,20]

The CARE-HF trial randomized 813 patients with NYHA functional class III–IV heart failure due to LV systolic dysfunction and cardiac dys-synchrony to medical therapy or CRT pacing therapy without an ICD. The primary endpoint was mortality or cardiovascular hospitalization. There were 82 deaths in the CRT group, as com-pared with 120 in the medical therapy group (20% vs 30%; $p < 0.002$).[21]

These data suggest – but do not prove – that in patients with an indication for pacing therapy and in whom excessive RV pacing (Cum% VP >40%) cannot be avoided, CRT could avoid or mitigate the detrimental side-effects of chronic RV pacing. The role of non-standard indications for CRT will be discussed in further detail in this chapter.

SELECTION OF PACING MODE IN SPECIFIC PATIENT GROUPS: TO PACE OR NOT TO PACE?

Patients with symptomatic bradycardia due to SND or AVB will need cardiac pacing. However, the key issue will be the selection of pacing mode, which will depend on (i) the integrity of AV conduction; (ii) the integrity of ventricu-lar conduction, and (iii) baseline LV systolic function.

Patients with symptomatic bradycardia due to SND and normal AV conduction

In this patient group, an atrial-based pacing mode with minimal or back-up ventricular pacing will probably be the most optimal pacing modality. Several pacing modalities could be applied to achieve this goal.

AAI pacing

As described above, AAI pacing has been shown to be superior to VVI pacing in patients with SND.[5] The disadvantage of this pacing mode is the risk of developing AVB or AF. Although the annual risk of AVB is low, the first manifes-tation is syncope in 50% of cases.[3,5] The risk of AF has varied in different clinical trials.[3–5,8–10]

Both developments will render AAI pacing inef-fective. For these reasons, single-chamber atrial pacemakers are not widely used.

Minimal ventricular pacing

Minimal ventricular pacing (MVP) is an atrial-based dual-chamber mode designed to pre-served normal AV conduction and ventricular activation. MVP can be also described as ADIR ('AAIR+'), with mode switching to DDDR during periods of AVB. Single dropped ventric-ular beats are permitted (Wenckebach behavior), while higher-level AV conduction failure causes mode switching to DDDR to prevent ventricular asystole. Tests for return of normal AV conduc-tion, by inhibiting ventricular pacing for one cycle, are conducted in a prespecified algorithm. If AV conduction is detected, the mode of opera-tion returns to MVP ('AAIR+').

In the MVP trial, 181 patients were random-ized to MVP or DDDR for 1 month, and then crossed over to the opposite mode for 1 month. MVP was associated with a mean absolute and relative reduction in Cum% VP (85.0% and 99.9%, respectively). There were no significant differences in the mean cumulative percentage of atrial pacing. Moreover, no adverse events were attributed to MVP (see Table 23.2).[22]

AV search hysteresis

AV search hysteresis automatically searches for intrinsic AV conduction and extends the AV delay by 10–100% to allow intrinsic conduction. The algorithm is designed to search for intrinsic conduction every x cycles (where x is a program-mable number from 32 to 1024). With AV search hysteresis, the device will function effectively in an AAIR mode, with mode switching to DDDR in the event of loss of AV conduction.

In the INTRINSIC RV study, 988 patients with a standard ICD indication were randomized to VVI-40 or DDDR 60–130 with AV search hys-teresis. The mean follow-up was 10.4 months. The primary endpoint, a composite of death or heart failure hospitalization, was observed in 32 patients (6.4%) in the DDDR AV search hys-teresis group versus 46 patients (5.1%) in the VVI group ($p < 0.001$ for non-inferiority analysis).

Table 23.2 Summary of effects of alternative pacing modalities in specific patient populations

Study	Pacing modality	Mean follow-up	Findings/comments
MVP trial[22] (N = 181) (ICD patients)	MVP vs DDD (crossover design)	1 month each modality	MVP was associated with a significant reduction in Cum% VP
INTRINSIC RV trial[23] (N = 988) (ICD patients)	VVI-40 vs DDDR 60–130 with AVSH	10.4 months	Significant reduction in Cum% VP in the DDDR AVSH with no significant differences in clinical outcomes
PAVE trial[24] (N = 184) (AF and AV junction ablation)	RV vs BiV	6 months	The BiV group had a significantly greater LVEF compared with the RV group
Leon et al[25] (N = 20) (AF and AV junction ablation)	Upgrade from RV to BiV pacing	17.3 months	Significant improvements in NYHA class, LVEF, reverse remodeling indices and heart failure
OPSITE[26] (N = 44) (AF and AV junction ablation)	LV vs RV	Acute preliminary data	LV pacing superior to RV pacing after AV nodal ablation
MIRACLE ICD II[28] (N = 186) (NYHA class II ICD patients with QRS≥130 ms)	CRT-on vs CRT-off	6 month	Significant improvements in reverse remodeling indexes, LVEF, and NYHA class
BLOCK HF	CRT-on vs CRT-off	Ongoing	Evaluating role of CRT in patients with LVEF ≤50%, and symptomatic bradycardia with different degrees of AVB
REVERSE[29]	CRT-on vs CRT-off	Ongoing	Evaluating role of CRT in patients with LVEF <40%, NYHA class I–II, QRS >120 ms
MADIT-CRT[30]	CRT-D vs ICD	Ongoing	Evaluating role of CRT in patients with LVEF <30%, NYHA class I–II, QRS >130 ms

AF, atrial fibrillation; AV, atrioventricular; AVB, AV block; AVSH, atrioventricular search hysteresis; BiV, biventricular; CRT, cardiac resynchronization therapy; Cum% VP, cumulative percentage of ventricular pacing; ICD, implantable cardioverter defibrillator; LV, left ventricular; LVEF, LV ejection fraction; MVP, minimal ventricular pacing; NYHA, New York Heart Association; RV, right ventricular.

Interestingly, the mean Cum% VP in the DDDR AV search hysteresis arm was 10%.[23]

Lowering the lower rate limit

Typically, the lower rate limit (LRL) for permanent pacing is programmed to 60–70 min^{-1}. In the DAVID trial, a backup LRL of 40 min^{-1} was associated with a significant reduction in Cum% VP. Similarly, patients with symptomatic bradycardia due to SND could potentially benefit from lowering the LRL to a rate of 50 min^{-1}. This approach has not been prospectively tested in clinical trials, but it makes intuitive sense.

Patients with symptomatic bradycardia due to AVB

In this group of patients, chronic RV pacing cannot be avoided and could induce ventricular dyssynchrony. A chronic Cum% VP >40% has been associated with a higher incidence of AF, heart failure hospitalization,[3–5,11] and ventricular arrhythmias.[14] The effects of ventricular dyssynchrony induced by RV pacing appear to be more dramatic in patients with baseline LV dysfunction or a previous history of heart failure.[11,14] It has also been shown that these adverse clinical outcomes are associated with concomitant atrial and ventricular remodeling.[2,6,15,16]

It is known that CRT has beneficial effects on clinical outcomes and reverse remodeling.[17-21] Due to these findings, there has been increased interest in evaluating the role of CRT in patients with high-grade AVB.

The PAVE trial compared chronic biventricular (BiV) pacing with RV ventricular pacing in 184 patients undergoing ablation of the AV node for the management of AF. The study endpoints were change in the 6-minute walk test, quality of life, and LVEF. Patient characteristics were similar in the two groups. At 6 months post ablation, patients treated with CRT had a significant improvement in 6-minute walk distance ($p = 0.04$). LVEF was significantly greater in the BiV group ($p = 0.03$). Patients with LVEF ≤45% or with NYHA class II–III symptoms receiving a BiV pacemaker appeared to have a greater improvement in 6-minute walk distance compared with patients with normal systolic function or class I symptoms.[24]

Leon et al[25] evaluated the effects of a BiV upgrade in 20 patients with severe heart failure (LVEF ≤35% and NYHA functional class III or IV) who had previously undergone AV junction ablation and RV pacing for the management of AF. The mean follow-up was 17.3 months. NYHA functional classification improved by 29% ($p < 0.001$), LVEF increased by 44% ($p < 0.001$), LV end-diastolic diameter (LVEDD) decreased by 6.5% ($p < 0.003$) and LVESD decreased 8.5% ($p < 0.01$). The number of hospitalizations decreased by 81% ($p < 0.001$).

The Optimal Pacing Site (OPSITE) study is a prospective, randomized trial comparing RV and LV pacing for patients with AF undergoing AV junction ablation. Acute preliminary data from 44 patients have been reported. Compared with RV pacing, LV pacing caused a 5.7% increase in LVEF and a 16.7% decrease in the mitral regurgitation (MR) score; the QRS width was 4.8% shorter with LV pacing. Similar results were observed in patients with or without systolic dysfunction and/or native LBBB. Rhythm regularization achieved with AV junction ablation improved LVEF with both RV and LV pacing.[26]

Hay et al[27] reported the acute hemodynamic effects of different pacing techniques in nine patients with heart failure, AF, and severe AVB.

Ventricular stimulation was applied to the RV (apex and outflow tract), to the LV free wall, and to both ventricles. BiV pacing improved systolic function more than pacing at either site alone ($p < 0.05$), and LV pacing was significantly better than RV pacing. However, only BiV pacing improved diastolic function (isovolumic relaxation). Sequential RV–LV stimulation offered minimal or no advantage over simultaneous RV–LV stimulation.

These findings suggest that patients with AVB, LVEF <45%, and NYHA functional class II–IV appear to benefit from CRT as compared with RV pacing alone. These data also suggest that in patients with AVB, BiV pacing may be superior to LV pacing. The benefit of CRT is not yet clear in patients with AVB and normal LVEF.

The BLOCK HF trial is prospectively enrolling patients with LVEF ≤50%, NYHA functional class I–III, a class I or IIa indication for a permanent pacemaker, and AVB or AV Wenckebach or PR > 300 ms when pacing at 100 bpm. All patients will receive a CRT pacemaker, with randomization to RV versus BiV pacing. The primary endpoint is a combined endpoint of overall mortality, heart failure-related urgent care, and changes in LV volumes.

Patients with symptomatic bradycardia and baseline ventricular dyssynchrony

In this group of patients, the goal of pacing is to improve ventricular synchronization while providing the necessary cardiac pacing. However, the role of CRT in patients with mildly depressed LV systolic function (LVEF 35–50%) and/or NYHA functional class I–II has not been elucidated.

The MIRACLE ICD II study was a randomized clinical trial of CRT in 186 NYHA class II heart failure patients on optimal medical therapy with LVEF ≤35%, QRS ≥130 ms, and a class I indication for an ICD. During a 6-month follow-up, there were significant improvements in ventricular remodeling indices, specifically LV end-diastolic and end-systolic volumes (LDEDV and LDESV: $p = 0.04$ and 0.01, respectively), LVEF ($p = 0.02$), and NYHA class ($p = 0.05$). No significant differences were noted in 6-minute walk distance or quality-of-life scores.

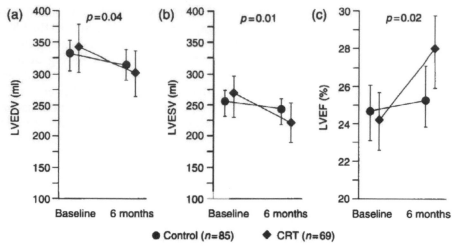

Figure 23.4 Change in left ventricular end-diastolic volume (LVEDV) (a), end-systolic volume (LVESV) (b), and ejection fraction (LVEF) (c) after 6 months of cardiac resynchronization therapy (CRT) or no pacing in the MIRACLE ICD II trial.

(Figure 23.4).[28] It is possible that longer follow-up would have provided further benefits as observed in CARE-HF (mean follow-up of 29.4 months), where CRT-P alone showed significant benefit on clinical parameters, reverse remodeling indices and mortality.[21]

As shown earlier, the detrimental effects of a high cumulative percentage of RV pacing, and therefore RV pacing-induced ventricular dyssynchrony, are time-dependent and modulated by the baseline LVEF. Thus, patients with mildly depressed LVEF (35–50%) and/or NYHA functional class I–II would probably need longer follow-up before significant clinical differences could be observed.

The REVERSE study is a prospective randomized clinical trial designed to establish whether CRT combined with optimal medical therapy can attenuate heart failure progression compared with medical therapy alone in patients with NYHA class I–II, QRS >120 ms, LVEF <40%, and an LVEDD >55 mm. Patients with a class I–II indication for ICD will receive CRT-D.[29]

The MADIT-CRT study is a prospective randomized clinical trial designed to determine if CRT-D will reduce the risk of mortality and heart events, as compared with ICD only, in patients with NYHA class I–II, QRS >130 ms, and LVEF <30%. Patients with a class I–II indication for ICD will receive CRT-D.[30] A summary of

the trials completed and ongoing regarding alternative pacing modalities is presented in Table 23.2.

FUTURE PERSPECTIVES IN DEVICE THERAPY

Patients with symptomatic bradycardia due to SND or AVB will need cardiac pacing. The selection of a particular device and selection of the pacing mode will depend on the integrity of AV conduction, the integrity of ventricular conduction, and baseline LV systolic function. Patients with symptomatic bradycardia due to SND and normal LV systolic function will benefit most from dual-chamber pacing with programming features that would allow preservation of intrinsic AV and ventricular conduction (MVP, AV search hysteresis, or lower LRL). It is still unclear whether or not patients with mildly depressed LVEF (35–50%) and preserved AV and ventricular conduction would benefit from a different pacing modality if a high Cum% VP can be avoided. The intuitive answer is no – but this requires further clinical studies.

Whether or not CRT will have a role in patients with a high Cum% VP and normal LVEF is not known at present. The role of CRT in patients with LVEF ≤50% and symptomatic bradycardia due to AVB is currently being evaluated in the BLOCK HF trial. The role of CRT in patients with LVEF <40% and NYHA functional class I–II is being evaluated in REVERSE and MADIT-CRT. The results of these clinical trials should provide the data that we need on the optimal use of CRT.

REFERENCES

1. Grines CL, Bashore TM, Boudoulas H, et al. Functional abnormalities in isolated left bundle branch block. The effect of interventricular asynchrony. Circulation 1989;79:845–53.

2. van Oosterhout MF, Prinzen FW, Arts T, et al. Asynchronous electrical activation induces asymmetrical hypertrophy of the left ventricular wall. Circulation 1998;98:588–95.

3. Sweeney MO, Hellkamp AS, Ellenbogen KA, et al. Mode Selection Trial Investigators. Adverse effect of ventricular pacing on heart failure and atrial fibrillation among patients with normal baseline QRS duration in a clinical trial of pacemaker therapy for sinus node dysfunction. Circulation 2003;107:2932–7.

4. Lamas GA, Lee KL, Sweeney MO, et al. Mode Selection Trial in Sinus-Node Dysfunction. Ventricular pacing or dual-chamber pacing for sinus-node dysfunction. N Engl J Med 2002;346:1854–62.

5. Andersen HR, Nielsen JC, Thomsen PE, et al. Long-term follow-up of patients from a randomised trial of atrial versus ventricular pacing for sick-sinus syndrome. Lancet 1997;350:1210–16.

6. Nielsen JC, Andersen HR, Thomsen PE, et al. Heart failure and echocardiographic changes during long-term follow-up of patients with sick sinus syndrome randomized to single-chamber atrial or ventricular pacing. Circulation 1998;97:987–95.

7. Andersen HR, Thuesen L, Bagger JP, Vesterlund T, Thomsen PE. Prospective randomised trial of atrial versus ventricular pacing in sick-sinus syndrome. Lancet 1994;344:1523–8.

8. Connolly SJ, Kerr CR, Gent M, et al. Effects of physiologic pacing versus ventricular pacing on the risk of stroke and death due to cardiovascular causes. Canadian Trial of Physiologic Pacing Investigators. N Engl J Med 2000;342:1385–91.

9. Lamas GA, Orav EJ, Stambler BS, et al. Quality of life and clinical outcomes in elderly patients treated with ventricular pacing as compared with dual-chamber pacing. Pacemaker Selection in the Elderly Investigators. N Engl J Med 1998;338:1097–104.

10. Toff WD, Camm AJ, Skehan JD; United Kingdom Pacing and Cardiovascular Events Trial Investigators. Single-chamber versus dual-chamber pacing for high-grade atrioventricular block. N Engl J Med 2005; 353:145–55.

11. Wilkoff BL, Cook JR, Epstein AE, et al. Dual chamber and VVI implantable Defibrillator Trial Investigators. Dual-chamber pacing or ventricular backup pacing in patients with an implantable defibrillator: the Dual Chamber and VVI Implantable Defibrillator (DAVID) trial. JAMA 2002;288:3115–23.

12. Wilkoff BL. Dual Chamber and VVI Implantable Defibrillator Trial Investigators. The Dual Chamber and VVI Implantable Defibrillator (DAVID) Trial: rationale, design, results, clinical implications and lessons for future trials. Card Electrophysiol Rev 2003;7:468–72.

13. Sharma AD, Rizo-Patron C, Hallstrom AP, et al. DAVID Investigators. Percent right ventricular pacing predicts outcomes in the DAVID trial. Heart Rhythm 2005; 2:830–4.

14. Steinberg JS, Fischer A, Wang P, et al. MADIT II Investigators. The clinical implications of cumulative right ventricular pacing in the Multicenter Automatic Defibrillator Implantation Trial II. J Cardiovasc Electrophysiol 2005;16:359–65.

15. Prinzen FW, Hunter WC, Wyman BT, McVeigh ER. Mapping of regional myocardial strain and work during ventricular pacing: experimental study using magnetic resonance imaging tagging. J Am Coll Cardiol 1999;33:1735–42.

16. Tse HF, Yu C, Wong KK, et al. Functional abnormalities in patients with permanent right ventricular pacing: the effect of sites of electrical stimulation. J Am Coll Cardiol 2002;40:1451–8.

17. Bradley DJ, Bradley EA, Baughman KL, et al. Cardiac resynchronization and death from progressive heart failure: a meta-analysis of randomized controlled trials. JAMA 2003;289:730–40.

18. Abraham WT, Hayes DL. Cardiac resynchronization therapy for heart failure. Circulation 2003;108:2596–603.

19. Bristow MR, Saxon LA, Boehmer J, et al. Comparison of Medical Therapy, Pacing, and Defibrillation in Heart Failure (COMPANION) Investigators. Cardiac-resynchronization therapy with or without an implantable defibrillator in advanced chronic heart failure. N Engl J Med 2004;350:2140–50.

20. Ellenbogen KA, Wood MA, Klein HU. Why should we care about CARE-HF? J Am Coll Cardiol 2005;46: 2199–203.

21. Cleland JG, Daubert JC, Erdmann E, et al. Cardiac Resynchronization-Heart Failure (CARE-HF) Study Investigators. The effect of cardiac resynchronization on morbidity and mortality in heart failure. N Engl J Med 2005;352:1539–49.

22. Sweeney MO, Ellenbogen KA, Casavant D, et al. The Marquis MVP Download Investigators. Multicenter, prospective, randomized safety and efficacy study of a new atrial-based managed ventricular pacing mode (MVP) in dual chamber ICDs. J Cardiovasc Electrophysiol 2005;16:811–17.

23. Olshansky B, Day J, Moore S. Is dual chamber programming inferior to single chamber programming in a implantable cardioverter defibrillator? Results of the INTRINSIC RV study. Program and Abstracts from the Heart Rhythm Society 2006 Annual Scientific Sessions, May 17–20, 2006, Boston, MA.

24. Doshi RN, Daoud EG, Fellows C, et al. PAVE Study Group. Left ventricular-based cardiac stimulation post AV nodal ablation evaluation (the PAVE study). J Cardiovasc Electrophysiol 2005;16:1160–5.

25. Leon AR, Greenberg JM, Kanuru N, et al. Cardiac resynchronization in patients with congestive heart failure and chronic atrial fibrillation: effect of upgrading to biventricular pacing after chronic right ventricular pacing. J Am Coll Cardiol 2002;39:1258–63.

26. Puggioni E, Brignole M, Gammage M, et al. Acute comparative effect of right and left ventricular pacing in patients with permanent atrial fibrillation. J Am Coll Cardiol 2004;43:234–8.

27. Hay I, Melenovsky V, Fetics BJ, et al. Short-term effects of right–left heart sequential cardiac resynchronization in patients with heart failure, chronic atrial fibrillation, and atrioventricular nodal block. Circulation 2004; 110:3404–10.

28. Abraham WT, Young JB, Leon AR, et al. Multicenter InSync ICD II Study Group. Effects of cardiac resynchronization on disease progression in patients with left ventricular systolic dysfunction, an indication for an implantable cardioverter-defibrillator, and mildly symptomatic chronic heart failure. Circulation 2004;110:2864–8.

29. Linde C, Gold M, Abraham WT, Daubert JC. REVERSE Study Group. Rationale and design of a randomized controlled trial to assess the safety and efficacy of cardiac resynchronization therapy in patients with asymptomatic left ventricular dysfunction with previous symptoms or mild heart failure – the REsynchronization reVErses Remodeling in Systolic left vEntricular dysfunction (REVERSE) study. Am Heart J 2006;151:288–94.

30. Moss AJ, Brown MW, Cannom DS, et al. Multicenter Automatic Defibrillator Implantation Trial–Cardiac Resynchronization Therapy (MADIT-CRT): design and clinical protocol. Ann Noninvasive Electrocardiol 2005;10(4 Suppl):34–43.

24

Cardiac resynchronization therapy in right bundle branch block

Antonio Berruezo and Ignacio Fernández-Lozano

Introduction • Epidemiology of basal conduction defects • Asynchrony • Biventricular pacing • Conclusions

INTRODUCTION

It is well established that left bundle branch block (LBBB) QRS morphology on the surface electrocardiogram (ECG) correlates with delayed activation of both endocardial and epicardial aspects of the left ventricle (LV) during normal sinus rhythm and during pacing from the apex of the right ventricle (RV).[1-3] Likewise, it is true that most LBBB QRS pattern patients with heart failure have a left intraventricular uncoordinated contraction as a result of an LV free-wall mechanical delay. Thus, the electrophysiological and mechanical bases for CRT in a case of LBBB are widely accepted and support the use of biventricular pacing in order to correct this electrical and mechanical asynchrony. However, little is known about the electrophysiological and mechanical effects of right bundle branch block (RBBB) in heart failure patients.

Cardiac resynchronization therapy (CRT) in heart failure patients with a prolonged QRS duration (mostly LBBB) has been demonstrated to improve symptoms and functional capacity and to reduce major morbidity.[4-8] Recently, a reduction in overall mortality[8,9] has also been demonstrated, due to fewer deaths both from worsening heart failure and from sudden death.[10]

Not only QRS morphology but also the duration of the QRS is important when considering heart failure patients to treat with CRT.

Data from some studies suggest that the longer the duration of the QRS interval, the more benefit can be expected from CRT. That is, in one of these studies,[10] only patients with a QRS duration >160 ms obtained a statistically significant reduction in all-cause mortality, although patients with a QRS duration <160 ms showed a trend toward reduction in all-cause mortality.

At present, the weight of evidence favors CRT treatment only for patients with LBBB. However, guidelines do not mention the morphology of QRS. In the American College of Cardiology/American Heart Association (ACC/AHA) guidelines, biventricular pacing is recommended in medically refractory, symptomatic New York Heart Association (NHYA) class III or IV patients with idiopathic dilated or ischemic cardiomyopathy, prolonged QRS interval (≥130 ms), LV end-diastolic diameter (LVEDD) ≥55 mm and LV ejection fraction (LVEF) ≤35%.[11] In the European Society of Cardiology (ESC) heart failure guidelines, ventricular dyssynchrony is considered to be present when the QRS width is ≥120 ms.[12]

EPIDEMIOLOGY OF BASAL CONDUCTION DEFECTS

It is known that the prevalence and prognostic value of intraventricular conduction defects, either RBBB or LBBB, increases with the age of the patient and the presence of hypertension, diabetes, coronary artery disease, and heart failure. Thus, basal conduction defects are markers of cardiovascular disease in the general population. On the other hand, RBBB is more prevalent that LBBB (24–113/1000 vs 6–57/1000, respectively, in the population aged >60 years).

The Framinghan study showed an increase in mortality and in the probability of developing cardiovascular disease in men, after adjustment for the influence of diabetes, hypertension, age, coronary artery disease, and heart failure, in patients with LBBB.[13] However, it has been proved that the presence of complete RBBB in patients without heart failure or pacemakers is as strong and independent a predictor of all-cause mortality as LBBB, even after adjustment for exercise capacity, nuclear perfusion defects and other risk factors. The relative risk with respect to the normal QRS duration patients was 1.5 (95% confidence interval 1.1–2.1).[14]

Basal conduction defects are much more frequent in patients with heart failure than in the general population. Approximately one-third of patients with heart failure have an increased QRS duration. In most heart failure patients (around 30%),[15] the ECG shows an LBBB configuration, indicating a delay in LV activation. An RBBB configuration is seen in the ECG pattern in 4–6% of heart failure patients[16,17] and up to 10% of CRT candidates.[7]

The global mortality of patients with heart failure and LBBB is greater than that of the patients with RBBB. In the Italian Network on Congestive Heart Failure (IN-CHF) registry, of a total of 5517 patients with heart failure, 659 (11.9%) died within the first year of follow-up. The global mortality of patients with LBBB was higher and significantly different from that of patients with RBBB (16.1% vs 1.9%, respectively).[16]

ASYNCHRONY

Mechanical asynchrony is the ultimate consequence of a number of different processes that may affect the spread of electrical impulses within the heart or other factors, such as the contractility of different segments of the ventricles.

The decrease of the contractility of segments of the LV could explain the presence of LV mechanical asynchrony, evaluated by means of echocardiographic parameters in patients with a narrow QRS complex.[18,19] In patients with heart failure, the decrease in LVEF is inversely proportional to the degree of asynchrony. Likewise, a *high* prevalence of LV mechanical asynchrony in patients with severe LV dysfunction has been demonstrated using echocardiography and other imaging techniques.[20,21] In addition, it has been shown that patients with a narrow QRS complex not only have asynchrony but also benefit from CRT.[22,23] Thus, if we assume that patients with narrow QRS and LV dysfunction may have left intraventricular asynchrony owing to a low LVEF, this must also be true for patients with RBBB.

It has been demonstrated that electrical activation of the epicardium of the LV free wall (registered from the LV electrode of a resynchronization device) in patients with a narrow QRS complex takes place earlier than in patients with LBBB, with respect to the onset of the QRS complex on the surface ECG. In this way, the electrical activation occurs after approximately 65% (range 23–99%) of the QRS duration in patients with narrow QRS (≤120 msec) and after approximately 90% (range 77–102%) of the QRS duration in patients with LBBB. The ranges suggest that some patients with narrow QRS may have some kind of 'hidden electrical asynchrony', quantitatively similar to that of LBBB patients. Additionally, the immediate effects (evaluated through echocardiographic techniques) of biventricular pacing in the LV do not differ between narrow QRS and LBBB patients.[24] Thus, the observed delay in LV activation in heart failure patients with a narrow QRS complex may also be present in RBBB patients.

In another study, Fantoni et al[25] characterized RV and LV endocardial activation in heart failure patients with RBBB and LBBB QRS morphology, using a three-dimensional (3D) non-fluoroscopic electroanatomic contact mapping system. The 3D mapping system allowed the assessment of electrical activation sequences with high spatial and temporal resolution. In this study, the investigators were able to demonstrate that the total endocardial activation time was significantly longer in patients with RBBB compared with LBBB. Also, they found that the activation times of the LV anterior and lateral regions were not significantly different between patients with RBBB and LBBB, regardless of the etiology. The authors suggested that the LV delay of activation was related to a more compromised hemodynamic profile and more severe clinical presentation of these patients compared with patients with LBBB. With respect to the ECG morphology of RBBB patients, they found that two-thirds of them showed a broad, slurred and notched R wave on leads I and aVL, together with a leftward axis deviation. Thus, delayed LV activation in heart failure patients presenting with RBBB can be non-invasively identified through the surface ECG. In these cases, the pattern defined by Rosenbaum et al[30] as 'RBBB masking LBBB' can be noted. It is not known whether the LV activation sequence is of similar degree in RBBB patients without LBBB masking. These mapping data are helpful in understanding the rationale for delivering CRT in heart failure patients with RBBB.

BIVENTRICULAR PACING

In the CRT trials, the ECG inclusion criterion has been the QRS width. Of the patients included in clinical trials up to 2004, 64% had LBBB and the rest had either RBBB or intraventricular conduction delay. Thus, the percentage is so low that it limits interpretation of the results.

In 2001, Garrigue et al[26] showed the results of a prospective study of 12 heart failure patients with complete RBBB with a QRS duration > 140 ms in whom a CRT device was implanted. After 1 year of follow-up, investigators concluded that only patients with a RBBB associated with a major left intraventricular asynchrony, detected echocardiographically (left intraventricular delay evaluated with Doppler tissue imaging), were likely to respond to pacing therapy.

With the addition of data from the MIRACLE ICD[27] and CONTAK CD[28] trials, Egoavil et al[29] identified 61 patients with RBBB, 34 of whom were randomized to CRT and 27 to a control group. The 3- and 6-month follow-up data analysis showed that CRT in RBBB patients only

improved NYHA functional class at the same level as the patients in the control group. The authors concluded that at present, CRT should not be recommended for heart failure patients with RBBB, until results of a prospective study with an adequate sample size are available (Table 24.1).

Finally, Fernández-Lozano et al[30] analyzed the results of a series of 17 heart failure patients with complete RBBB, from a total of 160 patients who underwent CRT. They considered as responders those patients who were alive and free of heart transplant or heart failure hospitalization and who improved at least 10% in the

Table 24.1 Outcome in 61 heart failure patients with RBBB who were randomized to a cardiac resynchronization therapy (CRT) group (n=34) or a control group (n=27): pooled data from the MIRACLE ICD and CONTAK CD trials

	At randomization	6 months	p
NYHA functional class:			
CRT	3.1	2.3	<0.001
Control	3.0	2.8	0.005
VO$_{2max}$ (ml/kg/min):			
CRT	12.7	12.4	0.85
Control	13	13.6	0.60
6-minute walk distance (m):			
CRT	284.1	339.4	0.08
Control	260.7	291.8	0.35
QoL score:			
CRT	51.8	37.7	0.053
Control	51.1	42.8	0.13
LVEF (%):			
CRT	27.2	29.0	0.54
Control	31.1	32.0	0.67
NE levels (pg/dl):			
CRT	623.1	412.1	0.10
Control	587.9	600.5	0.91

Baseline demographics did not differ between the CRT and control groups. With the exception of NYHA class, patients with RBBB according to a wide QRS did not derive significant benefit from CRT in any of the other parameters studied at 6 months. The results were consistent with a placebo effect

NYHA, New York Heart Association; VO$_{2max}$, peak oxygen consumption; QoL, quality-of-life; LVEF, left ventricular ejection fraction; NE, norepinephrine (noradrenaline)

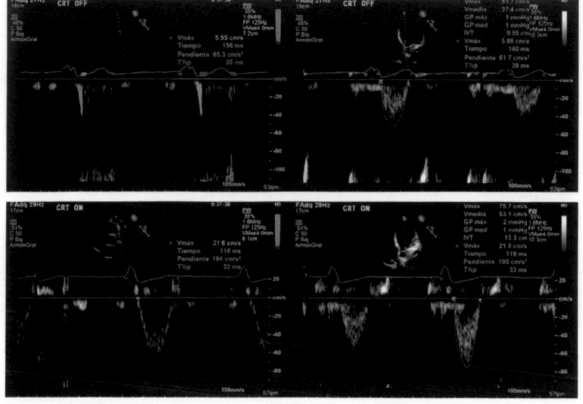

Figure 24.1 Echocardiographic Doppler measurements with the cardiac resynchronization therapy (CRT) device activated (CRT ON) and deactivated (CRT OFF). The patient was a 64-year-old man with dilated cardiomyopathy with right bundle branch block (RBBB) and III NYHA functional class III heart failure. The interventricular asynchrony (the difference between pre-ejection pulmonary and aortic times) with the CRT device deactivated was 16 ms (CRT OFF) and was reduced to 4 ms with the CRT device activated (CRT ON).

6-minute walk test. At 6 months of follow-up, 81% of LBBB patients and only 60% of RBBB patients improved with respect to the baseline. Analysis of the echocardiographic data showed that the greater the basal intraventricular asynchrony, the greater was the clinical improvement. Also, CRT showed an improvement in interventricular mechanical delay but not in intraventricular mechanical delay in the whole group of RBBB patients. An example of echocardiographic measurements of a patient with heart failure and RBBB in whom a CRT device was implanted is shown in Figures 24.1 and 24.2.

CONCLUSIONS

Not all patients with heart failure respond to CRT. At present, the benefit of CRT in RBBB heart failure patients has not been definitively demonstrated, although some electrophysiological, ECG, and echocardiographic data support the rationale and suggest a possible benefit in a proportion of them. However, in order to reduce the percentage of non-responder patients with CRT devices, it is convenient to evaluate either the presence of intra-LV conduction defects by means of ECG criteria or the presence of mechanical asynchrony by means of echocardiographic measurements.

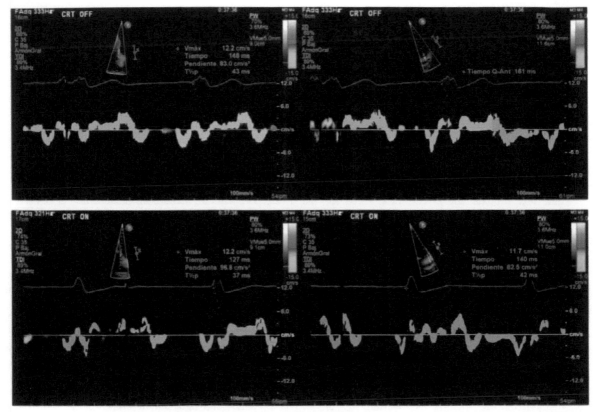

Figure 24.2 Echocardiographic tissue Doppler measurements with the CRT device activated (CRT ON) and deactivated (CRT OFF) in the same patient as in Figure 24.1. The left intraventricular asynchrony prior to implantation was only 13 ms (CRT OFF) and was not modified after the CRT device was activated (CRT ON).

REFERENCES

1. Vassallo JA, Cassidy DM, Marchlinski FE, et al. Endocardial activation of left bundle branch block. Circulation 1984;69:914–23.

2. Wyndham CRC, Smith T, Meeran MK, et al. Epicardial activation in patients with left bundle branch block. Circulation 1980;61:696–703.

3. Vassallo JA, Cassidy DM, Miller JM, et al. Left ventricular endocardial activation during right ventricular pacing: effect of underlying heart disease. J Am Coll Cardiol 1986;7:1228–33.

4. Auricchio A, Stellbrink C, Sack S, et al. Long-term clinical effect of hemodynamically optimized cardiac resynchronization therapy in patients with heart failure and ventricular conduction delay. J Am Coll Cardiol 2002;39:2026–33.

5. Abraham WT, Fisher WG, Smith AL, et al. Cardiac resynchronization in chronic heart failure. N Engl J Med 2002; 346:1902–5.

6. Cazeau S, Leclerq C, Lavergne T, et al. Effects of multi-site biventricular pacing in patients with heart failure and intraventricular conduction delay. N Engl J Med 2001;344:873–80.

7. Bristow MR, Saxon LA, Boehmer J, et al. Cardiac resynchronization therapy with or without an implantable defibrillator in advanced chronic heart failure. N Engl J Med 2004;350:2140–50.

8. Cleland JGF, Daubert JC, Erdmann E, et al. The effect of cardiac resynchronization on morbidity and mortality in heart failure. N Engl J Med 2005;352:1539–49.

9. Freemantle N, Tharmanathan P, Calvert MJ, et al. Cardiac resynchronisation for patients with heart failure due to left ventricular systolic dysfunction – a systematic review and meta-analysis. Eur Heart J 2006;8:433–40.

10. Cleland JGF, Daubert JC, Erdmann E, et al, on behalf of the CARE-HF Study Investigators. Longer-term effects of cardiac resynchronization therapy on mortality in

heart failure [the CArdiac REsynchronization–Heart Failure (CARE-HF) trial extension phase]. Eur Heart J 2006;27:1928–32.

11. Gregoratos G, Abrams J, Epstein AE, et al. ACC/AHA/NASPE 2002 Guideline Update for Implantation of Cardiac Pacemakers and Antiarrhythmia Devices: Summary article. A report of the American College of Cardiology/American Heart Association Task Force on Practice Guidelines (ACC/AHA/NASPE Committee to update the 1998 pacemaker guidelines). Circulation 2002;106:2145–61.

12. Swedberg K, Cleland J, Dargie H, et al. Guidelines for the Diagnosis and Treatment of Chronic Heart Failure: Full text (update 2005). The Task Force for the Diagnosis and Treatment of CHF of the European Society of Cardiology. Eur Heart J 2005;20:1115–40.

13. Schneider JF, Thomas HE, Kreger BE, et al. Newly acquired left bundle-branch block: the Framingham Study. Ann Intern Med 1979;90:303–10.

14. Hesse B, Díaz LA, Snader CE, Blackstone EH, Lauer MS: Complete bundle branch block as an independent predictor of all-cause mortality: report of 7073 patients referred for nuclear exercise testing. Am J Med 2001;110:253–9.

15. Kazan A, Barold S. Significance of QRS complex duration in patients with heart failure. J Am Coll Cardiol 2005;46:2183–92.

16. Baldasseroni S, Gentile A, Gorini M, et al. Intraventricular conduction deffects in patients with congestive heart failure: left but not right bundle branch block is an independent predictor of prognosis. A report from the Italian Network on Congestive Heart Failure (IN-CHF database). Ital Heart J 2003;4:607–13.

17. Wilensky RL, Yudelman P, Cohen AI, et al. Serial electrocardiographic changes in idiopathic dilated cardiomyopathy confirmed at necropsy. Am J Cardiol 1988;62:276–83.

18. Perez de Isla L, Florit J, García-Fernández MA, Evangelista A, Zamorano J, on behalf of the RAVE (Registro de Asincronía Ventricular en España–Spanish Ventricular Asynchrony Registry) study investigators. J Am Soc Echocardiogr 2005;18:850–9.

19. Kapetanakis S, Kearney MT, Siva A, et al. Real-time three-dimensional echocardiography. A novel technique to quantify global left ventricular mechanical dyssynchrony. Circulation 2005;112:992–1000.

20. Kerwin WF, Botvinick EH, O'Connell JW, et al. Ventricular contraction abnormalities in dilated cardiomyopathy: effect of biventricular pacing to correct interventricular dyssynchrony. J Am Coll Cardiol 2000;35:1221–7.

21. Yu CM, Yang H, Lau CP, et al. Regional left ventricle mechanical asynchrony in patients with heart disease and normal QRS duration: implication for biventricular pacing therapy. Pacing Clin Electrophysiol 2003;26:562–70.

22. Yu CM, Lin H, Zhang Q, et al. High prevalence of left ventricular systolic and disatolic asynchrony in patients with congestive heart failure and normal QRS duration. Heart 2003;89:54–60.

23. Gasparini M, Mantica M, Galimberti P, et al. Beneficial effects of biventricular pacing in patients with a 'narrow' QRS. Pacing Clin Electrophysiol 2003;26:169–74.

24. Turner MS, Bleasdale RA, Vinereanu D, et al. Electrical and mechanical components of dysssynchrony in heart failure patients with normal QRS duration and left bundle-branch block. Impact of left and biventricular pacing. Circulation 2004;109:2544–9.

25. Fantoni C, Kawabata M, Massaro R, et al. Right and left ventricular activation sequence in patients with heart failure and right bundle branch block. J Cardiovasc Electrophysiol 2005;16:112–19.

26. Garrigue S, Reuter S, Labeque JN, et al. Usefulness of biventricular pacing in patients with congestive heart failure and right bundle branch block. Am J Cardiol 2001;88:1436–41.

27. Young JB, Abraham WT, Smith AL, et al. Combined cardiac resynchronization and implantable cardioversion defibrillation in advanced chronic heart failure: the MIRACLE ICD trial. JAMA 2003;289:2685–94.

28. Higgins SL, Hummel JD, Niazi IK, et al. Cardiac resynchronization therapy for the treatment of heart failure in patients with intraventricular conduction delay and malignant ventricular tachyarrhythmias. J Am Coll Cardiol 2003;42:1454–9.

29. Egoavil CA, Ho RT, Greenspon AJ, Pavri BB. Cardiac resynchronization therapy in patients with right bundle branch block: analysis of pooled data from the MIRACLE and Contak CD trials. Heart Rhythm 2005;2:616–18.

30. Fernández-Lozano I, Escudier JM, Díaz Infante E, et al. Biventricular pacing in right bundle-branch block. Europace 2005;7(Suppl 1):64.

25

Cardiac resynchronization therapy in mildly symptomatic heart failure

John Rogers, Jigar Patel, and J Thomas Heywood

Introduction • Benefits of resynchronization • Prior trials in mild heart failure patients • Ongoing randomized trials • CRT for mildly symptomatic patients

INTRODUCTION

Despite significant advances in the pharmacologic treatment of left ventricular (LV) systolic dysfunction, morbidity and mortality remain high.[1] Device therapies, including pacemakers, implantable cardioverter–defibrillators (ICDs), and cardiac resynchronization therapy (CRT), have now been conclusively shown to improve symptoms and mortality when added to standard medical therapy.[2-8] ICDs are indicated for New York Heart Association (NYHA) class II and III patients, but most studies with CRT have required patients to have at least moderate symptoms (NYHA class III–IV).[9,10] This was a reasonable approach early on, because it allowed trials to be smaller, reserving this expensive therapy for those most likely to benefit.[11]

However, as CRT matures and attains more widespread acceptance, should it be offered to less symptomatic patients?[12] This issue becomes more pressing when an ICD is implanted for primary sudden death prophylaxis in a patient who would meet electrocardiographic (ECG) or echocardiographic criteria for LV dyssynchrony. In these cases, should the patients also have the 'third wire'? Only limited data exist about the efficacy of CRT in such patients. Fortunately, trials are underway that hopefully will answer this question definitively.

One major problem in designing trials to evaluate the effect of CRT for mild heart failure is the difficulty in distinguishing NYHA class II and class III patients. The differences between mild and moderate heart failure are subjective. Moreover, an individual patient can change NYHA class due to dietary indiscretion on the one hand or improved therapy on the other. Hence, although NYHA classification is a powerful predictor of mortality,[13] more objective markers of prognosis (LV size, brain natriuretic peptide (BNP), and QRS duration) may be better indicators for CRT therapy in the future. Thus, the studies described below are of great importance.

BENEFITS OF RESYNCHRONIZATION

Many benefits of CRT have emerged from the trials in advanced heart failure patients. For example, in physiologic studies, CRT has been demonstrated to acutely improve contractile force of the heart, as measured by the first derivative of LV pressure with respect to time, dP/dt.[14] CRT has also been shown to decrease the neurohormonal activation[15] that is a pathologic hallmark of heart failure. Perhaps because of this effect, positive remodeling has frequently been demonstrated, with randomized trials showing a significant decrease in LV volumes, and a concurrent increase in LV ejection fraction (LVEF).[4,7,16,17] This remodeling, along with coordinated contraction of the papillary muscles, can lead to decreased mitral regurgitation, which has also been a finding in randomized trials.[3,4,7,16,18]

Improvements in LV structure and function together with improved neurohormonal status, lead to improved symptoms of heart failure. For example, in the MIRACLE trial, the CRT group (vs the control group) had an average 6-minute walk distance 29 meters greater ($p = 0.005$), Minnesota Living with Heart Failure (MLWHF) score 9 points lower ($p = 0.001$), and peak oxygen consumption (VO_{2max}) 0.9 ml/kg/min greater ($p = 0.009$), with benefits occurring as early as 1 month after randomization.[4] Also, in CARE-HF, the NYHA class in the CRT group was 0.6 lower than in medical therapy ($p < 0.001$), and the MLWHF score was 10 points lower ($p < 0.001$).[8] In the COMPANION trial, 6 months after randomization, the CRT-only group had an average increase in 6-minute walk distance of 40 meters ($p < 0.001$) and a decrease in MLWHF score of 25 points ($p < 0.001$), and 61% experienced improvement in NYHA class ($p < 0.001$).[7]

Recent trials have also analyzed the effect of CRT on mortality. For example, the COMPANION trial randomized 1520 patients to optimal medical therapy, CRT only (Guidant CONTAK-TR), or CRT with defibrillator function (Guidant CONTAK-CD). After 14–16 months of follow-up, the COMPANION trial found that the CRT-only group had a 'marginally significant' reduction in the secondary endpoint of all-cause death (hazard ratio (HR) 0.76, 95% confidence interval (CI) 0.58–1.01, $p = 0.059$). After 12 months of follow-up, the CRT-only group experienced a significant reduction in the primary endpoint of death or hospitalization from any cause (HR 0.81, 95% CI 0.69–0.96, $p = 0.014$). Subsequently, in CARE-HF, 813 patients were randomized to receive either medical therapy or CRT-only (Medtronic InSync or InSync III). After 29 months of follow-up, the CRT group was associated with a significant reduction in death from any cause (HR 0.64, 95% CI 0.48–0.85, $p < 0.002$).

The impact of CRT on sudden death is less clear. In the COMPANION trial, the incidence of sudden death was not reduced with CRT only

(HR 1.21, 95% CI 0.7–2.07, $p = 0.50$).[19] Similary, in CARE-HF, the rate of sudden death was 32% in the medical therapy group and 35% in the CRT group (no confidence intervals were given). Before drawing conclusions from this data, it is worth recalling the ongoing difficulties with classification of mode of death, especially with regard to the definition of sudden death.[20] The definition used for sudden death in the CARE-HF trial was not documented, and in COMPANION, the definition of sudden death was 'observed or unobserved, but assumed to be instantaneous because of the clinical setting'.

Although sudden death may not be affected by CRT, this therapy may be beneficial as an adjunct to implantable defibrillators. For example, in a small trial of 18 patients who had their ICDs upgraded to CRTs with ICDs, it was shown that the frequency of ventricular tachycardia was decreased from 0.31 to 0.13 episodes per patient per month ($p = 0.59$).[21] Likewise, the frequency of ventricular fibrillation decreased from 0.083 to 0.004 episodes per patient per month ($p = 0.03$). As a consequence, the frequency of shocks from the ICD decreased from 0.048 to 0.003 episodes per patient per month ($p = 0.05$). Therefore, CRT can be viewed as a means of decreasing the burden of ICD discharges for the patient.[6]

PRIOR TRIALS IN MILD HEART FAILURE PATIENTS

Although most studies to date with CRT have been in advanced heart failure patients, two large trials have studied patients with mild heart failure. The first of these was CONTAK-CD, which randomized 581 patients with NYHA class II–IV heart failure, LVEF ≤35%, and QRS >120 ms, to CRT-on or CRT-off (Guidant Ventak CHF or CONTAK-CD).[6] In the CONTAK-CD study, 158 patients with NYHA class II were included. Between implantation and randomization, the clinicians were allowed to push aggressive medical therapy for 30 days. As a result, many of the baseline NYHA groupings changed before randomization, including 40% of those initially NYHA class III–IV who improved to class I–II prior to randomization.

Also of note, the population in CONTAK-CD differed from that in other CRT trials in that there were fewer ischemic etiologies (55% in CONTAK-CD vs 67% in other trials) and more beta-blocker use (63% vs 48% in other trials). The results of the CONTAK-CD trial showed that there was no difference between the CRT-on versus CRT-off groups in the composite endpoint of mortality, hospitalization for heart failure, and ventricular arrhythmias requiring therapy. For the NYHA class I–II groups, there was no improvement in 6-minute walk, MLWHF score, VO_{2max}, or LVEF. These results may have been influenced by lack of stability in NYHA groupings, difference in ischemic etiology, and beta-blocker use. Furthermore, because these patients had relatively mild symptoms, it may be difficult to demonstrate significant improvement in a small subset of patients. Nonetheless, there was evidence of reverse remodeling, with small but significant changes in LV end-systolic and end-diastolic diameters (LVESD and LVEDD) (Table 25.1). This positive remodeling may not have resulted immediately in improved symptoms, but may over time have prevented clinical deterioration. In addition, the duration of follow-up in CONTAK-CD was possibly too short to test this hypothesis.

The MIRACLE ICD II trial randomized 186 patients with NYHA class II, LVEF ≤35%, LVEDD ≥55 mm, and QRS ≥130 ms to receive CRT-ICD (Medtronic InSync ICD) on or off.[22] This trial ran concurrently with the MIRACLE ICD trial, with separate prespecified endpoints for the NYHA class II patients. MIRACLE ICD II showed that CRT improved the secondary endpoints of NYHA class by 0.18 ($p = 0.05$), of LV end-diastolic volume (LVEDV) by 41 ml ($p = 0.04$), of LV end-systolic volume (LVESV) by 42 ml ($p = 0.01$), and of LVEF by 3.8% ($p = 0.02$). Furthermore, the composite clinical status score improved in the CRT-on group vs the CRT-off

---

Table 25.1 Previous trials of CRT in mild heart failure

Trial	No. of patients	Endpoint	Results of therapy vs control
CONTAK-CD[6]	158	*Primary*	
		Composite mortality, hospitalization, VT	Hazard ratio 0.88 (NS)
		Secondary	
		Increase in 6-min walk	17 vs 10 ($p = 0.55$)
		Change MLWHF score	−1 vs −4 ($p = 0.26$)
		Improvement in VO_{2max}	0.2 vs 0.0 ($p = 0.77$)
		Change in LVEDD[a]	**−2.4 vs 0.0 ($p = 0.024$)**
		Change in LVESD[a]	**−3.2 vs −0.5 ($p = 0.014$)**
		Improvement in LVEF	4.7 vs 2.9 ($p = 0.16$)
MIRACLE ICD II[22]	186	*Primary*	
		Change in VO_{2max}	0.5 vs 0.2 ($p = 0.87$)
		Secondary	
		Change in 6-min walk	38 vs 33 ($p = 0.59$)
		Change in MLWHF score	−13.3 vs −10.7 ($p = 0.49$)
		Change in LVEDV[a]	**−41 vs −16 ($p = 0.04$)**
		Change in LVESV[a]	**−42 vs −14 ($p = 0.01$)**
		Change in LVEF[a]	**3.8 vs 0.8 ($p = 0.02$)**
		Change in mitral regurgitation (cm^2)	−1.7 vs −1.0 ($p = 0.25$)
		Change in Ve/VCO_2[a]	**−1.8 vs 0.5 ($p = 0.01$)**
		Change in NYHA class[a]	**−0.18 vs 0.01 ($p = 0.05$)**

Bold items are significant at a $p ≤ 0.05$ level.

MLWHF, Minnesota Living with Heart Failure; VT, ventricular tacharrhythmias requiring device therapy; NS, not-significant; LVEDD, left ventricular end-diastolic diameter (mm); LVESD, LV end-systolic diameter (mm); LVEDV, LV end-diastolic volume (ml); LVESDV, LV end-systolic volume (ml); Ve, minute ventilation; VCO_2, minute carbon dioxide production.

group (49% vs 36%; $p = 0.01$). However, the primary endpoint of change in VO_{2max} was no different between the two groups.

ONGOING RANDOMIZED TRIALS

It is clear from the above discussion that the experience of CRT in mildly symptomatic heart failure, although promising, is very limited. Because of the cost and the small, but not insignificant, morbidity associated with device implantation, it is imperative that more data be obtained. Two large randomized trials are currently underway that should provide much more data about the use of CRT in mildly symptomatic individuals with heart failure (Table 25.2).

The REVERSE (REsynchronization reVErses Remodeling in Systolic Left vEntricular Dysfunction) trial began in the summer of 2004 in over 100 sites in the USA, Canada,

and Europe.[23] The expected sample size is 512 patients, who will be followed for 5 years, with an expected study duration of 87 months. A combined ICD/CRT device (Medtronic) will be implanted and then CRT will be activated on a 2:1 basis in a blinded fashion. LV epicardial leads will not be allowed, and patients will have atrioventricular (AV) delay optimization by echocardiography prior to discharge from their implant hospitalization. In the USA and Canada, therapy will be blinded (CRT-on or CRT-off) for 12 months, following which CRT will be activated in all patients. In Europe, therapy will be blinded for 24 months. Enrollment for REVERSE was completed in September 2006. Twelve month follow-up is expected to be completed for all patients by October 2007.

The primary endpoint of REVERSE will be a composite endpoint of mortality, hospitalization for heart failure, discontinuation of double-blind treatment with CRT, or worsening

Table 25.2 Ongoing trials of CRT in mild heart failure

Trial	Projected No. of patients	Study start	Projected duration	Inclusion criteria	Endpoint
REVERSE[23]	512, with 2:1 CRT-on vs CRT-off	Summer 2004	87 months	LVEF ≤40%	*Primary* Composite of mortality, hospitalization, discontinuation of blind treatment, deterioration of functional status *Secondary*
				QRS ≥120 ms	Increase in 6-min walk
				LVEDD ≥55 mm	Change in MLWHF score
				NYHA class I or II	Change in NYHA class
				Stable medical regimen	Change in LVESV
MADIT-CRT[27]	1820, with 3:2 randomization	December 2004	45 months	LVEF ≤30%	*Primary* Death or HF event *Secondary*
				QRS ≥130 ms	Change in LVEDV
				Sinus rhythm	Change in LVESV
				Ischemic heart disease, NYHA class I–II	Multiple heart failure events
				Non-ischemic, NYHA class II	
				Stable medical regimen	

MLWHF, Minnesota Living with Heart Failure; LVEDD, left ventricular end-diastolic diameter (mm); LVESD, LV end-systolic diameter (mm); LVEDV, LV end-diastolic volume (ml); LVESDV, LV end-systolic volume (ml).

functional status. There are a number of secondary endpoints that will be evaluated as well, including LVESV index after 12 months of blinded therapy, changes in NYHA class, change in quality-of-life scores, and change in 6-minute walk distance. The aim of the trial, rather than focusing on patient improvement, will be to demonstrate that CRT stabilizes and slows progressive remodeling because patients enrolled in REVERSE will have little or no symptoms of heart failure.

Major inclusion criteria for REVERSE were NYHA class I or II heart failure, QRS duration ≥120 ms, LVEF ≤40%, LVEDD ≥55 mm (or 2.8 cm/m^2 body surface area) and a stable medical regimen. Major exclusion criteria for REVERSE were NYHA class III or IV symptoms within 90 days, admission for heart failure within 90 days, atrial fibrillation, atrial flutter, creatinine >3.0 mg/dl, and significant hepatic abnormalities.

One substudy already planned for REVERSE will investigate the effect of optimizing interventricular timing. In the CRT-on group, echocardiographic tissue Doppler imaging will be used to measure the time to peak systolic contraction of basal septal and basal free walls of the LV. The optimum interventricular timing for each patient will be identified by testing each offset from −20 (right ventricular (RV) lead first by 20 ms) to +20 (LV lead first by 20 ms), searching for the setting that produces the shortest delay between time to peak systolic contraction of the LV walls. The large, randomized trials completed so far have not optimized the interventricular timing of the CRT devices, because of lack of this feature in devices and lack of uniformity in the procedure. Interventricular timing has been shown to improve stroke volume, dP/dt, and exercise capacity, so the standardized use of this technique in the REVERSE trial may produce a more impressive response.[1,24-26]

The other ongoing large trial for mild heart failure patients is MADIT-CRT (Multicenter Automatic Defibrillator Implantation Trial).[27] In this trial, the recruitment goal is 1820 patients. Patients will be randomized 3:2 to receive CRT-ICD or ICD only, and the follow-up will average 20–33 months, continuing until a common study termination date. All devices implanted for this study will be manufactured by Guidant Corporation, and the study will be administered by the University of Rochester.

The primary endpoints of MADIT-CRT are death or heart failure event (e.g., acute decompensated heart failure requiring hospitalization or outpatient treatment with intravenous diuretics, inotropes, or nesiritide). Deaths will be classified according to cause, such as sudden death. Secondary endpoints will include LVESV (measured by echocardiography while CRT is turned off) at 12 months, LVEDV (also measured while CRT is turned off), and the rate of multiple heart failure events.

Major inclusion criteria for MADIT-CRT include ischemic heart disease and NYHA class I or II symptoms for the previous 3 months, or non-ischemic heart disease and NYHA class II for the previous 3 months. Patients must also have LVEF ≤30% within 14 days prior to randomization, QRS ≥130 ms, sinus rhythm, and stable optimal pharmacologic therapy. Major exclusion criteria are NYHA class III or IV symptoms in the previous 3 months, coronary artery bypass grafts or intervention in the previous 3 months, and non-ischemic cardiomyopathy with NYHA class I symptoms. As of June 2006, approximately 630 patients had been enrolled in MADIT-CRT. Enrollment has been rather slow in this study – perhaps because clinicians may prefer not to risk the randomization of their patients with a wide QRS to the group which receives on ICD without CRT therapy.

CRT FOR MILDLY SYMPTOMATIC PATIENTS

CRT has so far been a therapeutic option for patients with moderate heart failure despite optimal medical management. In these patients, CRT has the potential to improve symptoms and reduce mortality. It is known that even asymptomatic patients with reduced LVEF have increased mortality.[28] Since one of the benefits of CRT is reverse remodeling and improved systolic function, it may be of benefit in these less symptomatic patients. This hypothesis is supported by the MIRACLE ICD II and CONTAK-CD trials, in which CRT produced reverse remodeling in a period as short as

6 months. These trials were limited by several factors, one of which was that NYHA class II patients were analyzed primarily as a subgroup of the more symptomatic patients. Also, the major benefit of CRT in NYHA class I and II patients has been reverse remodeling, but only over some time will the reduced chamber volumes, improved LVEF, and decreased mitral regurgitation translate to improved outcomes. This may explain the lack of clinical efficacy in the small trials so far – the follow-up has been too short to detect clinical improvement, despite positive remodeling.

The ongoing trials are specifically targeting NYHA class I–II patients, and are incorporating new techniques such as interventricular timing optimization. The two large trials currently underway should be expected to meet secondary endpoints such as reverse remodeling. However, the primary endpoints may be more difficult, since the event rate in NYHA class I and II patients in REVERSE and MADIT-CRT (all of whom have defibrillators) should be quite low. In SCD-HeFT, mortality in those with ICDs was only 5.8% per year.[10] In a recent report, Parkash et al[29] found a 1-year mortality rate in low-risk patients (NYHA class I–II, normal renal function, age < 80 years, and sinus rhythm) of <5%. Thus, the challenge will be to follow such patients for a sufficiently long period to demonstrate prolonged clinical stability rather than improved symptoms. On the positive side, these studies will be much longer than previous trials, with the REVERSE trial having a follow-up of 12 months for patients in the USA and Canada and 24 months for European patients, and MADIT-CRT a follow-up of 20–33 months.

The primary endpoints of both studies will include death and hospitalizations, but REVERSE will also include change in functional status or the need to activate CRT in control patients. The primary endpoint goal is subtly different – that fewer patients will *worsen* with CRT compared with control – whereas most other heart failure trials have depended on mortality and hospitalization to drive their clinical endpoints. Therefore, the chief aim of this trial is not to improve symptoms but rather to stabilize patients with LV dysfunction, and hence prevent disease progression. These two studies will

help determine if positive results with surrogate endpoints can translate into meaningful clinical outcomes, such as reduced mortality, hospitalization, or prolonged clinical stability.

In a few short years, CRT has brought a new realm of therapy to patients significantly limited by heart failure. On the other hand, this therapy is expensive, does not always work, and carries some risk. The two ongoing trials will answer two important questions. Does the incremental cost associated with CRT in patients receiving defibrillators produce clinically significant results? Can CRT bring about longer clinical stability than pharmacologic therapy alone? Our patients and those of us who care for them anxiously await the results of these landmark trials.

REFERENCES

1. American Heart Association. Heart Disease and Stroke Statistics – 2005 Update. Dallas, TX: American Heart Association, 2005.

2. Auricchio A, Stellbrink C, Sack S, et al. Pacing Therapies in Congestive Heart Failure (PATH-CHF) Study Group. Long-term clinical effect of hemodynamically optimized cardiac resynchronization therapy in patients with heart failure and ventricular conduction delay. J Am Coll Cardiol 2002;39:2026–33.

3. Cazeau S, Leclercq C, Lavergne T, et al. Multisite Stimulation in Cardiomyopathies (MUSTIC) Study Investigators. Effects of multisite biventricular pacing in patients with heart failure and intraventricular conduction delay. N Engl J Med 2001;344:873–80.

4. Abraham WT, Fisher WG, Smith AL, et al. MIRACLE Study Group. Multicenter InSync Randomized Clinical Evaluation. Cardiac resynchronization in chronic heart failure. N Engl J Med 2002;346:1845–53.

5. Young JB, Abraham WT, Smith AL, et al. Multicenter InSync ICD Randomized Clinical Evaluation (MIRACLE ICD) Trial Investigators. Combined cardiac resynchronization and implantable cardioversion defibrillation in advanced chronic heart failure: the MIRACLE ICD trial. JAMA 2003;289:2685–94.

6. Higgins SL, Hummel JD, Niazi IK, et al. Cardiac resynchronization therapy for the treatment of heart failure in patients with intraventricular conduction delay and malignant ventricular tachyarrhythmias (CONTAK CD). J Am Coll Cardiol 2003;42:1454–9.

7. Bristow MR, Saxon LA, Boehmer J, et al, for the Comparison of Medical Therapy, Pacing, and Defibrillation in Heart Failure (COMPANION) Investigators.

Cardiac-resynchronization therapy with or without an implantable defibrillator in advanced chronic heart failure. N Engl J Med 2004; 350:2140–50.

8. Cleland JG, Daubert JC, Erdmann E, et al, for the Cardiac Resynchronization-Heart Failure (CARE-HF) Study Investigators. The effect of cardiac resynchronization on morbidity and mortality in heart failure. N Engl J Med 2005;352:1539–49.

9. Moss AJ, Zareba W, Hall WJ, et al, for the Multicenter Automatic Defibrilator Implantation Trial II Investigators (MADIT II). Prophylactic implantation of a defibrillator in patients with myocardial infarction and reduced ejection fraction. N Engl J Med 2002;346: 877–83.

10. Bardy GH, Lee KL, Mark DB, et al. Sudden Cardiac Death in Heart Failure Trial (SCD-HeFT) Investigators. Amiodarone or an implantable cardioverter–defibrillator for congestive heart failure. N Engl J Med 2005;352: 225–37.

11. Calvert MJ, Freemantle N, Yao G, et al. CARE-HF Investigators. Cost-effectiveness of cardiac resynchronization therapy: results from the CARE-HF trial. Eur Heart J 2005;26:2681–8.

12. Wang TJ, Evans JC, Benjamin EJ, et al. Natural history of asymptomatic left ventricular systolic dysfunction in the community. Circulation 2003;108:977–82.

13. Bouvy ML, Heerdink ER, Leufkens HG, Hoes AW. Predicting mortality in patients with heart failure: a pragmatic approach. Heart 2003; 89: 605–9.

14. Bleasdale RA, Turner MS, Mumford CE, et al. Left ventricular pacing minimizes diastolic ventricular interaction, allowing improved preload-dependent systolic performance. Circulation 2004;110:2395–400.

15. Erol-Yilmaz A, Verberne HJ, Schrama TA, et al. Cardiac resynchronization induces favorable neurohumoral changes. Pacing Clin Electrophysiol 2005;28:304–10.

16. Linde C, Leclercq C, Rex C, et al, on behalf of the Multisite Stimulation Cardiomyopathies Study Group. Long-term benefits of biventricular pacing in congestive heart failure: results from the Multisite Stimulation in Cardiomyopathy (MUSTIC) study. J Am Coll Cardiol 2002;40:111–18.

17. Stellbrink C, Breithardt OA, Franke A, et al. PATH-CHF (PAcing THerapies in Congestive Heart Failure) Investigators; CPI Guidant Congestive Heart Failure Research Group. Impact of cardiac resynchronization therapy using hemodynamically optimized pacing on left ventricular remodeling in patients with congestive heart failure and ventricular conduction disturbances. J Am Coll Cardiol 2001;38:1957–65.

18. Fukuda S, Grimm R, Song JM, et al. Electrical conduction disturbance effects on dynamic changes of functional mitral regurgitation. J Am Coll Cardiol 2005;46:2270–6.

19. Carson P, Anand I, O'Connor C, et al. Mode of death in advanced heart failure: the Comparison of Medical, Pacing, and Defibrillation Therapies in Heart Failure (COMPANION) trial. J Am Coll Cardiol 2005;46:2329–34.

20. Narang R, Cleland GF, Erhardt L, et al. Mode of death in chronic heart failure: a request and proposition for more accurate classification. Eur Heart J 1996;17: 1390–403.

21. Ermis C, Seutter R, Zhu AX, et al. Impact of upgrade to cardiac resynchronization therapy on ventricular arrhythmia frequency in patients with implantable cardioverter–defibrillators. J Am Coll Cardiol 2005;46: 2258–63.

22. Abraham WT, Young JB, Leon AR, et al. Multicenter InSync ICD II Study Group. Effects of cardiac resynchronization on disease progression in patients with left ventricular systolic dysfunction, an indication for an implantable cardioverter–defibrillator, and mildly symptomatic chronic heart failure. Circulation 2004;110: 2864–8.

23. Linde C, Gold M, Abraham WT, Daubert JC; REVERSE Study Group. Rationale and design of a randomized controlled trial to assess the safety and efficacy of cardiac resynchronization therapy in patients with asymptomatic left ventricular dysfunction with previous symptoms or mild heart failure – the REsynchronization reVErses Remodeling in Systolic left vEntricular dysfunction (REVERSE) study. Am Heart J 2006;151:288–94.

24. Leon AR, Abraham WT, Brozena S, et al. InSync III Clinical Study Investigators. Cardiac resynchronization with sequential biventricular pacing for the treatment of moderate-to-severe heart failure. J Am Coll Cardiol 2005;46:2298–304.

25. van Gelder BM, Bracke FA, Meijer A, Lakerveld LJ, Pijls NH. Effect of optimizing the VV interval on left ventricular contractility in cardiac resynchronization therapy. Am J Cardiol 2004;93:1500–3.

26. Sogaard P, Egeblad H, Pedersen AK, et al. Sequential versus simultaneous biventricular resynchronization for severe heart failure: evaluation by tissue Doppler imaging. Circulation 2002;106:2078–84.

27. Moss AJ, Brown MW, Cannom DS, et al. Multicenter Automatic Defibrillator Implantation Trial – Cardiac Resynchronization Therapy (MADIT-CRT): design and clinical protocol. Ann Noninvasive Electrocardiol 2005;10(4 Suppl):34–43.

28. The SOLVD Investigators. Effect of enalapril on mortality and the development of heart failure in asymptomatic patients with reduced left ventricular ejection fractions. N Engl J Med 1992;327:685–91.

29. Parkash R, Stevenson WG, Epstein LM, Maisel WH. Predicting early mortality after implantable defibrillator implantion: a clinical risk score for optimal patient selection. Am Heart J 2006:151;397–403.

30. Rosenbaum MB. Types of right bundles branch block and their clinical significance. J Electrocardiol 1968; 1(2):221–229.

Cardiac resynchronization therapy in patients with narrow QRS

Bàrbara Vidal, Marta Sitges, and Lluís Mont

Introduction • QRS duration and cardiac resynchronization therapy • Mechanical versus electrical dyssynchrony • Intraventricular dyssynchrony and response to CRT • Benefit from CRT in patients with advanced heart failure and narrow QRS • Summary

INTRODUCTION

Several studies have shown that a wide QRS, mainly with a left bundle branch block (LBBB) morphology, is a marker of poor prognosis in patients with advanced heart failure.[1,2] There is a linear correlation between a QRS duration and age, with worse functional class, worse left ventricular ejection fraction (LVEF), more severe mitral regurgitation (MR), and shorter diastolic filling time of the left ventricle (LV). In general terms, the wider the QRS, the more severe is the ventricular dysfunction.[1,3]

QRS DURATION AND CARDIAC RESYNCHRONIZATION THERAPY

Previous studies have shown that about 30% of patients with heart failure show a wide QRS (90% of them with LBBB).[4,5] Cardiac resynchronization therapy (CRT) has proven to be effective in improving mortality and exercise capacity in patients with wide QRS, systolic LV dysfunction, and advanced heart failure.[6–8] The rationale behind CRT is the possibility of correcting an electrical delay created by a given conduction disturbance, by pacing areas with late activation within the LV. It has been taken for granted that a wide QRS is a surrogate

for electrical dyssynchrony that in turn would induce mechanical dyssynchrony in the ventricular contraction. Accordingly, established indications for CRT are based on the QRS width.[9–11]

On the other hand, it is well established from the results of several multicenter international randomized trials that, using this type of criteria for candidate selection, there is a constant proportion (approximately 30%) of non-responders among patients treated with CRT.[12,13] It has been suggested that a percentage of non-responders may be attributable to the fact that patients may show a wide QRS but do not have mechanical dyssynchrony in ventricular contraction, and therefore CRT is useless simply because there is no myocardium to resynchronize. Therefore, several authors have underlined the importance of demonstrating mechanical dyssynchrony by imaging techniques before implanting a CRT device, in order to improve the clinical outcomes after CRT. Imaging techniques, not only can demonstrate mechanical dyssynchrony, but can also delineate the extent of the scar tissue not amenable to resynchronization.[14]

Due to its wide availability, high temporal resolution (allowing the study of rapid events during the cardiac cycle), and low cost, echocardiography has been the most frequently used imaging technique is the investigation of mechanical dyssynchrony.[15] The methodology used for assessing cardiac dyssynchrony with echocardiography is not the subject of this chapter and has been reviewed elsewhere;[16] here, we simply point out that it is based mainly on the analysis of segmental ventricular motion with tissue Doppler imaging (TDI) techniques, three-dimensional (3D) echocardiography, or, more recently, 2D velocity imaging. However, no single parameter is currently considered the gold standard for defining cardiac mechanical dyssynchrony. Other techniques, such as magnetic resonance imaging (MRI), may also play a role in the study of dyssynchrony and tissue viability. Although some studies are beginning to clarify what is the most powerful echocardiographic parameter to detect dyssynchrony and to predict response to CRT,[17] the integration of multimodality cardiac imaging and the global integration of several echocardiographic parameters to assess dyssynchrony will probably be necessary in the future for optimal patient selection.[18]

MECHANICAL VERSUS ELECTRICAL DYSSYNCHRONY

The presence of a wide QRS in patients with dilated cardiomyopathy (DCM) of any etiology has been considered to be a marker of delayed electrical activation of some regions of the myocardium. This delay induces inter- and intraventricular dyssynchronous contraction and relaxation resulting in less efficient performance of the LV.[19] This concept has been challenged by the observation that not all patients with a wide QRS show mechanical dyssynchrony (Figure 26.1), whereas a proportion of patients with narrow QRS do. Some authors have suggested that the presence of extracellular deposits, a loss in the number of myocytes, or ultrastructural lesions may induce delayed mechanical contraction without showing electrical changes on the surface ECG.[20]

The correlation between QRS width and LV performance has been studied by Leclerq et al[21] in a canine model with LBBB and ventricular dysfunction. They observed that biventricular pacing and LV pacing alone induced the same

hemodynamic improvement in dP/dt and aortic pressure, despite LV pacing producing a wider QRS. They therefore concluded that there was no correlation between QRS duration and mechanical response.

A series of echocardiographic studies have also analyzed the correlation between QRS width and the presence of mechanical dyssynchrony (Table 26.1). Several methods have been used – this may be a limitation, since there is no single standardized echocardiographic measurement to diagnose inter- and intraventricular dyssynchrony. Yu et al[22] found a high percentage of intraventricular dyssynchrony in patients with heart failure and wide QRS (73%) using tissue Doppler imaging; however, they also found dyssynchrony in 51% of those patients with narrow QRS. Breithardt et al[23] also performed an echocardiographic study of the cycle of inward and outward displacement of each region of the endocardial wall and the presence of dyssynchrony in patients with advanced heart failure and wide QRS included in the PATH-CHF trial. They found that some patients showed synchronous contraction between the septal and lateral walls despite a wide QRS, and that the lack of dyssynchrony (defined as a lack of correspondence between the phase angles of the regional displacement curves) was a predictor of a lack of response.

Ghio et al[1] analyzed the presence of dyssynchrony in a series of 158 consecutive patients with low LVEF (<35%). Patients were classified into three groups according to QRS width. Group 1 comprised 61 patients with normal QRS width, group 2 included 21 patients with LBBB and a QRS duration of 120–150 ms, and group 3 included 76 patients with QRS >150 ms. Interventricular dyssynchrony (defined by the presence of an intraventricular mechanical delay >40 ms) was present in 12%, 52%, and 72% of these groups, respectively. Intraventricular dyssynchrony (defined by the presence of one or more differences >50 ms) among regional pre-ejection periods assessed with TDI velocities was present in 30% of patients with narrow QRS, 57% of group 2 patients, and 71% of group 3 patients. Therefore, although the proportion of patients with dyssynchrony is higher in those with a wide QRS, a significant proportion of

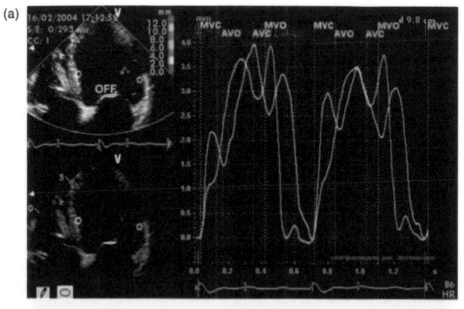

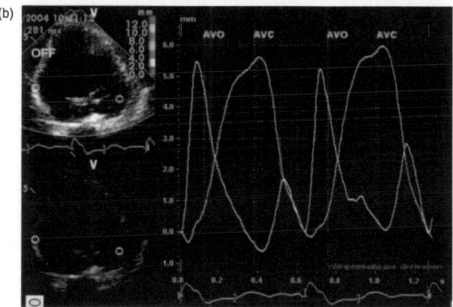

Figure 26.1 Tissue Doppler-derived displacement of the lateral (green) and septal (yellow) walls from an apical four-chamber view in two patients with dilated cardiomyopathy and left bundle branch block. (a) In this patient, there is a high degree of superposition of both curves, indicating that there is little intraventricular asynchrony – at least between these two walls. (b) In this patient, there is no superposition in either curve, indicating the presence of significant intraventricular asynchrony.

patients with a narrow QRS also show interventricular and, particularly, intraventricular dyssynchrony. In a similar study, Yu et al[24] analyzed 200 subjects by TDI. Patients were again divided into three groups: heart failure and narrow QRS ($n = 67$), heart failure and wide QRS ($n = 45$), and normal patients ($n = 88$). The authors used a complex measurement of systolic and diastolic asynchrony assessed by the maximum difference in time to peak myocardial

Table 26.1 Prevalence of left ventricular asynchrony in patients with heart failure and narrow QRS

Study	n	Parameter	Cut-off (ms)	Prevalence of dyssynchrony (%)		
				QRS <120 ms	QRS 120–150 ms	QRS >150 ms
Bleeker et al[39]	90	TDI (septal to lateral)	60	27	60	70
Bleeker et al[25]	64	TDI (septal to lateral)	60	33	–	–
Yu et al[24]	112	Ts (12-segment)	100	51	73	–
Ghio et al[1]	158	TDI	50	29.5	57.1	71
Perez et al[38]	296	M-mode TDI	130	40	61	
			50	38	40	

TDI, tissue Doppler imaging; Ts, Maximal difference in time to peak myocardial systolic contraction.

systolic contraction and early diastolic relaxation obtained in 12 segments. The prevalence of intraventricular systolic asynchrony was present in 51% of the narrow-QRS patients and 71% of the wide-QRS patients. Bleeker et al[25] studied a series of 64 consecutive patients with narrow QRS and heart failure with low LVEF (<35%). They assessed dyssynchrony with TDI, calculating the delay in peak systolic velocities between the septum and the lateral wall. A septal-to-lateral wall delay >60 ms was used as a cut-off value for defining the presence of intraventricular dyssynchrony, which was present in 33% of patients, in a similar proportion to that observed in the studies by Ghio et al[1] and Yu et al.[24] An example of mechanical dyssynchrony in a patient with DCM and narrow QRS is shown in Figure 26.2.

Despite the fact that dyssynchrony is more frequently observed in patients with a wide QRS, it can be absent, and, conversely, it may be present in 30% of patients with LV systolic dysfunction and a narrow QRS – a proportion consistently observed in several studies. The conclusion is that by applying only the QRS criteria for selection of patients for CRT, patients with a narrow QRS and mechanical dyssynchrony that would potentially respond to CRT remain currently excluded from the therapy.

INTRAVENTRICULAR DYSSYNCHRONY AND RESPONSE TO CRT

In order to evaluate whether the presence of mechanical dyssynchrony detected by echocardiography has clinical relevance, it is necessary to demonstrate that patients with mechanical dyssynchrony actually have a better clinical outcome after CRT than those without it. First of all, it has been shown that intraventricular mechanical dyssynchrony is a predictor of bad prognosis among patients with heart failure, independently of QRS width and LVEF.[26–28] On the other hand, several authors have observed with different echocardiographic methods, ranging from simple assessment with M-mode[29] to more sophisticated 3D echocardiography and TDI analyzing up to 16 segments, that the presence of mechanical dyssynchrony is a predictor of LV reverse remodeling and of a better clinical response after CRT in patients with LV systolic dysfunction.[19,30–32]

The demonstration of the non-linear relationship between electrical (QRS width) and mechanical cardiac dyssynchrony and the observation of the prognostic implications of at least mechanical intraventricular asynchrony in patients with heart failure has led to the hypothesis that mechanical dyssynchrony should actually be used as a selection criterion for CRT, independently of QRS duration. Although at present there are insufficient data to support this hypothesis, some studies have already used this criterion for patient inclusion.[33]

BENEFIT FROM CRT IN PATIENTS WITH ADVANCED HEART FAILURE AND NARROW QRS

Although a number of studies are currently being completed, data on the utility of CRT in patients with narrow QRS and heart failure

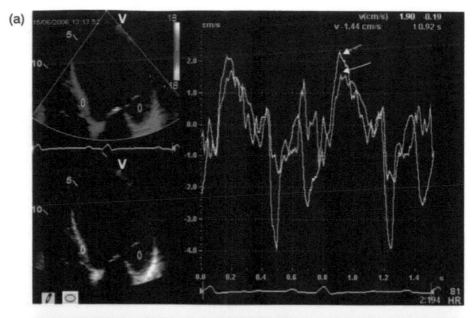

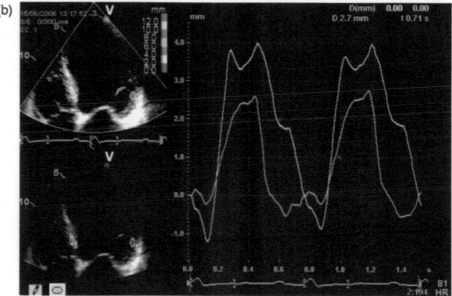

Figure 26.2 Tissue Doppler-derived velocity and displacement curves from the apical four-chamber (a,b) two-chamber (c,d) views in a patient with idiopathic dilated cardiomyopathy and narrow QRS (120 ms). There are almost no delays in the peak systolic velocities of the lateral (green) and septal (yellow) walls (arrowheads in (a)) and there is a high degree of superposition in the displacement of both walls (b). In the two-chamber views, however, there are significant delays in the peak systolic velocities of the anterior and inferior walls (90 ms, (c)) and there is little superposition of the curves of displacement (d) of both walls. Therefore, this patient did have intraventricular assynchrony despite having a narrow QRS, specifically between the inferior and the anterior walls but not between the lateral and septal walls. *continued*

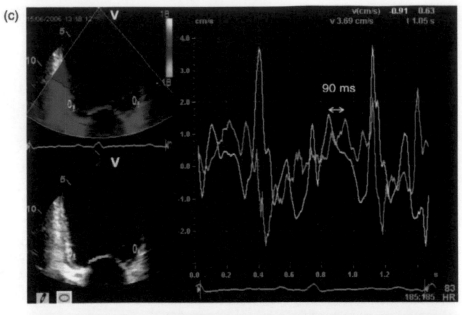

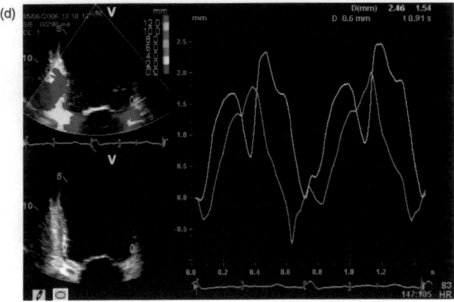

Figure 26.2 —cont'd

are still scarce (Table 26.2). Yu et al[22] described a good response to CRT in patients with intermediate QRS duration (120–150 ms): at 3 months' follow-up, patients showed a significant improvement in the 6-minute walk test and in NYHA functional class, with significant LV reverse remodeling. However, it could be argued that these patients may not have a strictly normal or narrow QRS.

Achilli et al[34] prospectively studied a group of 52 consecutive patients with LVEF <35% and evidence of interventricular and intraventricular dyssynchrony. Interventricular dyssynchrony was defined as an interventricular delay >20 ms. Intraventricular dyssynchrony was considered present when the time from QRS onset to maximum LV posterolateral wall inward displacement (Q-LW) was greater than the time from

Table 26.2 Response to cardiac resynchronization therapy in patients with heart failure and narrow QRS

Study	n	Follow-up (months)	Mean QRS (ms)	Asynchrony assessment	Clinical response	Hemodynamic response	Echocardiographic response
Gasparini et al[40] QRS 120–150 ms	30	11	130 ± 115		↓NYHA FC ↑6MWT	↑LVEF	↓ LV volumes ↓ LV diameters
Achilli et al[34] QRS <120 ms	14	18 ± 9	110 ± 11	(+) inter/intra-ventricular	↓NYHA FC ↑6MWT	↑LVEF	↓ LV diameters ↓ Mitral regurgitation
Turner et al[35] QRS<120 ms	8	Acute	100	(+) inter/intra-ventricular	↓NYHA FC	↑LVEF	↓ Mitral regurgitation
Yu et al[22] QRS 120–150 ms	27	3	134 ± 14		↓NYHA FC ↑6MWT	↑LVEF dP/dt	↓ LV diameters ↓ LV volumes ↓ Mitral regurgitation

LVEF, left ventricular ejection fraction; NYHA FC, New York Heart Association functional class; 6MWT, 6-minute walking test.

QRS onset to the beginning of the transmitral filling interval and when Q-LW > 9.9 corrected units (a measure derived from analysis of normal subjects). There were 14 patients with narrow QRS treated with CRT, and their clinical outcome was compared with that observed in a group of 38 patients with wide QRS, also treated with CRT. Baseline characteristics were similar in both groups. At 6 months' follow-up, there was no difference in the magnitude of LV reverse remodeling between the groups, with significant reductions in ventricular diameters, volumes and mitral regurgitation and a significant improvement in LVEF. The distance reached in the 6-minute walk test also improved in both groups. Finally, the magnitude of improvement in inter- and intraventricular dyssynchrony was also similar in the two groups.

Response to CRT in patients with narrow QRS was analyzed in another small study by Turner et al[35] in a series of eight patients with NYHA functional class III–IV and a normal QRS duration. CRT reduced NYHA functional class (from 3.4 to 1.8; p <0.001), improved LVEF (from 36.1 ± 7% to 38.4 ± 7%; p <0.05), reduced the severity of mitral regurgitation, and improved inter- and intraventricular dyssynchrony.

More recent reports have led to similar conclusions, although in small series. Bleeker et al[36] performed a case–control study including 33 patients with advanced heart failure (NYHA functional class III), severe systolic LV dysfunction and narrow QRS, and 33 patients with similar characteristics but with a wide QRS. The indication for CRT was based on a delay between septal and lateral peak systolic velocities >65 ms. The narrow-QRS group showed less septal-to-lateral delay (110 ± 8 ms vs 175 ± 22 ms).[41] At 6 months' follow-up, both groups showed an improvement in NYHA functional class and reverse LV remodelling by echocardiography. Cazeau et al[37] also reported a series of patients with narrow QRS (mean 120 ± 19 ms). The probability of clinical response to CRT was 70% in those patients having at least one of the following basal parameters defining dyssynchrony: a left atrioventricular filling time <40% of the cardiac cycle, an interventricular delay >40 ms, or a pre-ejection aortic time > 140 ms.

A large study is presently being conducted to analyze the echocardiographic predictors of response to CRT (the PROSPECT study).[17] This study will enroll approximately 300 patients in up to 75 centers. Centers outside the USA may enroll patients with a narrow QRS if there is echocardiographic evidence of LV dyssynchrony. The results from this study may add some data relevant to the issue of the utility of CRT in patients with heart failure and narrow QRS.

SUMMARY

The classic QRS duration criteria used to identify candidates for CRT may be less sensitive and specific than echocardiographic or imaging measurements of mechanical cardiac dyssynchrony. Whether selection for CRT should be based in mechanical dyssynchrony measurements rather than on QRS duration remains to be established by studies involving a larger number of patients. Furthermore, standardized and feasible echocardiographic criteria to evaluate dyssynchrony are needed.

REFERENCES

1. Ghio S, Constantin C, Klersy C, et al. Interventricular and intraventricular dyssynchrony are common in heart failure patients, regardless of QRS duration. Eur Heart J 2004;25:571–8.

2. Baldasseroni S, Opasich C, Gorini M, et al. Left bundle-branch block is associated with increased 1-year sudden and total mortality rate in 5517 outpatients with congestive heart failure: a report from the Italian Network on Congestive Heart Failure. Am Heart J 2002;143:398–405.

3. Kashani A, Barold SS. Significance of QRS complex duration in patients with heart failure. J Am Coll Cardiol 2005;46:2183–92.

4. Aaronson KD, Schwartz JS, Chen TM, et al. Development and prospective validation of a clinical index to predict survival in ambulatory patients referred for cardiac transplant evaluation. Circulation 1997; 95:2660–7.

5. Shamim W, Francis DP, Yousufuddin M, et al. Intraventricular conduction delay: a prognostic marker in chronic heart failure. Int J Cardiol 1999;70:171–8.

6. Cazeau S, Leclercq C, Lavergne T, et al. Effects of multisite biventricular pacing in patients with heart failure and intraventricular conduction delay. N Engl J Med 2001;344:873–80.

7. Auricchio A, Stellbrink C, Block M, et al. Effect of pacing chamber and atrioventricular delay on acute systolic function of paced patients with congestive heart failure. The Pacing Therapies for Congestive Heart Failure Study Group. The Guidant Congestive Heart Failure Research Group. Circulation 1999; 99:2993–3001.

8. Abraham WT, Fisher WG, Smith AL, et al. Cardiac resynchronization in chronic heart failure. N Engl J Med 2002;346:1845–53.

9. Gregoratos G, Abrams J, Epstein AE, et al. ACC/AHA/NASPE 2002 Guideline Update for Implantation of Cardiac Pacemakers and Antiarrhythmia Devices: Summary article: a report of the American College of Cardiology/American Heart Association Task Force on Practice Guidelines (ACC/AHA/NASPE Committee to Update the 1998 Pacemaker Guidelines). Circulation 2002;106:2145–61.

10. Hunt SA. ACC/AHA 2005 Guideline Update for the Diagnosis and Management of Chronic Heart Failure in the Adult: a report of the American College of Cardiology/American Heart Association Task Force on Practice Guidelines (Writing Committee to Update the 2001 Guidelines for the Evaluation and Management of Heart Failure). J Am Coll Cardiol 2005;46:e1–82.

11. Krum H. The Task Force for the Diagnosis and Treatment of Chronic Heart Failure of the European Society of Cardiology. Guidelines for the Diagnosis and Treatment of Chronic Heart Failure: Full text (update 2005). Eur Heart J 2005;26:2472; author reply 2473–4.

12. Bradley DJ, Bradley EA, Baughman KL, et al. Cardiac resynchronization and death from progressive heart failure: a meta-analysis of randomized controlled trials. JAMA 2003;289:730–40.

13. Diaz-Infante E, Mont L, Leal J, et al. Predictors of lack of response to resynchronization therapy. Am J Cardiol 2005;95:1436–40.

14. Bleeker GB, Kaandorp TA, Lamb HJ, et al. Effect of posterolateral scar tissue on clinical and echocardiographic improvement after cardiac resynchronization therapy. Circulation 2006;113:969–76.

15. Bax JJ, Ansalone G, Breithardt OA, et al. Echocardiographic evaluation of cardiac resynchronization therapy: ready for routine clinical use? A critical appraisal. J Am Coll Cardiol 2004;44:1–9.

16. Bax JJ, Abraham T, Barold SS, et al. Cardiac resynchronization therapy: Part 2 – Issues during and after device implantation and unresolved questions. J Am Coll Cardiol 2005;46:2168–82.

17. Yu CM, Abraham WT, Bax J, et al. Predictors of response to cardiac resynchronization therapy (PROSPECT) – study design. Am Heart J 2005;149:600–5.

18. Breithardt OA, Breithardt G. Quest for the best candidate: How much imaging do we need before prescribing cardiac resynchronization therapy? Circulation 2006; 113:926–8.

19. Bax JJ, Marwick TH, Molhoek SG, et al. Left ventricular dyssynchrony predicts benefit of cardiac resynchronization therapy in patients with end-stage heart failure before pacemaker implantation. Am J Cardiol 2003;92:1238–40.

20. Weber KT, Anversa P, Armstrong PW, et al. Remodeling and reparation of the cardiovascular system. J Am Coll Cardiol 1992;20:3–16.

21. Leclercq C, Faris O, Tunin R, et al. Systolic improvement and mechanical resynchronization does not require electrical synchrony in the dilated failing heart with left bundle-branch block. Circulation 2002;106:1760–3.

22. Yu CM, Fung JW, Chan CK, et al. Comparison of efficacy of reverse remodeling and clinical improvement for relatively narrow and wide QRS complexes after

cardiac resynchronization therapy for heart failure. J Cardiovasc Electrophysiol 2004;15:1058–65.

23. Breithardt OA, Stellbrink C, Kramer AP, et al. Echocardiographic quantification of left ventricular asynchrony predicts an acute hemodynamic benefit of cardiac resynchronization therapy. J Am Coll Cardiol 2002;40:536–45.

24. Yu CM, Lin H, Zhang Q, Sanderson JE. High prevalence of left ventricular systolic and diastolic asynchrony in patients with congestive heart failure and normal QRS duration. Heart 2003;89:54–60.

25. Bleeker GB, Schalij MJ, Molhoek SG, et al. Frequency of left ventricular dyssynchrony in patients with heart failure and a narrow QRS complex. Am J Cardiol 2005;95:140–2.

26. Xiao HB, Roy C, Fujimoto S, Gibson DG. Natural history of abnormal conduction and its relation to prognosis in patients with dilated cardiomyopathy. Int J Cardiol 1996;53:163–70.

27. Gottypaty V. The resting electrocardiogram provides a sensitive and inexpresive marker or prognosis in patients with chronic heart failure. J Am Coll Cardiol 1999;33(Suppl):145A.

28. Bader H, Garrigue S, Lafitte S, et al. Intra-left ventricular electromechanical asynchrony. A new independent predictor of severe cardiac events in heart failure patients. J Am Coll Cardiol 2004;43:248–56.

29. Pitzalis MV, Iacoviello M, Romito R, et al. Ventricular asynchrony predicts a better outcome in patients with chronic heart failure receiving cardiac resynchronization therapy. J Am Coll Cardiol 2005;45:65–9.

30. Kapetanakis S, Kearney MT, Siva A, et al. Real-time three-dimensional echocardiography: a novel technique to quantify global left ventricular mechanical dyssynchrony. Circulation 2005;112:992–1000.

31. Sogaard P, Egeblad H, Kim WY, et al. Tissue Doppler imaging predicts improved systolic performance and reversed left ventricular remodeling during long-term cardiac resynchronization therapy. J Am Coll Cardiol 2002;40:723–30.

32. Zhang Q, Yu CM, Fung JW, et al. Assessment of the effect of cardiac resynchronization therapy on intraventricular mechanical synchronicity by regional volumetric changes. Am J Cardiol 2005;95:126–9.

33. Cleland JGF, Daubert J-C, Erdmann E, et al. The effect of cardiac resynchronization on morbidity and mortality in heart failure. N Engl J Med 2005;352:1539–49.

34. Achilli A, Sassara M, Ficili S, et al. Long-term effectiveness of cardiac resynchronization therapy in patients with refractory heart failure and 'narrow' QRS. J Am Coll Cardiol 2003;42:2117–24.

35. Turner MS, Bleasdale RA, Mumford CE, Frenneaux MP, Morris-Thurgood JA. Left ventricular pacing improves haemodynamic variables in patients with heart failure with a normal QRS duration. Heart 2004;90:502–5.

36. Bleeker G, Van der Wall EE, Steendijk P, et al. Cardiac resynchronization therapy in patients with narrow QRS. Heart Rhythm 2006;3(Suppl):AB43-5.

37. Cazeau S, Leclerq C, Paul V, et al. Identification of potential CRT responders in narrow QRS using simple echo syssynchrony parameters: preliminary results of the DESIRE study. Heart Rhythm 2006;3(Suppl): AB43-4.

38. Perez de Isla, Florit J, Garcia–Fernandez MA, et al. Prevalence of echocardiographically detected ventricular asynchrony in patients with left ventricular systolic dysfunction. J Am Soc Echocardiogr 2005; 18(8):850–9.

39. Bleeker G, Schalij M, Molhoek S. Relationship between QRS duration and left ventricular dyssynchrony in patients with end-stage heart failure. J Cardiovasc Electrophysiol, 2003;15:544–549.

40. Gasparini M, Massimo M, Galimberti P, et al. Beneficial effects of biventricular pacing in patients with narrow QRS. PACE 2003;26(pt. 11):169–174.

41. Bleeker GB, Van der Wall EE, Steendijk P, et al. Cardiac resynchronization therapy in patients with a QRS complex ≤120 ms. Heart Rhythm 2006;3(5) (Suppl 1):S90.

Index

T - #0492 - 071024 - C344 - 246/189/16 - PB - 9780367388607 - Gloss Lamination